Bone,
Breath, &
Gesture

Bone, Breath, & Gesture

Practices of Embodiment

Edited by

Don Hanlon Johnson

1995

North Atlantic Books
Berkeley, California

California Institute of Integral Studies
San Francisco, California

Bone, Breath, and Gesture

Published by
North Atlantic Books
P.O. Box 12327
Berkeley, CA 94712
and
The California Institute of Integral Studies
765 Ashbury Street
San Francisco, California 94117

This is issue #51 in the *Io* series.

Cover art: Copperplate engraving by Jan Wandelaer, from Bernard
    Seigfried Albinus, *Tabulae Sceletiet Musculorum Corporis Humani* (Leyden,
    The Netherlands: J. & M. Verbeek, 1747)
Cover and book design by Paula Morrison
Printed in the United States of America

Bone, Breath, and Gesture is sponsored by the Society for the Study of Native Arts and Sciences, a nonprofit educational corporation whose goals are to develop an educational and crosscultural perspective linking various scientific, social, and artistic fields; to nurture a holistic view of the arts, sciences, humanities, and healing; and to publish and distribute literature on the relationship of mind, body, and nature.

Library of Congress Cataloging-in-Publication Data

Bone, breath, and gesture : practices of embodiment / edited by Don
    Hanlon Johnson.
        p. cm.
    Includes bibliographical references.
    ISBN 1-55643-201-1
    1. Mind and body therapies.   2. Chronic pain—Treatment.
    I. Johnson, Don, 1934– .
    RC489.M53B66   1995
    616.5'3—dc20   95-3876
                                                                        CIP

1 2 3 4 5 6 7 8 9 / 99 98 97 96 95

Grateful acknowledgment is given to the following individuals and institutions who have freely contributed material to this volume:

Judith Aston for "Three Perceptions and One Compulsion," and to Joan Skelly and Judith Pollock who helped her edit.

Bonnie Bainbridge Cohen and Nancy Stark Smith for excerpts from *Sensing, Feeling, and Action.* This material first appeared in *Contact Quarterly Dance Journal: A Vehicle for Moving Ideas.*

Elizabeth A. Behnke for "Matching."

Elizabeth Beringer for her interview with Ilse Middendorf.

Emilie Conrad Da'Oud for "Life on Land."

Rosemary Feitis, Jan Davis, and Alan Demmerle for excerpts from *Ida Rolf Talks about Rolfing and Physical Reality.*

Eleanor Criswell Hanna for Thomas Hanna, "What Is Somatics?" and for his interviews with Carola Speads and Mia Segal.

Feather Whitehouse King for Mary Whitehouse, "The Tao of the Body."

Elaine L. Mayland for excerpts from her book *The Rosen Method.*

Meta Publications for excerpts from Moshe Feldenkrais, *The Elusive Obvious.*

Ilse Middendorf for excerpts from her book *The Perceptible Breath: A Breathing Science.*

Ilana Rubenfeld for her interview with Irmgard Bartenieff.

Joan Schirle for her interview with Marjory Barlow.

The Charlotte Selver Foundation for the article by Elsa Gindler and for John Schick's interview with Charlotte Selver.

Carola Speads for excerpts from her *Ways to Better Breathing.*

David Zemach-Bersin for his interview with Gerda Alexander.

Deane Juhan for excerpts from *Job's Body.*

And to the following photographers: Louise Gund for the photo on p. ix, Lionel Delevingne for pp. 109 and 137, Ron Thompson for p. 149, Vera Orlock for p. 183, Carolyn Caddes for p. 239, Mark Diekhans for p. 315, Joel Gordon for p. 339, and Karen Zurlinden for p. 353.

Table of Contents

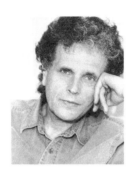

Introduction

Don Hanlon Johnson

THIS CENTURY HAS witnessed an incomprehensible savaging of flesh. Its global and local wars, genocides, politically directed torture and famine, terrorist attacks, the selling of children and women into prostitution, and personal wanton violence to family members and street victims would be more than enough evidence for a non-terrestrial to condemn us for criminal disregard for the muscle fibers, fluids, and neural networks within which we live. An alien visitor might not notice, however, that these painfully tangible wounds to the body politic are symptomatic manifestations of highly abstract ideas that rapidly gained a disproportionate amount of physical power. While violence and greed have always been a part of human life, this century stands out for its sophisticated political, religious, and scientific justifications for sacrificing human lives in favor of complicated abstractions. Palpable values of caring for infants and the aging, feeding the hungry, caring for the sick, nurturing the sources of intelligence found in explorations of bodily feeling and movement hold the lowest possible places on scales of values motivating actual social choices.

Although muffled by the din of those dominant voices, there has been a steady resistance building among innovators who have devoted their lives to developing strategies for recovering the wisdom and creativity present in breathing, sensing, moving and touching. They worked quietly, wrote very little. Typically, they spent their lives outside the vociferous worlds of university and research clinic. This series of volumes gathers these voices from out-of-print writings, unpublished lectures, as well as some new writing by teachers who have never before been published.

The outlines of this movement of resistance can be discerned as early as the middle of the last century when a number of people began to question the dominant notions of the body and healing.

A typical example is Leo Kofler. He was born in 1837 in Austria and started training for his life's work as an organist and choirmaster at eleven years old. In 1860, he was afflicted by tuberculosis, a disease which had taken several of his relatives including three sisters. From that time on, his breathing, his livelihood, was in jeopardy. He emigrated in 1866 for a job at the German Lutheran Church in Newport Kentucky. Anna, his oldest and favorite sister who had been the picture of perfect health when he left Austria, sent him a photograph in 1876 showing how afflicted she had become. She died three years later. "But I love this life," he wrote of her death, "for the sake of the work that I do, and I love my work for the sake of my life and that of my dear wife and children. I did not wish to die, and I fully made up my mind to fight death."[1] He set upon a life's work of studying the nature of breath, both from the standpoint of anatomical studies and practical exercises. By 1887, having gained the position of organist and choirmaster of St. Paul's Chapel in Manhattan, a position in which he remained for the rest of his life. He had healed himself and developed a method for teaching others how to free restrictions to the breath which he described in his book *The Art of Breathing*.

Two German women, Clara Schlaffhorst and Hedwig Andersen, came to New York to study with him. When they returned to Germany they translated his book, which had rapidly gone out of print in English, into German. That translation is now in its thirty-sixth edition. Inspired by his method, they founded the Rotenburg school, where Elsa Gindler, who inspired the work of a number of people in this volume, eventually studied.

Like Kofler, the innovators in this volume embarked on their various paths of discovery when they bumped up against problems that were insoluble by methods then available in medicine, dance, exercise, and psychology.

Many were faced with a physical dysfunction or illness which threatened their life and work, and for which their physicians could offer no relief. Gindler had tuberculosis; F. M. Alexander had chronic laryngitis; Gerda Alexander had rheumatic fever; Moshe Feldenkrais, Bonnie Bainbridge Cohen and Judith Aston had severe accidents leaving crippling bone fractures.

Others found a gap between the luminosity they found in bodily awareness and the sterility of existing methods of teaching exercise, dance, and physical manipulation. Charlotte Selver was drawn to seek out Gindler in frustration at the lack of imagination and spontaneity in the teaching of Gymnastik. As a young woman, Ilsa Middendorf found depths of spiritual insight in breathing that had no match in the formalized techniques then popular in Berlin. Ida Rolf felt that physical therapists, chiropractors, and osteopaths failed to appreciate the revolutionary consequences for human consciousness inherent in a balanced body.

These pioneers in embodiment are typically a feisty lot, unwilling to take at face value a poor medical prognosis, a dull exercise class, ordinary states of consciousness. Rejecting the bleakness of conventional wisdom, they have chosen to survive outside the mainstream, like artists often struggling to make a living by doing something other than their heart's work. Marion Rosen and Carola Speads worked for years as physical therapists; Bonnie Bainbridge Cohen as an occupational therapist; Emilie Conrad Da'Oud as a fashion model and night club entertainer; Moshe Feldenkrais as a professor of engineering. Many of their students now live as quiet outlaws, neither psychologists, nor physical therapists, nor physicians, though bearing resemblances to all of those officially sanctioned professionals. Those few who, like Marion Rosen and Bonnie Bainbridge Cohen, have gone through the process of gaining an academic degree or a professional license typically do it not primarily for interest in the material itself—psychology, osteopathy, medicine—but for the sake of protecting their practices and giving their clients access to third party payments.

Kofler and his Rotenburg heirs are not an isolated esoteric school. There is an unbroken lineage from him and a handful of European and American contemporaries to a large number of teachers practicing today throughout the world. Every teacher represented in this volume is connected with every other one in an identifiable web of interconnections. If one examines the history of any one of the seemingly fragmented methods of contemporary embodiment practices, one is taken back to 1800's New England; Kirksville, Missouri; Melbourne, Australia; Wuppertal and Munich in Germany; and Vienna. This lineage is not simply the abstract one of theory, created by a common readership of key texts. There are several teachers in the San Francisco Bay Area, for example, who can trace back the succession of their teachers directly to teachers in that earlier period.

This long history gives the lie to the common misperception that the methods found within this community are not well founded in scientific research, that they are "new age" and "alternative" to more reliable methods of Western biomedicine and psychology. Any of the practices mentioned in this collection has a longer history of clinical work behind it than does psychoanalysis, any of the younger psychotherapies, or physical medicine. Many suffering from chronic physical pain, for example, have been attracted to these works because of countless reports of their successes in these kinds of afflictions. While biomedicine can point to many empirical studies of its practices for dealing with chronic pain, their ironic conclusions point increasingly to the failure of drugs, surgery, and physical therapy to alter the course of such widespread complaints as back pain, arthritis, headaches, and repetitive motion syndrome.[2]

Yet it is true that it has been difficult to engage in the kind of widespread dialogue that is needed to produce significant reflection and reliable research on the efficacy of these works. The tenacious split between mind and body infects even those who vigorously criticize it. One of its most widespread manifestations is in an institutional split between theory and practice. The dazzlingly skillful work, representing lifetimes of study, observation, trial, error and reflection represented in this volume is given short shrift by academic scholars, medical researchers, educators and funders. Schools of embodiment practices are relegated to new age self-help techniques, in a dismissal sometimes abetted by practitioners within the field who are unaware of the full riches of their own heritage. Such widespread failures to grasp the full meaning of these practices are similar to misunderstandings encountered by teachers of ancient systems of meditation and the martial arts. Tai chi chuan, acupuncture, hatha yoga and vipassana, for example, are ancient complex systems of educating many aspects of the person. They include mental and imaginative practices, dietary prescriptions, ethical norms, hands-on techniques, movement exercises, and methods for sensing various flows of energy in the body. In the West, one or another element—needles, moxibustion, concentration on breathing, a morselized movement sequence, a particular herbal formula—is lifted out of its holistic contexts. A small fragment of these rich traditions is subjected to a reductionist empirical study by a medical or psychological researcher from a major university and proposed to the media world as a promising new alternative, given a new name and often franchised

It is no surprise that the community represented in this volume is not well understood. Its principal teachers have worked hard to break the hold of supposedly rational verbosity on the quieter intelligence of flesh. With the exception of a few innovators and their heirs—Wilhelm Reich, Edmund Jacobson, and Walter Cannon, for example—they write little, and often in fragments, close to the logic of bones interlocking with each other without a proliferation of unnecessary adhesions. Identifying the harmony of voices of the tradition is similar to the tasks facing scholars of other traditions that have existed on the margins of the dominant culture. Feminists have had to ferret fragments of women's wisdom out of diaries and bundles of old letters found in dusty attic trunks. Pre-colonial tribal Americans and African Americans have had to go into the nooks and crannies of small towns and remote areas to seek out living memories of the ancient wisdom traditions pulverized by the onrush of EuroAmerican development.

Despite the many lines of alliance, both practical and theoretical, between the people in this community and those of older cultures, I have included, except for one Australian, only Western Europeans or North Americans of European origin. The pie might have been sliced otherwise. For example, I can imagine a volume on embodied breath that would include Ilsa Middendorf, Elsa Gindler, hatha yoga, taoism, and Russian hesychasm. My choice for the present volume is based on the fact that those other communities have already initiated vital moves to gather their lost and damaged sources of wisdom. They are already far ahead of our community in articulating the wisdom they have to offer a traumatized social body. We in this community have more basic work to do to become more fit to join our voices with resistant strains from these other traditions.

A similar reason prompted my exclusion of representative writings from the schools of progressive relaxation, autogenic training, and classical manipulative osteopathy, despite their common inspiration with the ones represented here. These three schools of practical work evolved within the American university world, and already enjoy a rich theoretical and empirical body of literature.[3]

Not having easy access to their common origins, Feldenkrais, Alexander, Trager, and Hakomi practitioners, Rolfers, Rosen workers, Sensory Awareness teachers, and their co-workers from other schools think of themselves as isolated from one another, and more unique or special than they are. They often compete by exaggerating their own claims, and devaluing the work of others engaged in the same basic task of regaining a measure of fleshy sanity. Ida Rolf and Charlotte Selver, for example, can seem so far apart that it would be impossible to speak of them as sharing a similar vision: Dr. Rolf with her elbow probing people's *fasciae latae* edging them towards her ideal of perfection; Ms. Selver eschewing any form of intrusion into one's natural unfolding. And yet, when compared to the dominant philosophy of our culture, they stand out as fighting in favor of a common vision of the meaningfulness of our flesh, bones, and eyes.

During the past two decades, a few of us have made efforts to bring to awareness the unity of vision existing among these many schools of work, with the aims of initiating more careful philosophical and empirical reflection, improving our educational standards, and taking a public stance in favor of the needs of the body increasingly at risk. In 1977, the late Thomas Hanna initiated the journal *Somatics*, which has provided a forum for many different teachers to speak of their work. He wrote a series of essays, the first of which is reproduced in this volume, offering the first definition for the common vision of this field. He gave it the name "Somatics," adding the significant final "s" to distinguish it from the commonly used adjective, "somatic." "Somatic" as in "psychosomatic" has been used to mean the physicalistic body as distinct from the mind or soul of a person; or to designate the musculoskeletal frame as distinct from the nervous and visceral systems of the body, and from the cranium. Hanna recovered the older Christian mystical use of the term, whose source is in the New Testament. Paul distinguishes between the Greek word *sarx* , which has the sense of "a hunk of meat," from *soma,*, which Paul used to designate the luminous body transformed by faith. Hanna argued that it was the sarcal body, gross and mechanistically conceived, separate from mind and imagination, that dominated Western thought and medicine. In his view, the teachers of embodiment practices were recovering a hidden sense of the wise, imaginative and creative body, thus creating a "Somatics," what Edmund Husserl, the founder of modern phenomenology called "somatology."[4]

For over thirty years, Esalen Institute in Big Sur has provided a climate in which teachers of these various schools can interact, and in which students have been able to study many different methods. Innovators like Robert Hall, Richard Strozzi Heckler, Bonnie Bainbridge Cohen, Ron Kurtz and Ilana Rubenfeld synthesized approaches from many different schools. The first Somatics graduate programs were established at Antioch University West (now at California Institute of Integral Studies, the co-publisher of this series), Naropa Institute, and Ohio State University. Elizabeth Beringer and David Zemach-Bersin founded Somatic Resources which published a number of out-of-print books by authors in this field, and sponsored many international teachers coming together to give trainings. Richard Grossinger and Lindy Hough of North Atlantic Books have published a modest line of texts in the field.[5] In 1987, a group of European practioners founded an international professional society of Somatics practioners, which has held yearly congresses throughout the world attended by hundreds of teachers and practitioners. In 1992, Esalen's founder Michael Murphy published his encyclopedic *The Future of the Body* which outlines the history of these various movements and documents the research behind them.[6]

These various moves towards an integrated field are justified by the fact that the innovations created by this quirky group are not haphazard and idiosyncratic, though to the outsider—sometimes even to the insider—they often appear as a proliferation of methods and therapeutic approaches. Underlying the various techniques and schools, one finds a desire to regain an intimate connect with bodily processes: breath, movement impulses, balance and sensibility. In that shared impulse, this community is best understood within a much broader movement of resistance to the West's long history of denigrating the value of the human body and the natural environment. The resistance comes from many quarters: psychoanalysis, poetry and literature, American pragmatism, European phenomenology, feminism, marxism, tribal and non-Western activists and intellectuals. The unique contribution of the people in this volume is the development of practical strategies for effecting a return to the healing intelligence of the body. Just as solar engineers and organic farmers have demonstrated alternatives to the energy and agricultural technologies that have alienated us from the earth, these somatics innovators have challenged the dominant models of exercise, manipulation, and self-awareness that alienate people from their bodies. They have developed alternative ways of moving, touching, and being aware that bring us closer to the wisdom inherent in the ancient structures of collagen, nerve fiber, and cerebrospinal fluid, thus, the subtitle of this series of books, "Practices of Embodiment."

This volume is devoted to the most basic teachings of this tradition: about experiencing (Section I), about the personally meaningful intricacies of bodily structure and function (II), and about recovering the many possibilities of body movement (III). Section IV is a collection of beginnings of a field theory of these works, followed by a bibliography, a list of pilot studies of various methods, and information about how to contact various schools. The second volume contains the voices of those like Wilhelm Reich, Alexander Lowen, Nina Bull, Gerda Boyesen, Lillemor Johnsen, Stanley Keleman, Ilana Rubenfeld, Robert Hall, Ron Kurtz and Eugene Gendlin, who have articulated the implications of embodiment for the revisioning of psychology. The third volume will deal with the flowering of these approaches into skilled means for altering the course of bodily development, demonstrated in narratives of actual work with individuals.

Perhaps the significance of drawing together the various voices that make up this community of embodiment practices can best be understood in reference to its polar opposite, the schools of systematic political torture—not the wanton violence of urban gangs and psychopaths, but the meticulously calculated abuse of the body aimed at transforming the consciousness of the tortured into submission to the regime of the agents of the torture. These sciences and schools are sanctioned by governments, including our own, which offers favored governments training in torture at certain of our military bases. The teachers are physicians and psychologists expert in how to use sophisticated technologies to keep people alive at the margins of death with the maximum amount of pain. It is an impolite topic, rarely discussed in mainstream media or in the conference rooms of major American foundations, and yet its existence, like the omnipresence of radioactive substances is everywhere.[7] In 1987, when I first joined with a small group of people to initiate a healing center in San Francisco for survivors of such torture, I was asked by funding agencies to estimate the population in need. I guessed that there were 700 in the Bay Area. By the time of this writing, I would say that the number is closer to 40,000 from Central America, Brazil, Cambodia, Burma, Tibet, Haiti, South Africa, China, Iran, the former USSR. Even this number does not include those still alive from the Holocaust, or the many families who themselves have been permanently damaged by the torture of their loved ones. Add the numbers of prostituted children, the lower class men used as fodder for war, the women and children who are abused by personally violent men and one can begin to sense the climate of pervasive abuse to the flesh.

To clean up such an atmosphere we need a strong public voice on behalf of the sensitivity of flesh, the sacredness of nature, the importance of health and affection over religious and political ideologies and over stark greed. We hope that this volume will help weave together the tens of thousands of visionaries who are deeply devoted to the wisdom of material reality, and will increase the likelihood of joining somatics practitioners more effectively together with community organizers, tribal peoples, ecologists, artists, and others, who are struggling to be heard over the bloated bellowings of those who would continue the old savaging of flesh under the guise of an obscure superior knowing.

Notes

1. *The Art of Breathing As the Basis for Tone Production* (7th Revised Edition. New York: Edgar S. Warner and Co., 1901; available in the Lincoln Center Library), 15, 16.

2. For example, the body of empirical research of Dr. Richard Deyo of the University of Washington Medical School, which has recently appeared in the popular press, gives a dreary picture of the various mainstream strategies that are used for the relief of chronic back pain, most of which, according to his studies, have no evidence to support their predictive success. Cf. Michael Von Korff, ScD; William Barlow, Ph.D.; Daniel Cherkin, PhD; and Richard A. Deyo, MD, MPH, "Effects of Practice Style in Managing Back Pain," Ann Intern Med. 1994; 121: 187–195.

3. Despite the fact that these methods were developed in the United States by Edmund Jacobson (progressive relaxation), Johannes Schultz (autogenic training), and Andrew Still (osteopathy), their original genius is found more intact in Europe than here where they have been digested and fragmented by the dualistic medical world within which they grew up.

4. *Ideas Pertaining to a Pure Phenomenology and to Phenomenology and to a Phenomenological Philosophy.* Third Book. *Phenomenology and the Foundations of the Sciences.* Trans. Ted E. Klein and William E. Pohl. (The Hague: Martinus Nijhoff, 1980), p. 2, 3. Cited by Elizabeth Behnke, "On the intertwining of phenomenology and somatics," *The Newsletter of the Study Project in Phenomenology of the Body,* 6:1 (Spring, 1993), 11.

5. Richard Grossinger's classic *Planet Medicine* (Berkeley: North Atlantic, 1995) brilliantly situates these somatics practices within the vast history of healing approaches.

6. Michael Murphy, *The Future of the Body: Explorations into the Further Evolution of Human Nature* (Los Angeles: Jeremy Tarcher, 1992).

7. Elaine Scarry's uncomfortable book, *The Body in Pain: The Making and Unmaking of the World* (New York: Oxford, 1985), is a good introduction to this anti-therapy of scientifically generated pain.

1.

Coming To Our Senses

Elsa Gindler

*T*he late Elsa Gindler (1885–1961) is known throughout the world for having created a radically simple way of working with experience, *a Western form of meditation, in which participants learn simply how to pay attention—to eating, standing, walking, speaking, lifting a stone. Her school flourished between the two wars in Berlin. Partly in reaction to Nazi demands, she refused to give her work a name. Sometimes she called it "Human Work," or "Unfolding at a later stage of life." All of her writings save this one were destroyed when her studio was burned by Nazi soldiers during the final months of the war. Her teachers have disseminated her work throughout the world. The best known are Dr. Lilly Ehrenfried who took the work to France, and Carola Speads and Charlotte Selver who brought it to the United States.*

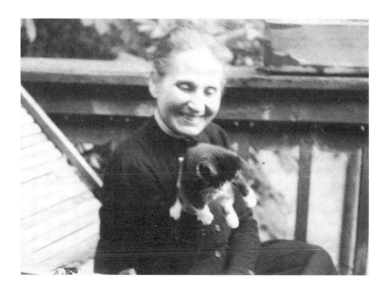

Gymnastik for People
Whose Lives Are Full of Activity

Elsa Gindler

IT IS DIFFICULT for me to speak about *Gymnastik* because the aim of my work is not the learning of certain movements, but rather the achievement of concentration. Only by means of concentration can we attain the full functioning of the physical apparatus in relation to mental and spiritual life. We therefore advise our students from the very first lesson that our work must be pursued consciously; it can only be entered into and understood through consciousness.

Now it becomes ever more and more apparent to all of us that we do not quite keep up with our lives—that the balance of physical, spiritual and intellectual forces is disturbed. In most cases this disturbance already begins to happen in the school years. Then, beyond the problems of school and puberty, problems in family relationships and profession—and perhaps misfortune—bring us difficulties with which we can no longer cope. We no longer lead our lives thoughtfully and sensitively. We become rushed and allow confusions around and within us to accumulate in such a way that they get the upper hand at very inappropriate moments.

Inadequacy dominates us in general and in particular. Daily there are the same, small, endless, infinitely important mishaps. In the morning we are not rested and therefore get up just that much too late to permit ourselves to take care of our body with the calmness and quickness which would fill us with well-being and vigor. It is not without reason that we say, "I must bathe, I must brush my teeth (drink coffee, go to the theater, a party, etc.)" instead of, "I am going to brush

Translated by The Charlotte Selver Foundation. *Somatics* August/Winter 1986–87, pp. 35–39.

my teeth, etc." These expressions reveal something important—that we do everything in order to be finished with it, and then the next thing that must be done comes along. If a room is cleaned for the purposes of getting through with it, it looks different from the room that has been cleaned with the sense of having it clean and orderly. And how extraordinary: the success is so much greater with the latter yet no more time is needed. On the contrary, we become able to reduce the time for a task while substantially increasing the quality of the results.

We also come into a state that is more human because, when a task is executed thoughtfully, and when we are contented with ourselves in the doing, we experience consciousness. By that I mean consciousness that is centered, reacts to the environment and can think and feel. I deliberately avoid defining this consciousness as soul, psyche, mind, feeling, subconsciousness, individuality, or even the "body-soul." For me, the small word "I" summarizes all this. And I always advise my students to replace my words with their own (those words which they use in talking to themselves) in order to avoid getting a knot in their psyche and having to philosophize for hours about what was really meant. In that same time they could be doing something useful.

It may be regarded as a somewhat presumptuous to wish to approach the attainment of consciousness by means of *Gymnastik*. And it really is! We are always embarrassed when this work is called *Gymnastik*. Most people have become accustomed to regard *Gymnastik* as certain exercises, so the first question put to us is always about our "typical exercises." To this we can only reply that our work is not *Gymnastik* in the ordinary sense, which certainly does not bring about consciousness: what does is the mind that is present and concentrated on situation.

In general people think, "When I have learned the relaxation exercises I am relaxed; if I can do the breathing exercises I can breathe; when I do the swinging exercises I work with *élan*; and when I have learned how to correct bow-legs or knock-knees, they will be straight." This is not true, and we invariably see failure resulting from this naive opinion.

It is clear that merely learning and doing these *Gymnastik* exercises cannot lead to the attainment of full consciousness. How do we get closer to that? Simply by using all our spirit and feeling in bringing our body closer to be a responsive instrument for living. We see to it that our students do not learn an exercise; rather, the *Gymnastik* are a means by which we attempt to increase intelligence. When we breathe, we do not learn fixed exercises, rather, exercises are the means of our getting acquainted with the workings of our lungs, either through inducing or releasing holdings. When we become aware that our shoulder-girdle is not in a position where it works easily we do not put it into the correct position from without. That does not really help anything, for as soon as the person is busy with something else he forgets his shoulder-girdle. Admittedly these are people who can clench and hold it in just the "right" place, but then that's just what it looks like—like clenching.

Usually we start a course by asking our students what they want to work on. In the beginning the result is shocking. Either nobody says anything, or somebody says, "You should get rid of my stomach," and other similar requests. The first stumbling-block is when I answer that I would not think of getting rid of someone else's stomach; the person would have to do that for himself.

Let us assume it has been decided to work on the shoulder girdle. We carefully examine it as to detail of form and usage. With the help of a skeleton we find out how it can best fulfill its function. We compare our functioning with that of the skeleton and then work to find out what has to happen within ourselves to come closer to such functioning.

In most instances, and especially during the beginning sessions, we work blindfolded so that each person is trying, by himself, to determine from where the holding of a wrong position originates, and what hinders the shoulder-girdle from finding the right position. Suddenly, each student is working in his own fashion. That means that each one in the class works differently, with a pervading concentration and quiet that would be envied in many lecture halls.

The leader notices at once where something goes amiss. He sees, for instance, how some students have a talent for always choosing the most difficult and problematic tasks. It is the business of the leader to point out that one reaches an objective by using the simplest and easiest experiments. In each course, however, we work with completely different exercises, inventing new ones as it goes along.

In this manner we accomplish something essential. The student begins to feel that he is in charge of himself. He suddenly feels that if he wishes he can work on his whole body in the same manner that he worked on his shoulder-girdle. His consciousness of self is heightened, he is no longer confused by the range of the subject matter, he is encouraged. This is a state which cannot be attained by exercises alone, regardless of how thought-out they may be.

So much for our way of working. Now to the areas of learning, which are breathing, relaxation, and tension—words often misused as are all beautiful things in the world. As long as they remain just words, they create mischief; as soon as they are imbued with experience they become great mediators of life.

One of the most delicate and difficult areas of our work is breathing. As we can see among small children and animals, every movement can increase and deepen breathing. Among adults, however, whose physical, spiritual, and mental processes are no longer governed by the unity of consciousness, the relationship between breathing and movement is disturbed. And almost all of us are in this situation. Regardless of whether we want to speak, make a small movement, or think, we impede breathing. Even while resting we impede it. We need only to consider how freely the neck emerges from the trunk of most animals, and, in a quiet moment, compare our own neck to theirs. Usually we will find that our neck is being pulled considerably inward from the middle of the body, approximately from the diaphragm. When this interconnection is observed for a longer time, it will be noticed that this cramping is quite arbitrary and that when one lets it go, one suddenly feels that the neck can be held much more freely. The constriction in the airstream through the neck (that occurs in almost everyone) suddenly ceases, and one feels much freer. At any time when this can be consciously permitted one feels not only that movements will not disturb the breathing, but can increasingly deepen it. Instead of becoming tired, one becomes refreshed by work. If this were translated to living, we would become more and more refreshed and productive the more demands are made upon us.

Actually, we imagine life to be that way, and we see over and over again that people who accomplish the most are fresher than those who do nothing. And if we observe successful people we can often see that they display a wonderful flexibility in reacting, in constantly changing from activity to rest. They have flexible breathing, or functional breathing. This is not easily attainable. Our students repeatedly confirm with little satisfaction that they need only think of an activity to feel how they immediately become rigid and impede their innate capacities. One is so used to doing it that it is difficult to abandon this nonsense.

In difficult situations—for example in marital quarrels or with the unexpected appearance of one's employer—we see that this gasping for breath and cramp in the diaphragm and stomach regions assumes frightening dimensions. Breathing stops, or a breath is hastily drawn, and the situation—which probably demands our greatest responsiveness—is hopelessly lost. We all know this condition well: embarrassment, anxiety, ill-humor, confusion in the mental and spiritual realms; trembling or an embarrassed fidgeting with arms and legs in the physical realm. If one is already conscious of how cramping—or constriction— can be eliminated by becoming aware of it, one is suddenly equal to the situation. The breath flows more freely, the mental confusion abates, one can make use of one's capacities.

It is clear that we cannot begin by working with large movements if even the smallest cause interference with the natural flow of breathing. One must first come to know—through observing oneself—just what one does with breathing while brushing one's teeth, while putting on one's socks, or while eating. So we begin by attempting to waken in our students an understanding of what happens in these daily performances. Then we have them try to make any movement without interfering with breathing. This requires so much work that one could probably stay with it forever. The main playground for this practice, however, is not the class session—there the release of constricted breathing is attained relatively easily and quickly. It is in life outside the classroom where we must notice how breathing becomes constricted in response to the most trivial causes; it is there where the tendency to constriction must be overcome. Simply noticing the constriction already brings help, and the oftener we notice it, and the more we accustom ourselves to investigating whether it is not perhaps an interference with breathing, the more easily and naturally it will be relieved. Small happenings allow us more time to do this than the big ones, but in any case we will begin to feel the beneficial effects as soon as breathing is released, noticing that rigidity immediately vanishes. It is this which we have to experience: how at the moment natural breathing is permitted we get the feeling of life. In addition, constricted breathing is closely related to unhealthy physical tension; we can never reach physical ease if the activity of breathing is not simultaneously freed of all constriction.

We must recognize and sense the connection between breathing and bodily movement, and bring about their correlation. In doing so we begin to understand that the demands made upon us by life are not so overwhelmingly difficult, that they can be carried out with greater economy of strength, without our usual maximum effort and turmoil.

Holding one's breath during exhalation is one of the more familiar interferences with breathing. Its counterpart frequently occurs during inhalation, manifesting itself as a kind of sucking in of air. Good undisturbed breathing happens involuntarily. We can, however, influence breathing willfully, thereby modifying it and diverting it from its natural course. This occurs when we do not wait for inhalation to be stimulated on its own through physical impulse, and when we do not permit exhalation to occur completely.

If one wishes to carry breathing all the way to completion, it is necessary to be able to carry through the four phases of breathing: inhalation, pause, exhalation, pause. These pauses and the conscious feeling of them are of the greatest importance. The pause, or rest, after exhalation must not be lifeless. It should never be a matter of holding the breath. On the contrary, it should most closely resemble the pause we experience in music—which is the vital preparation for what is to follow. It is wonderful to see how inhalation emerges from this living pause. There is an opening of the cells: the air enters easily and silently and we feel fresh and toned up.

What happens, though, if we do not wait until the lungs have opened up? And when do we wait for it? Immediately after exhalation, we often take in air arbitrarily and try to pump the lungs full of air before they ask for it. This is utterly inappropriate. We soon feel how the course of air in the lungs falters, and there occurs a thick feeling around the breast bone, the air is dammed up in the large bronchi and there is pressure and closure in the small ones. The air does not and cannot enter the lungs freely because the small lung vesicles have not yet opened. And it is these that must be supplied with oxygen while breathing. Access to them, the smallest bronchia, is provided by vessels more delicate than hair, so naturally the attempt to press the dammed-up air into them must fail. In addition, it often occurs that the air vesicles, at the time when the air is prematurely pumped in, have not yet emptied themselves of the old supply of air. They now do that, and the air stream trying to work upward and outward from inside collides with the air being pumped in from the outside so that there occurs a kind of piling up, and the result is a pressed, constricted feeling. But if we wait for the opening of the smallest vesicles we thereby permit a pause to occur completely. Then, as soon as the vesicles become empty, they suck in air automatically. The air then easily penetrates the smallest, hair-fine vessels. Nowhere does congestion occur, and nowhere is there a sensation of thickness or of lack of air. We do not need to bring into action any special activity for inhalation.

This is the difference between the breathing that occurs when the lungs and vesicles are open and breathing which occurs through the arbitrary inhalation of air. The difference for movement is very significant. If movement is undertaken during arbitrary breathing—i.e., while air is being pumped in—it will not be alive and will get no feeling of movement. If the movement occurs with open breathing, the movement becomes alive.

For releasing people from constrictions, only those movements can be fruitful which are connected with conscious and spontaneous breathing or, to state it more specifically, with breathing which happens through open vessels. Anything else would be more likely to disturb the collaboration between breathing and movement and to increase the habit of excessive and inappropriate effort. This is an additional reason compelling us to carefully assess any movements to be used in releasing constriction. For example, it makes running for which much inhalation of air is necessary, seem unsuitable. The tendency is to pull in air—which does not help supply the lungs with air, nor assist in eliminating the deficiency of oxygen resulting from running. If we practice running in our work, we start by doing so for such a short time that we can run with open breathing, then gradually increase the time.

An adequate supply of air is necessary and helpful in every task. It is not possible to swim or even float quietly without the ability to provide the lungs with air. In jumping, the jump succeeds quite differently, and even its form is different, if one has prepared oneself through "opening" for it. One can see this also among animals. Cats prepare for their leaps; no ladybug or bird flies up without making itself light through filling up with air. We can gradually come close to this if we observe ourselves continually in daily life, preferably on minor occasions. Thinking about it, alone, will not bring us a step closer. We must just open our senses to these phenomena.

When the student has learned to react with breathing to the small stimuli, and has come to improved functioning of the lungs, a new task emerges spontaneously—that of bringing the entire lungs to more working. Almost all of us use only a small part of the lungs in breathing. If this small part functions well, as has been described, we can accomplish much in life. However, in our work it is clearly shown that, if we engage the full capacity of the lungs in working, we can increase our efficiency significantly. And here begins the education in exhalation. It must take place without pressure, it must be elastic, it must be like the gentlest breeze, and it must bring about the greatest possible emptying.

In the course of these considerations we have often used the word "constriction" or "cramping" and must go into this topic in greater detail. I have tried to show to what a great extent constriction is bound up with disturbances in breathing and these, once again, with disturbances in the psychic realm. Releasings, or relaxations, are hence utterly dependent upon our being able to create a living image of the state of relaxation and of realizing it through suitable exercises.

For us relaxation is that condition in which we have the greatest capacity of reacting. It is a stillness within us, a readiness to respond appropriately to any stimulus. We read that the Arabs have a capacity through which, after long hours of trekking through the desert, they can lie motionless on the sand for ten minutes, and in this ten minutes to regenerate themselves so that they are then able to continue walking for hours longer. This is an example of relaxation. We hear that top businessmen often remain utterly motionless for a moment while directing all their senses inward. Then, suddenly, they seem to awaken and make decisions that are uniquely right. It is clear that in this moment of being in themselves relaxation has taken place. This is the kind of relaxation we are seeking. It can be most readily reached through the experience of gravity.

It is gravity which our limbs must learn to feel and understand. Indeed, every cell in us must once again become able to respond to gravity. Who of us, for instance, is truly relaxed as we lie in bed before going to sleep—responding to gravity as does a sleeping animal? When we attempt to feel the weight everywhere in the body, even in the head, we get into a state where nature takes over the work for us. To the extent that we can come to a way of lying in which this state is possible, natural breathing will occur—not arbitrary breathing with great movements of the chest, but a quiet breathing where the breath flows imperceptibly back and forth and brings sleep.

As for standing—real standing—we must feel how we give our weight, pound for pound, onto the earth, and how in doing so the feet become steadily lighter. Here is a paradox: the more weighty we become the lighter we become and the quieter we become.

In sitting we must be upright. As long as we slouch, we disturb all the internal functions. When one straightens up, one can feel how breathing immediately becomes quieter and more satisfying. It can often be observed how people who are bored or fatigued, in order to come to themselves, take a good strong stretch out of the crooked position. In sitting the joints will be freely movable, and there will be plenty of room for the stomach to function and for the spine to stretch itself to its full extension. If we then swing the torso forward at the hip joints, there is an expansion of the upper portion of the lungs, the same expansion we find so beneficial in swimming and especially in walking against the wind.

Now a word about tension, our third area of study. It may seem that tension comes off rather poorly in our work, but I must say that it only seems that way. Healthy tension is for us in the greatest contrast to constricting. We gladly give ourselves a work-out, but we do not wish to wear ourselves out—and that is where the difference lies. In reality, whoever is truly able to relax is also capable of healthy tension. This we perceive as the beautiful changeability of energies that react to every stimulus, increasing and diminishing as required. Above all, it includes the strong feeling of inner strength, of effortlessness in accomplishment—in short, a heightened *joie de vivre*. Healthy tension as we understand it is the possibility of overcoming the greatest obstacles with the greatest ease through the power of heightened breathing.

Generally speaking, in all of this, the most essential things we have to keep in mind are: that any correction made from without is of little value, and that each of us must try to gain understanding for the special nature of our own constitution in order to learn how to take care of ourselves.

Charlotte Selver

Charlotte Selver came to the United States in 1938 as a refugee, and soon managed to earn a living teaching the Gindler work in New York, her early students including Fritz Perls, Alan Watts, and Erich Fromm. She has had a major influence on Humanistic Psychology and was the first person to lead workshops at Esalen Institute. The radical simplicity of her work led to her being invited to be a regular teacher of Zen students. At the time of this writing, she is ninety-four years old and still traveling to Europe, Maine, and Mexico teaching her work to which her vitality and acuity are better testimony than any possible research could yield.

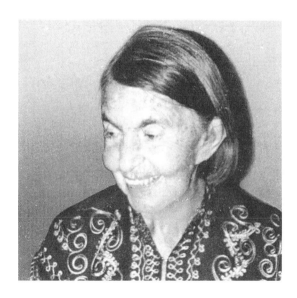

Interview with Charlotte Selver

John Schick

This interview was conducted with Charlotte at her home in early June, 1987, two months after her eighty-sixth birthday. At the time, she had just finished conducting a three-month study group at Green Gulch Farm in Muir Beach, California. As I talked with her, she was preparing for a trip to Europe two days hence.

Schick: This spring you've celebrated your eighty-sixth birthday, and I'm wondering, do you sense your approach to the work maturing or changing in any way?

Selver: It changes every day because it's no method, it's always meeting new whatever reality brings, whatever at the moment is acute. But I do think that the enormous difficulties in the world situation, the problem of starvation, the political injustices, the persecutions and all that is happening now, has augmented my desire to let people open their eyes and open their hearts for others in the world and become active in that what is necessary today. I do see the danger that when people become very involved in studying breathing, for instance, or becoming quiet, that this will become their world, so that they lose connection with all that is happening in the world, and by that narrow their own viewpoints and their participation with life.

Schick: Has this become a deep concern of yours?

Selver: It's my concern and I try as much as possible wherever I can during the work to find ways to let people feel what is happening in

---

John Schick, "Interview with Charlotte," *The Sensory Awareness Foundation Newsletter* (Winter, 1987), 2. (Available from The Sensory Awareness Foundation, 273 Star Route, Muir Beach, CA 94965.)

the world. for instance, I have sometimes taken articles from the newspapers which describe a condition in a certain country and I ask my students to read it and to feel what they read. I have tried to open their hearts for what is happening with the hope that it is in some way possible for them that they become active and play a positive role in the world, instead of just keeping their attention on their study and in the narrow room of their friends and interests.

Schick: Do you consider this development of a person's responsiveness toward all life to be an important aspect of this work?

Selver: This is what the work is about. When one studies human nature and really experiences what is given; when one takes it seriously to see, to listen, and to feel, then it is obvious that the wish will come to contribute to a world which makes it possible that more and more people can be open for that what they experience, and lose their aggressions, and feel with others, and listen to others, and speak their mind, and act their mind. The greatest influence on me was the way Elsa Gindler lived. She was there for everybody. She was conscious of the influence which poverty and oppression had on so many people. The way she went through the Hitler time; working; hiding people who were persecuted, sharing her very meager rations with them, helping them to get out of the country, even at the risk of her own life, all this has been working in me.

Schick: Are there any other changes in approach which you notice?

Selver: Yes, it has become more a question of communication, of the quality and clarity of communication. One very important part of this is that people speak directly out of their experience and not speak *about* what they experience. But that when they speak, they relive their experience, and by that the way of speaking becomes more direct and more precise, more fully backed by their experience. One of the things which is difficult to bring about is that people learn to differentiate between sensation and emotion. Most of those who come to our work have been in psychoanalysis, or have worked with psychotherapists, and they slide very easily into the emotional experience rather than into the sensory experience. So to keep the keel straight is very important, that people don't mix it up. Of course, very often in a sensory experience emotions come up and they should not be suppressed, but one would have to feel the difference between the two.

Schick: Have the kinds of people who come to study with you changed over the years?

Selver: Oh, yes. When I first started out in New York, I often had people come to me who had kinks in themselves. Now, most people come because they are interested in the work itself, and they come to see how far they can trace their own abilities.

Schick: What would you say are some of the important questions which occupy you now concerning the work?

Selver: How it is that we can help people to become more awake, and how, after they begin to wake up, they learn to trust their own sensations. And how it is that they can discover that they really can see, and hear, and sense; and that this alone can be a very powerful agent in one's life. One can learn not to restrict one's view; to feel oneself as a member of this planet we all live on. It's important that people learn to stop circling around themselves and instead to become open to the world and active. When I started to study with Elsa Gindler, I was very deeply impressed by her including the whole cosmos in her work. she made us conscious of the fact that every person has his potentials, and how very important it is that we make it possible that more and more people can develop these potentials.

Schick: This is a theme we keep returning to; it's clear that this whole question of a person's responsiveness to the larger world in which she lives is a very important one for you.

Selver: *Yes, it's extremely important.*

Schick: Why do you think it is that this responsiveness is lacking in so many people today?

Selver: Many people feel they are too weak for such a task, but in the moment in which a person wakes up and becomes more ready, and by this I mean more willing, they will discover in themselves a boundless amount of energy. So the work is partly to discover what amount of energy is needed for every given task and to allow that this energy can be expressed unhindered. This is what it means to be potent. And this potency goes hand in hand with seeing more, hearing more, feeling more, and being more in touch with what happens. Some people think that they get so sensitive they can't stand it. Do you realize that one *can* stand it? But this has something to do with being able to stand. People have usually learned from other people what to think, and we are not going this way because we feel that the person has all the abilities to find out for himself. He doesn't have to look to other people to be told what is right. This possibility of discovering gradually that one can trust one's own reactions can be a very powerful event.

Schick: So, you try to provide your students with questions which they must investigate on their own?

Selver: Yes, that's right. This is very important, this is the only way to create a healthier society. The basis in our work is that when one gradually begins to go into each activity anew, one loses one's habitual stance. And this approaching each activity anew means a person who is awake and changeable. When one becomes more awake, when one loses one's restrictions, the organism becomes a very movable and elastic entity. The more one loses the tendency to protect oneself, the more one becomes trustful of one's own abilities ... with all this comes movability and elasticity. So that one does not always toot into the old horn, but rather learns to approach every situation anew, more and more new. so gradually as people are more with what they are doing, they become more reactive. The tendency to withhold gives up by itself. No one has to do it, it happens on its own.

Schick: So it's partly a question of becoming more awake, of becoming more responsible ...

Selver: The first thing is one must have occasions to discover that one can trust oneself.

Schick: Do you try to provide such occasions in the classes?

Selver: *This is the practice.* While people are attending to the given task, the attitudes which they bring with them clearly show. At first, only other people see it, but by and by, people feel it themselves, and then they discover how they acquired these attitudes. Most of the time it's something they acquired long ago. It takes patience and time to discover what the gesture says. For instance, the gestures of people who always want to be graceful, this kind of false gesture [indicates gesture], or people who are afraid, or aggressive. They discover it in themselves. When I am used to shouting and then I begin to hear, to listen, my voice lessens because it's not necessary to shout in every occasion. It's not always agreeable what one finds. It's a beginning of a new beginning.

It has nothing to do with criticism, or feeling guilty, or anything like that, but just in quiet and openness to feel what belongs to the moment and what doesn't. I remember when I was for the first time with Gindler, I was just a guest, and she asked, "Do you feel that you are going through space?" "Do you feel the air around you?" "Do you really want to jump?" "Do you use the floor as a springboard?" I had been studying gymnastics and had never heard such questions. I was amazed! In my studies up until I met Gindler, I had been learning something entirely apart from reality. I was taught certain things and I learned them, but I never came more in contact with my environment and my own inner capacities and so one.

Schick: So for you it all started with Gindler ...

Selver: The very first time I visited Gindler and heard her ask questions of her students, I realized this was the work I had to go into.

Schick: And you are still working at it in your eighty-sixth year.

Selver: I am fascinated by it. It's my dish.

Carola Speads

Unlike Charlotte Selver who applies Gindler's work to every human activity—sitting, reading the newspaper, eating, singing, touching—Carola Speads, also a refugee from 1930's Germany to New York, has devoted her teaching to the experience of breathing.

Interview with Carola Speads

Thomas Hanna

Somatics: The work that you do in Physical Re-education comes from the teachings of Elsa Gindler, the famous Berlin physical educator. But did this work originate with Gindler or was her teaching part of an earlier tradition?

Speads: Elsa Gindler was a student of *Gymnastik*. This was a kind of body work that began around 1900. Its two great proponents in Germany were Hede Kallmeyer of Berlin and Bess Mensendieck, the American living in Hamburg. Kallmeyer was somewhat more artistic in her approach; Mensendieck, being married to a doctor, not surprisingly had a more medical viewpoint.

But the common feature of the various systems of *Gymnastik* was that they were originally developed for women—men only got into it later. Previously, the only system of physical education in Germany was created for men. It emphasized muscle building and was almost a preparation for military training. It was Mensendieck and Kallmeyer who introduced *Gymnastik* in Germany and Elsa Gindler studied with Kallmeyer in Berlin.

Mensendieck was an American. At a certain point in her work she wanted to publish a book using pictures in the nude. At the time this was, of course, impossible. So she went to Germany, and did her work and publications there and in Holland.

Eventually there were many teachers of *Gymnastik* all over Germany, each with a wrinkle of her own, and that made it into different "schools." But Gindler was a central figure in this movement throughout Germany and was president of the "German Association

Thomas Hanna, Ph.D. *Somatics* Spring/Summer 1981, pp. 10–13 of *Gymnastik* Teachers." Because of my early involvement in this movement I helped in the organizing of the association which brought together all the different schools of *Gymnastik*. These schools were, by the way, freestanding institutions, totally separate from the public school system, which taught the old tradition of physical education. But *Gymnastik* was closely supervised and licensed by the authorities.

These schools were quite revolutionary. My parents were, for example, appalled that I wanted to teach in this area, so much so that they refused to even mention it to others, they were so embarrassed. My mother said, "I don't know how anybody could be interested in others' flat feet!" And I told her I had no interest in flat feet, but was concerned with something quite different.

But then something special happened in 1925. The biggest German film company, the U.F.A., came out with a film that showed the nature of this kind of body work. I participated in the film and did some editing work for my school's part in it. Abruptly, *Gymnastik* became quite famous and everybody knew all about this new form of physical education.

Somatics: What was it that Mensendieck and Kallmeyer had in common?

Speads: You must remember that their two systems were at the very beginning of this movement. Both had studied with Genevieve Stebbins in America. People did not so much *follow* their systems as become provoked by this new approach. I think of them as the grandparents of this kind of work, Mensendieck had somewhat the spirit of a suffragette. Her attitude toward other teachers was that nobody else was right—she was a devil in that respect. Kallmeyer was a much more gentle and allowing teacher.

Somatics: What was it that drew you into training in this new area?

Speads: At that time in Germany there was a youth movement called the *Wandervogel*. It was progressive and I belonged to it. The *Wandervogel* had a group of older students who served as leaders on hikes and other activities. We found out that almost all these leaders were taking mysterious classes in something called *Gymnastik*, but they never mentioned it to us younger ones. We became quite curious, so three or four of us decided that if it was good enough for them it was good enough for us, so we made an appointment to have a lesson with one of these *Gymnastik* teachers to find out what it was all about. We had a private lesson. I forgot what we actually did but I remember that when we were lying on the floor resting the thought suddenly came to me that to teach others to experience what I had just experienced was truly something worth doing. It became my life vocation. From that point onward I was "hooked," and I never ceased to take lessons as long as I lived in Germany.

I took these lessons for my own interest and enjoyment. What I was learning from my teacher was so important to me that I persuaded her to start her own school for training teachers, which she did. her name was Anna Herrmann. This was during the early 1920s when inflation was so terrible in Germany. My father was well-to-do and quite generous, but he did not like giving me money to pursue such a funny profession. He wanted me to be a lady.

After one year of training with Anna Herrmann I told her that I hated to continue accepting money from my father, since he made such a face every time he gave it to me. I asked her what I should do? And she said, "Why don't you teach?" So after having had one year of training, I started to train other teachers as my own training continued. So, you see, I started quite early in the most important part of this work while I was still in my early twenties.

Somatics: And at this time you had not yet heard of Elsa Gindler?

Speads: Oh no. All along I knew of her. I had some friends who had been trained by her, so what she was doing was not unfamiliar to me. But as Anna Herrmann's school grew, she had less and less time to further me and the other young teachers who had later been added to her staff. We felt that we needed advanced training. So I took some lessons with Sophie Ludwig, one of Elsa Gindler's teachers. She mentioned to me that Elsa Gindler was to be giving a special summer course for her teachers, and would I like to join it? And I said I would.

So I met Gindler and worked with her that summer. I was the only outsider; the others were all her teachers. And as soon as I saw what she was doing I knew that this was exactly what I had always been striving for. From that time on I worked with no one else.

Gindler's teaching had both similarities with Herrmann's work and dissimilarities, but it was quite different from *Gymnastik* in that its emphasis was not on exercise per se. She had no interest in repeating things over and again in the attempt to obtain perfect movements. Instead, her emphasis was to find out what was wrong with what you did and what could be done to change it.

Somatics: So there was a therapeutic as well as educational goal involved in Gindler's approach?

Speads: Yes, this was always involved. Like the *Gymnastik* teachers, she was certainly concerned to improve one's carriage, balance, coordination, dancing ability, etc., but what distinguished her teaching was her interest in the effect of this work on the total person—not just the person's body.

Even so I must point out that at the beginning she was absolutely untouched by any interest or knowledge of psychology. I, myself, was familiar with psychoanalysis and was curious to know, for example, why able-bodied people could have exactly the same training in tumbling as others and yet never quite succeeded in doing it. What was the hidden factor that made them unable to perform? Obviously, it was something other than the physical. But when I raised such questions with Gindler she did not understand at first in what I was interested. She said, "What is matter? Isn't our work good enough for you?" But that was only at first—later, she also became interested in the psychological implications of her work.

One of the marked differences in Gindler's style of teaching was the amount of talking involved. We discussed things a great deal—almost as much as we did practical work. And this was always in a group situation. She did not do individual work with students but almost without exception, worked with groups. Lots of groups. She would begin at 8:00 in the morning, teach classes until about 2:00 P.M., then spend most of the dinner time talking with troubled students, then begin her classes again at 4:00 and continue until 10:00. She was a woman of enormous energy. She was never married, so had her total time available for her work.

Her classroom was very large—four times the size of my studio here in New York—and there were thirty or more students in every class. She was an intense woman, quiet-spoken: when she spoke in class you could hear a pin drop. When there was a problem in movement she would always remind us that by sensing ourselves, being aware of ourselves, changes would begin to occur if we were ready to allow changes to happen.

I studied with her every day, six days a week from Monday through Saturday. It was a sustained, intense experience, searching for one's best functioning. In her later years she always said that she was not "training" anybody, she was doing research, and if we wanted to participate in this research, fine. She was not responsible for giving us a whole or complete "course." She was going to pursue what *she* was interested in working on. And this is what she did every day for the whole year.

Somatics: Elsa Gindler was said to have once described her work as *Arbeit am Menschen* (work for the whole human being). Is this sustained, daily experimentation in bodily self-awareness what she meant by that?

Speads: Yes. It was an on-going research experience in one's own bodily functioning in the course of which one learned how to improve one's movement abilities. And Gindler had a wonderful way of coaxing you along in exploring movement. She made it easy. Some people, for example, are afraid to jump; they can hardly jump at all. And I remember how she started on this problem by having two students hold a long rope while others jumped over it. At first she would have them hold it almost next to the floor, jiggling it a little. No one had a problem with that. And gradually she would have it raised higher, an eventually we were all jumping up and down off chairs with no problem whatsoever.

Somatics: Was Elsa Gindler a tall woman? In the picture of her usually published she looks somewhat gaunt.

Speads: Oh no. She wasn't in the least gaunt. She was a woman of medium stature and very stout—almost as wide as she was tall. She had a thyroid problem. But medical knowledge of this condition was limited at that time, and she refused to have any medical treatment for the condition. she said, "I know my body and function quite well as I am, so why should I risk medical treatment simply for the sake of beauty?" So she never did anything about it.

Another thing about her: she was an extraordinarily generous woman. Anna Herrmann did not have much respect for her young teachers, but Elsa Gindler had. She not only asked me to teach at her school, she even shared her classes with me. For a while I started and finished the school year for her so she could have time for vacations. She gave courses elsewhere during the summer. And we also taught groups alternately. She would tell me how nicely I had brought them along. That was wonderful of her. And wonderful for a young teacher's confidence.

During her early years, Elsa actually did training—but that was in Gymnastik. Later, when she did her own experimental work she ceased to do formal training. Students came to her from all walks of life. Teachers from other schools of *Gymnastik* as well as physiotherapists, dancers, actors, musicians, medical specialists from orthopedists to psychoanalysts, as well as housewives and students.

All these people came to her because she was way beyond what anyone else was doing. Hers was a developing work, and everyone could see how far in advance she was. And what she did was effective. In terms of the level and quality of her work no other of the many movement schools could compare.

What happened was not just correction, nor was it only education and improvement: basically a change of lifestyle occurred. Remember that teachers in the field made up only a small portion of her classes. The great mass of her students were lay-persons from all walks of life. They are the ones who sought the changes that were made possible through her work.

Somatics: Was Elsa Gindler Jewish?

Speads: No, she was not. But also she had no sympathy with the Nazis. I remember once that during the 1930s a large national magazine wanted to do a major piece on Elsa Gindler and her school And she told them she had no school; that it was simply a small research center of no general interest whatsoever. And so she avoided any public identification with the Nazi regime.

At one point the Nazis required all gymnastic schools to include in their program a two week program of Nazi indoctrination, and all the working teachers had to take the course also. At this point, Gindler officially declared that hers was not a school so she had not to organize such a course. She would have nothing to do with the Nazis.

Somatics: Even though Gindler did not "train" teachers, still a number of teachers—like yourself—became teachers of *Arbeit am Menschen?* Were there very many to carry on this tradition?

Speads: Elsa Gindler acknowledged me and a few others to teach in her name. Presently there are Gindler representatives in Europe: in Germany, France, England, Switzerland, also here in the United States, and probably in more countries.

Somatics: How was it that you came to the United States?

Speads: My husband and I were both Jewish but, fortunately, he was a Czech citizen. In 1937 he was taken into protective custody, and when he was released in 1938 we immediately took a train to Czechoslovakia. Because we had Czech passports we were allowed to travel freely. Then we moved to France waiting to get into the United States on the immigrant quota, which happened in 1940.

We came first to New York briefly, then to Cleveland where we had some good friends, then returned to New York. From the beginning I continued teaching. No one knew of Gindler or *Arbeit am Menschen,* so I called the work, "Physical Re-education." I do not care too much for the word "physical," because this work goes much farther than that, but it is as good as certain high falutin' terms which do not suit my taste. And it is "education": it is continuing, follow-up movement—education one receives after one's *first* education as infant and child—so it's "Re-education."

A friend of mine who is a psychoanalyst once suggested that I entitle my work somatoanalysis, since I dealt as much with the mind as the body. From the very beginning, I knew that this type of work had to do with much more than the mere physiological—not that my work or Gindler's was ever clinical the sense of working with psychotics or very emotionally disturbed people.

In New York I have worked both with groups and individuals. Certainly, people will come to me often when they have pain or some kind of bodily problem, but very quickly we evolve beyond that focus. many dancers will come to me, especially after some injury. Someone will tell them that before they begin their dance training again they should work with me.

Sometimes that leads them to make very interesting discoveries. I remember a dancer who was injured falling off a horse. She had been coming to one of my classes and one day, while everyone was standing on one leg while doing something else with the other leg, she said in a loud voice, "Who's nuts? Me or you? Here I've been training in dance since I was sixteen, and one of the greatest problems I've had is standing on one leg while moving the other. And here I am in a class for lay-people, and I and *everybody* else can do it!" This gives you an idea of how different from the average way of exercising this approach is. Happenings like this were constant in Gindler's classes and in mine and in all of the other Gindler teachers.

Somatics: Is there an association of Gindler teachers, or any formal organization for continuing this tradition and teaching others?

Speads: No, that has never occurred. Gindler, herself, had no concern about forming a group or school—or even naming it. Even the expression, *Arbeit am Menschen*, is something I rarely heard her use, and she would certainly not have imposed that name on others. That was not her way.

It is a matter of concern to me that this tradition is not being continued by teachers who have had long-term training in this. It takes long years of intensive study, such as was the case for me in Berlin, in order to even begin understanding this work. All teachers in this field had to take three years of intensive, full-time training before they could pass the exam and be licensed.

Nowadays people seem to think that a few months of training in a bodily discipline is sufficient for them to understand the human body and be able to work with it. This is nonsense. A few months or even a full year of training is only a drop in the bucket. It is not enough. Most people have neither the time, nor the money, nor the dedication to spend the time necessary to understand and be truly prepared to teach.

Somatics: What, then, is to become of this tradition of Elsa Gindler? Is there nowhere some effort to continue it?

Speads: I think that in Berlin they are still doing some training. My colleague, Sophie Ludwig, wrote me that she had an assistant now, so that means that at least one new person has been trained. There may be more. But we have not seen each other for a long, long time, so I don't know exactly what is going on over there.

Sophie was dear friend of Elsa's. They lived together. And Sophie became the inheritor of Gindler's and Heinrich Jacoby's materials. Sophie, I should mention, was my very first teacher in the Gindler method. We still keep in contact. Her teaching, however, is not in the original building where Gindler worked. That building burned. It was bombed three days before the end of the Second World War, and everything of Gindler's—records, research notes, photographs—were destroyed. After the war, Gindler's former students began sending her their notes, photos, etc. so she could reconstitute her research materials. And Elsa resumed her teaching and continued until her death in 1967.

Somatics: Did you ever see Elsa Gindler again?

Speads: Yes, I always stayed in contact with her and met her often. The first time seventeen years after I last saw her in Berlin. In 1955 she wrote to me that she was going to give a summer course in Bavaria, and would I come, because it would probably be the last summer course she would ever give—as it turned out, it wasn't—and so I said yes, I would be delighted to come.

And what was so interesting was that I got there, and it was as if I had never left—not only in terms of our personal rapport, but in the way both she and I taught. After all those years I found that she used the same comparisons and examples that I had come to use during my work in New York. It was amazing. There was no distance between us, no time loss whatsoever.

After that, I would go and meet her almost every other year in Europe. The last time I saw her was the summer before she died. She was in her seventies. My husband and I flew over. We met in Zurich where she had waited three days for my arrival. Months later we heard that she was in the hospital. She had an ulcerated colon. During the war she had suffered considerably from malnutrition. Those photos you mentioned, with her looking "gaunt" were probably from that time.

Somatics: Do you know the family background of Elsa Gindler?

Speads: Gindler came from a working class background. I don't know what her father did, but I heard that her mother was a laundress.

Moreover, she was not a well-educated person. Being from the working class, she attended the usual free public schools until she was fourteen. That was the end of her formal education. I believe that was why she never wrote about her work. During those last years I asked her about that. I said, "Now that you are retired, why don't you write a book about your teachings?" But she declined. She said it was "too difficult a process."

There is, of course, more to it than that. The heart of her work was the experience of it—and that itself cannot be described. But some aspects of it can be talked about. In my book, *Breathing: The ABCs,* I have tried to explain the process that one must go through in order to experience and learn about oneself—in this case about oneself breathing. This book is only one stone in the edifice of our work. There are many other aspects and I hope that I shall be able to write about them.

Somatics: If you were limited to a few words, how would you describe the way in which your teacher, Elsa Gindler, approached human movement?

Speads: Gindler made the point that humans first explore and acquire their movement skills during infancy and childhood. These are natural movement skills born into the human system. But adults will find that these natural movements are, for varying reasons, interfered with. Thus, it behooves adults to become aware of these interferences and strive to remove them, so that movements will happen in the natural way they should.

But Gindler's work was not only concerned with the quality of human movement. Her work aimed at the development of the total personality. This was the reason why so many persons of such diverse backgrounds and interests came to study with her, and this is the reason why they come to study with me.

Ways to Better Breathing (Excerpts)

Carola Speads

Introduction

Years ago during a discussion about breathing, someone said to me, "Do breathing work? Why? Don't we all breathe?" Of course we do. But the *quality* of our breathing is the point in question, *not the fact* that we breathe. The quality of our breathing determines the quality of our lives: Health, moods, energy, creativity—all depend on the oxygen supply provided by our breathing. But the pressures of our modern-day life have created an almost literally breath-less culture. How many of us are really living in a state of adequate respiration? Even in the so-called healthy person, overtension (hypertension), flabbiness (hypotension), excitement and worry, as well as temperature changes and air pollution, may provoke shallow, irregular, or forced breathing.

Helping you to become aware of your breathing and teaching you how to have its full support are the aims of this book. Here I will present the basics—the ABC's of breathing work—rather than a compendium of all possible approaches. But just as you can go on to read anything once you have mastered the alphabet, you will find that these ABC's of breathing will enable you consciously to relate to your breathing and to help yourself when in need.

Some of the effects you will become aware of when doing breathing work successfully are an increase in circulation, normalization of tonus (the basic tension existing independent of voluntary action), and clearer thinking with a positive change in mood. With such results, you will know that your breathing has been changed more than superficially.

Great Neck, NY: Felix Morrow, 1986, pp. xvii–15

Breathing work is built upon the premise of the total unity of the human being. Its results prove the interrelation of body, mind, and emotions. Whether your breathing functions satisfactorily or whether it has been disturbed, not only your physical well-being is affected, but you as a total person benefit or suffer. Your breathing determines whether you are at your best or whether you are at a disadvantage. As you progress with your breathing work, you realize again and again how much you are influenced by any variation in your breathing—positively when it supports you adequately, or negatively when there is interference with the free flow of your breath.

Because interferences with breathing vary as much as individuals do, breathing work has to be geared to individual needs. There is no set routine to be followed. Whatever you do to help your breathing has to fit your very personal condition at the moment. Each of us has unique ways of using breathing well or of disturbing it. To try to help yourself by fixed exercises would be not only boring but also inefficient. An immense variety of approaches are necessary for successful breathing work. They make procedures and results continually new, exciting and interesting. Since all our activities depend on breath supply, you will acquire not only a mastery of a technique, but a mastery of life.

Your breathing needs have to be met in whatever state you are— at rest, in movement, when you feel peaceful, or when you are upset. Working, playing, or sleeping, your breathing should support you adequately. You need breath to perform tasks without becoming worn out, breath to bear up under adversity, and breath to recuperate from strain. If you succeed in letting your breathing adjust itself freely, your body will function properly, your mind will be clear, and your emotions will not overpower you.

Let us examine now what breathing really does. It is the means by which the body eliminates waste gases (among them carbon dioxide) and replenishes itself with fresh gases (among them oxygen), using the blood as a carrier to and from the lungs, where the exchange takes place. Therefore the well-being of your entire body depends on, and is influenced by, your breathing.

As an organic process, breathing is self-regulatory, controlled by the involuntary nervous system that safeguards its functioning. How, then, can it be interfered with, and how are we able to disturb it?

The explanation is that breathing, unlike other involuntary functions, is also partially under the influence of the voluntary nervous system; for instance, muscles, tendons, and joints have an influence on it. So do our thoughts and emotions. Any of these factors can and do affect our breathing. Figure 1 shows the manifold interdependences between breathing and various organs of the body. Effects occur in either direction, from the breathing on the organs or from the organs on the breathing. You will now understand the importance the quality of your breathing has for a good state of bodily and emotional well-being.

This book is *not* going to teach you to breathe (you have done this since you were born). It will focus only on breathing malfunctions, those predicaments involving the *quality of your breathing.* And it will deal only with the difficulties of the so-called healthy person, not those caused by disease of the breathing apparatus. (However, sick people can benefit from several of the experiments if they do them under the supervision of a doctor.)

My purpose is to help you experience how your breathing is working at a given moment, to feel whether and in what way it may have been interfered with, and, most important of all, to show you what can be done to let your breathing function adequately again.

A Note on the History of Breathing Work

The importance of breathing has been acknowledged throughout the history of mankind. In the East, the care of breathing was always an integral part of the religions of the Tibetans, Indians, Chinese, and Japanese. It was a feature of the cults of the ancient Egyptians. The ancient Hebrews used the word *wind*, the breath, in context with *soul.* The Bible emphasizes that God, creating Adam, "breathed into his nostrils the breath of life; and man became a living soul." This double meaning of "breathing" extends into modern English usage. The Latin verb *spirare*—to breathe—is used concerning breathing in the words *respiration*—our continuous breathing; *expiration*—our last breath; and in the other sense, concerning our souls and minds, it is contained in the words *spirit* and *inspiration*. The ancient Greeks used the word *diaphragm* to indicate the mind, as well as for breathing. The pneuma (breathing) theory dominated both the healing arts and philosophy during the first century A.D. In most religions, chants and spoken prayers (intense exhalations) for the "unordained," and special breathing training for the priests, were and still are the rule. All over the world — in fairy tales, legends, in secret societies — breathing plays a significant role.

In the West, in the second half of the nineteenth century, interest in breathing was renewed through the teaching of François Delsarte in Paris. Delsarte, having lost his singing voice through poor instruction, turned to the exploration of movement. Simultaneously he undertook the study of breathing. Eventually breathing work became an integral part of his system of movement education.

After the Franco-Prussian War of 1870–71, Delsarte's system was brought to the United States by his American student, Steele Mackay. Genevieve Stebbins and other teachers who had studied with Mackay spread the Delsarte method in this country. Stebbins achieved such success that word of her work spread to Europe. The German Hede Kallmeyer heard about it and came to new York to study with Stebbins. She taught Delsarte's method in Germany, eventually evolving her own system.[1]

Around 1910, Elsa Gindler, one of the most outstanding teachers in the field of physical re-education (in German, *Gymnastik*), became familiar with Delsarte's work through her studies with Hede Kallmeyer. Breathing work became part of her method as well as of all other systems of physical reeducation from 1900 to the present. It was Elsa Gindler who raised the standard of breathing work. She applied it to the highly original ideas she had developed in her movement work; body awareness as the basis, and experimenting as the procedure, instead of the mechanical approach that was generally followed in breathing work then and is still most often used today.

Delsarte's system was not the only method of breathing work that was relayed back and forth across the Atlantic. There was a second, no less important, influence on breathing work that passed from the United States to Europe.

The Swiss Leo Kofler, who worked as organist and choirmaster at Saint Paul's Chapel, Trinity Parish, in New York around 1877, developed a system of breathing and voice training. His book, *The Art of Breathing,* was translated into German in 1897 by Clara Schlaffhorst and Hedwig Andersen. It became the basis on which these two founded their Rotenburger Breathing School, which still flourishes in Germany today. The book is regularly brought up to date and still appears in new editions.[2]

I studied breathing with several of the German schools, but I am most deeply indebted to Elsa Gindler. My own method developed during my many years of teaching in Berlin and, since 1940, in New York City. In both countries I found a real need for breathing work. It greatly benefited all my students, whether they needed their breath professionally as musicians, actors, or teachers, for heavy physical work, or simply for everyday life.

Nowadays breathing work is part of all physical re-education programs abroad, and its importance to one's general well-being is fully recognized. Only recently has an interest developed in the United States in the role of breathing as an integral element of our bodily and emotional equilibrium. I hope this book will contribute to the growth of this interest and lead its readers to an understanding of how essential an adequate breathing support is and how caring for our breathing will enhance the quality of our lives.

Chapter 1:
The Role of Habits and the Best Way of Breathing

What causes poor breathing? What interferes with the quality of our breathing? Our way of life, of course. The stresses of modern times—war, crime, political unrest and upheaval, noise, air pollution, general and personal changes too sudden and too far-reaching for easy adjustment, mechanization threatening our sense of value as an individual—these are only a few of the difficulties that disturb our breathing.

Our breathing is affected by everything that happens to us—physical or emotional strain, injury, frustration, and even great success. Anything that goes on in us and around us has a simultaneous effect on our breathing. The free flow of air is hampered, exhalation is tampered with, and inhalation becomes insufficient. Breathing, a self-regulatory function, has the capacity to recover from strain and malfunctioning automatically as soon as the situation that cause the disturbance is over. Unfortunately, what usually happens is that instead of allowing our breathing to return and get back to normal in due time, we tend to interfere. Unconsciously and unintentionally, we often cling to the changed ways of breathing even after the events that brought on the disturbance have passes. At first this altered manner of breathing lasts for short periods, then for longer ones. Eventually it becomes habitual, and our breathing never regains its original undisturbed flow. For example, when you are startled by a sudden noise, you hold your breath, a perfectly normal reaction. The next time this happens, feel how long it takes you to let your breathing return to normal. Chances are you tend to hold onto the changed way of breathing well past the "emergency."

The experiments in this book will make you aware of how frequently a disturbed way of breathing is maintained after the initial disturbance has subsided. Most people are unaware that they do this. And, of course, only by becoming aware of poor habits can one try to overcome them.

Good breathing habits should be established early in life. Mothers and all those who care for infants should be alert to the processes of breathing recovery. Most people who pick up a baby in distress think they can lay the infant down as soon as he has stopped crying. But they should hold the baby closely, continuing to pat his back and comfort him, until he draws a deep breath. Only then has the infant's breathing normalized itself, and only then should you lay him down. This is a process so easy to observe that anyone alerted to it cannot possible miss it. Good breathing habits, instead of poor ones, would thus be promoted.

To sum up: Our breathing reacts to any impact on us. We hold our breath when shocked, we restrain it under stress, and it is stimulated by joy. It is certainly not the aim of breathing work, nor is it possible, to have one's breathing unaffected by life or to avoid life's problems. On the contrary, contact with your breathing will make you more open to life's experiences. It will give you the resilience to cope with life's challenges and to enjoy its pleasures. You will learn to overcome the weariness that follows periods of poor breathing, to restore loss of energy, and you will experience full vitality as an unavoidable consequence of fuller breathing. You will be more aware of the vacillations in your breathing. You will learn how to induce changes in your breathing to overcome strain.

Acquiring this skill, though, can be a long process. It is not easy to overcome or change ingrained habits. We can rarely change habits from one moment to the next; most often we overcome them only gradually. Therefore you need to give yourself enough time. But since breathing work is so gratifying in all its phases, you will not mind the time involved nor the patience and perseverance needed.

Because of the diversity of influences on our breathing, it is obvious that there cannot be one best way of breathing. I emphasize this because as soon as people become aware of the inadequacy of their breathing habits, they invariably ask, "Now, what is the best way of breathing?" or "How should I breathe?" There is no *one* way of breathing that is *the* right way or *the* best way to be aimed at for all times. We breathe in many ways, and many ways of breathing may be appropriate. Breathing is right not when it functions all the time in one particular "ideal" manner, but when it works in a way that lets it freely adjust, changing its quality according to our needs of the moment, so that it will adequately support us as we face the diverse challenge of our lives. Running requires a different kind of breathing from sleeping, alertness for an important interview a different quality of breathing from that for a casual chat with a friend. Anger will make us breathe differently from serenity. A certain kind of breathing may be right for one situation but inadequate for another. Sometimes a very full breath will be appropriate; other times a much shallower one. There is just no one best way of breathing.

Chapter 2: Method of Working

If you riffled through the pages of this book before you started to read it, you may have wondered what "breathing experiments" could be.

Most physical education systems use exercises to achieve their aims. These involve executing predetermined, fixed sequences of activities. Improvement is expected to be gained by repetition. The more you repeat the exercises, the better, supposedly, the result.

Such a mechanistic approach is futile as far as breathing is concerned. Changes in the quality of breathing have to be achieved in a totally different way, through experimentation.

Breathing varies continuously, automatically and perfectly adjusting to our activities, provided we do not interfere. Though we often do interfere with these adjustments, we cannot inhibit these changes altogether. Breathing remains an involuntary, self-regulatory function. It changes not only with physical activity but also with every emotional impact; both pleasure and pain are mirrored in our breathing.

Breathing being so variable, it would be impossible to invent the multitude of exercises necessary for the innumerable shadings in the quality of our breathing. And, of course, one could not begin to remember and repeat them!

Further, breathing is basically a self-regulatory function. You cannot possibly exercise something that is self-regulatory. Only willful actions can be repeated or "exercised."

We cannot "make" breathing as we can "make" a movement. Breathing can only be provoked, coaxed, induced to change on its own. This can be done by certain beneficial stimuli. After providing a stimulus, we must try to let the reactions to it develop as freely as possible. These reactions will be involuntary. They happen *to* us: we cannot make them; we can only try to let them through. This way of working with breathing is what is called "experimenting."

The experiments described in Part II of this book are a series of proved stimuli to breathing. I say "proved" so that the word *experimenting* will not convey the idea that what is going to happen when you do an experiment is totally unknown. In a general way, the reactions to a specific stimulus can be foreseen. However, the actual course of the processes that ensue, the sequence in which changes take place, and time involved will vary greatly. Reactions will depend on the momentary physical condition of the individual, on his or her mood, as well as on his or her experience of becoming aware of processes related to breathing and of letting changes in breathing through. You will understand that in spite of acquired experience and skill, you will not react as quickly or as easily to a stimulus when you are tired as when you are rested, when you have a headache as when you don't , when you are upset as when you are happy. These are only a few of the variables involved. And certainly do not underestimate the resistance against any kind of change that most of us have, which also greatly influences the process.

Most beginners need a good deal of time to become aware of their reactions to a stimulus and to let these reactions develop freely. At first, responses may develop only partially and slowly. However, once you have done the experiments more often, you will recognize one of the most rewarding features of breathing work, which is to experience how quickly reactions to a stimulus can set in and how thoroughly far-reaching the changes in the quality of your breathing become in a surprisingly short period of time. A student who planned breathing work during her summer vacation gave the following report: "Oh, well, I didn't have to do anything. Whenever I felt my breathing, I just let it recover, and my breathing was fine!" But to be able to let one's breathing recuperate and change that easily and that fast is the result of long work and experience.

When doing experiments, you need feedback. In breathing work, you rely on your body sense (kinesthetic sense), which enables you to become aware of yourself—not only to feel the position of your body in space but also to become aware of its condition. The sensations delivered inform you of the state of your breathing and of your reactions to the experiments. Like any of your senses, it can be highly developed and then used with greater efficiency. The more you use your body sense, the more developed it will become. Just as the trained musician hears details in a piece of music that the ordinary listener does not, you will find yourself sensing ever more about your breathing as soon as you begin consciously to use your body sense.

Unfortunately, intellectual development, not the development of our body sense, is emphasized in our culture. The body sense is usually applied in reference to pain. A new student proved this to me when answering my question as to what she could feel of her breathing, by saying, "Nothing aches." As if we should be aware only of discomfort! Thus many people are deprived of enjoying their own well-being. And they do not become aware early enough when something does begin to go wrong, and thus miss an opportunity to prevent serious trouble.

Movement is one way of activating our body sense. But we move less than prior generations did. Machines have taken over so much of the work for which bodily action was formerly needed, depriving us of many opportunities to develop our body sense. Sports, if done at all, usually involve the body in too specialized a way to give the variety of movement needed. And all too often sports training is so mechanical that it does not develop any sensing of the body at all.

Feeling yourself when experimenting does not mean that all you have previously learned about breathing is useless. Any scientific knowledge will be helpful in understanding your reaction to the experiments. Your first sensations when you begin to feel your breathing may be hazy and diffused. This should not be surprising, as most people are not in the habit of sensing their breathing at all. As you progress, however, you will become aware with great clarity of innumerable variations in the quality of your breathing and of exactly how your breathing reacts to specific experiments. Eventually it will be easy for you to become aware of your breathing.

At first, the end results of your work will be the easiest to feel. You will sense that your breathing is different from when you began the experiment. Later on, breathing sensations will become clear and irrepressible. As you become more skilled, you will be able to feel breathing changes as they are occurring. This is important. It is much easier to give in to these changes the moment you feel they are trying to break through. The more adept you become at feeling your breathing and allowing it to change, the faster and more far-reaching the impact of the experiments will be. This will shorten the time of your recovery from poor breathing states in your daily life. Not only will it make your everyday hustle less strenuous, but it will also enable you to enjoy all pleasant moments to the hilt.

Chapter 3: Sensations Related to Breathing

The sensations experienced when doing the experiments are often misinterpreted. They are never sensations of breathing itself. They are only *sensations related to breathing.* In their healthy state, neither diaphragm, lungs, nor the exchange of gases can actually be felt. What we do sense are the effects of breathing, influences of the breathing process on the body, changes that take place in relation to breathing. When people say, "I feel my lungs filling with air," they are not really feeling their lungs. What they feel is a widening of the chest cage as it accommodates the incoming air. This is a sensation related to filling of the lungs, but not the feeling of the lungs themselves. Such feelings and impressions initiated by the breathing process are the tools used in breathing work.

Sensations related to breathing can be felt in areas close to the lungs, such as the nose, mouth, chest, and abdomen, or farther away, in the arms or legs. The sensations in the extremities are mainly of circulatory influences derived from changes in breathing. In addition, you cannot miss feeling changes in your emotional states during your breathing work and afterward.

To explain this further, here are a few examples of sensations you may become aware of that are related to your breathing. First, you may feel the flow of air around your nose or mouth—just a little puff or a large amount of air. Breathing may be fast and shallow or slow and deep. You may feel irregularities in rhythm. You may experience sensations of frustration or satisfaction, as, for instance, the feeling of relief when an inhalation finally gets through (or "over the hump," as my students call it.) Or you may become aware of a sensation of depth in breathing ("It is streaming as if out of a deep well," a student once commented).

As these few examples demonstrate, the sensations related to one's breathing are of an infinite variety. Because you cannot foretell what sensations may occur, breathing work is endless interesting. Every time you do an experiment, your awareness will increase, and often you will experience new sensations or variations on familiar ones. I hear comments and expressions of amazement about this all the time.

Surely, like my students, you, too, will respond to the experiments with ever-renewed surprise: "I have never felt *that* before" or "I have felt it before, but *never quite like this."*

Chapter 4: Breathing Pause

Everyone knows that we breathe rhythmically. Most people assume that our breathing functions in a two-part rhythm: exhalation-inhalation. This is not so. At some point during your breathing work, you will discover that the breathing rhythm has three components: exhalation—pause—inhalation. The pause fulfills a double purpose: a resting from the effort of the inhalation and a rallying of the energy needed for the next inhalation. The pause, therefore, is not an idle period when nothing is happening; it is a vital phase in the breathing process.

The duration of the pause is significant. If we interfere with the length of the breathing pause, shortening it even slightly, we find ourselves feeling "rushed" and "pressured," that well-known state that interferes so often with our sense of well-being and is such a generally acknowledged burden in our daily lives. We have all experienced how strained this kind of breathing leaves us. We pay dearly for it in inefficiency, weariness, and irritability.

When starting breathing work, you may not immediately have any feel for the pause in your breathing. You may not be able to sense it for quite a while, neither in the checkups (described in Chapter Ten) nor during the experiments. But one day you will become aware of it, probably quite suddenly. It may confuse you or make you uncomfortable when suddenly you sense a delay before an inhalation sets in. but if you are anticipating such an occurrence, it will lose most of its confusing or irritating quality. Once this first confusion has passed, you feel tremendously relieved whenever experiencing the pause in your breathing rhythm.

Once the three-part rhythm of your breathing has reestablished itself, you will cherish it very much. A full-length pause in your breathing rhythm gives great relief, eradicates the feeling of being under pressure, and has a calming effect not only on your breathing but on your whole person, physically as well as emotionally.

But do not try to "do" or "make" the pause willfully. Because breathing is an involuntary process, you could never intentionally make the pause right. Its duration varies as your breathing changes, adjusting itself to the manifold tasks confronting you. The rhythm of your breathing, of which the pause is a phase, has to reestablish itself on its own. It is a part of the continuous, though varying, rhythm of your breathing.

Chapter 5: Speed of Recovery of Breathing

To anyone who works alone with this book, the speed with which he or she can achieve an improvement in breathing is important. The time varies greatly from individual to individual. The change can occur very quickly or very slowly. There are no rules, but certain factors do play a role in the time element.

Obviously, an inexperienced person will need more time to let breathing recover than will someone with experience. Occasionally, however, even when trying an experiment for the first time, a beginner can achieve a remarkably different, more satisfying way of breathing rather quickly.

Weather conditions also influence progress. Moderate temperatures and low humidity are favorable for breathing work and are time-cutting factors. On hot, humid days, it takes considerably longer to let your breathing up to par. Air pollution inevitably restricts breathing and prolongs the recovery period. The higher the pollution level and the longer it lasts, the more confined your breathing becomes. Then much more time is needed to recover from the shallow breathing and to eliminate dust and other pollutants so that deeper breathing can set in again. Do not try to breathe deeply outside in a heavy smog. But do make up for the shallow breaths taken outdoors when you are inside again.

The speed with which your breathing can recover is also greatly influenced by your emotional condition. If you are upset, unhappy, anxious—even overjoyed—you will need considerably more time for your breathing to recover than when you are in a placid mood.

The greatest obstacle to a quick breathing recovery is illness. It need not even be a serious illness. If you are just not feeling well, have a headache, or are getting a cold, you will find that your reactions to an experiment will be considerably delayed. At such times, be patient but persistent. Eventually you will succeed. I want to emphasize again that no one can foresee exactly what the sequence of reactions in breathing work will be, that there are no fixed rules—once in a while you may experience the opposite. You should always be prepared for the unexpected. For example, even when you are not well, change may come rapidly, as if your breathing had waited for the chance to be freed!

To sum up: Any day you start an experiment, you should allow whatever time it may take to let your breathing change. Because you reacted fast one day does not necessarily mean that you will react as quickly the next. Be flexible, let nature work at its own speed, and you will recuperate in the fastest way possible for you.

Notes

1. Anyone interested in exploring the development of the Delsarte System in the United States should refer to Ted Shawn's *Every Little Movement* (New York: M. Witmark and Sons, 1954), which contains an extensive bibliography.

2. Leo Kofler, *The Art of Breathing as the Basis of Tone Production* (New York: Edgar S. Werner, 1889, 1890, 1893; 1st German ed., Cassel, Germany: Baerenreiter Verlag, 1897; 23rd ed., 1966).

Marion Rosen

*M*arion Rosen was also a student of Gindler and a Jewish refugee, but unlike the others, came to the US by way of Siberia ending up in the San Francisco Bay Area. Living in Munich she was influenced by close friends who were psychoanalysts and by her own teachers in a sophisticated form of physical therapy. She has developed a subtle, gentle hands-on work that has proven of immense value particularly to people who have suffered physical and emotional abuse, and to people in recovery from addiction.

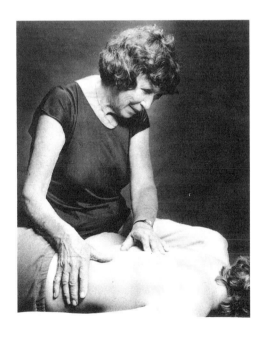

The Rosen Method (Excerpts)

Elaine Mayland

Chapter 1: Biography of Marion Rosen

There was a very awful day in Germany, the 9th of November, 1938, when the Nazis went around to Jews' houses and would smash the houses and some of the men were taken to concentration camps. That was a very, very frightening evening. The night before this happened, I had a dream, and there was a big, big sky, and there was a woman's face; a very lovely woman filled the whole sky, and she said, "Don't worry, I'll look after you." And that was all, that was the end of the dream. I just let myself be directed wherever it went, wherever the way opened up.

—Marion Rosen

Marion's European Beginnings

Marion Rosen was born in Nuremberg, Germany in 1914. Her father's import-export business prospered in the years immediately following World War I, and the family lived in moderate affluence. Marion was the third of four children; she had an older brother and sister and a younger sister.

In Marion's memories, her mother was a great collector of people. She had a fondness for music and musicians, art and artists, ideas and philosophers, learning and professors, commerce and shopkeepers, and people "from the street." She became friends with those who could expand her interests; she often entertained them at home.

Marion, as a small child, was sickly, suffering from recurrent sore

---

Elaine Mayland, *The Rosen Method*. 1–20 (published privately 1991)

throats and bouts of asthma. As she grew older, her health improved. By age fourteen she was already five feet nine inches tall and enjoyed swimming, horseback riding, hiking, bicycling, skiing, and above all, dancing. She had a burning desire to become a professional dancer but was told that she could not because she was too tall. She remembers her childhood fondly as carefree and fun-filled, with the single exception of her embarrassment about her height.

The political climate in Germany changed drastically during Marion's teenage years. Despite her mother's atypical lifestyle, she was rearing Marion and her sisters "to marry rich men and have children." Marion's father once said he had enough money so that none of his children would have to work. Matters in Germany worsened after Hitler's election, and it became obvious that Marion and her sisters would have to support themselves after all. By the end of her teenage years Marion had tried her hand at typing, shorthand, cooking, and housework, but wasn't good at any of them. She had a talent for languages and had thought she might become an interpreter, but she was not admitted to university because she was Jewish. This barrier was confusing to her because although Jewish by birth she had been brought up Lutheran.

In Marion's words:

I tried different things to do because it was obvious that I had to leave Germany, and I would have to earn a living. I couldn't think for the life of me how. I was brought up not to wash my own stockings, or if my bicycle needed air in the tires, I would have a man do it for me. I was really not a very practical person.

I was on a hike in the mountains with some friends and we stayed there overnight. When I came home in the morning, my mother was lying down because she had broken her ankle. She greeted me and said, "I have found a person who will train you."

She had in mind the woman she met when she broke her ankle and who had helped her until the doctor came. Usually I wouldn't have listened to her, thinking it was just another one of her fanciful ideas, but I said, "Who?"

She said, "Well, there are two people here, and one is a Mrs.

Lederer who works in New York. She does breathing and relaxation work with Karen Horney, and she could employ you if you wanted to go over there. Her friend is here with here, a Mrs. Heyer who lives in Munich who said she would like to meet you, and if you two get on together, she might like to train you!"

A few minutes later I met both women and took an immediate liking to them. Mrs. Heyer asked me if I would like to train with her. I said yes, and that was all.

Lucy Heyer was a masseuse, a dancer, the wife of Dr. Gustav Heyer (a colleague and former student of Dr. Carl Jung), and a student of Elsa Gindler. Elsa Gindler was the principal investigator then working on the integration of physical and personal development. She is generally considered the forerunner or "grandmother" of today's breathing and relaxation techniques.

The Heyers were part of a group of people in Munich using massage, breath work, and relaxation in conjunction with psychoanalysis as practiced by Jung and others. The group discovered that by synthesizing their several disciplines, the treatment time for psychoanalysis could often be dramatically reduced. Patients came to Dr. Heyer from all over Germany when it became known he was achieving results in far less time than other psychiatrists. It was this fertile, experimental clinical setting that Marion entered to begin her two-year apprenticeship with Lucy Heyer.

Although the Heyers were by then divorced, they still worked together. Psychoanalysis was left to Dr. Heyer and his colleagues; Mrs. Heyer and Marion conducted the breathing and massage sessions in near silence.

Marion remembers, "Sometimes the patients would cry and sometimes they would have pain or lose their pain, but always it was the analyst who did the talking."

Marion once interrupted her two-year study with Lucy Heyer to go for six months to the Tavistock Clinic in London, where her brother was completing his psychiatric residency. She obtained work at the clinic and began to put into practice the techniques she had studied in Germany, and again, the patients she treated lost their symptoms.

However, the London doctors, who were finding their patients improving much more quickly than they expected, had no approach for dealing with the asymptomatic patient within the psychoanalytic framework. Further, as Marion was not good at promoting her work, she returned to Germany, feeling herself a failure, to complete her training with Mrs. Heyer. Mrs. Heyer considered Marion her most gifted pupil.

By the time she finished her training with Mrs. Heyer, Marion's parents had fled Germany for England. Her older sister had married and gone to Switzerland. Marion and her younger sister went to Sweden to wait for American visas.

The waiting period was a difficult time, as Marion had only a letter of introduction from Lucy Heyer, no legal status, and was living with her sister in the home of a friend of their father. Marion's sister obtained a work permit, and the two of them lived on the sister's small earnings. Marion needed to occupy her time while waiting for her visa. Her visa was two years in coming. Marion remembers:

> First I went to somebody who was teaching dance and asked if I could watch. I said I could massage and maybe do some exchange. As luck would have it, the dance teacher had an incredibly sore ankle. I gave her three treatments, and it improved greatly. She was interested in me after that. Then I gave her a treatment for lumbago on the afternoon before she had an evening performance. From then on I was allowed to come and go as I pleased at the dancing school. I spent a lot of my time there watching the dancers.

Dance was not the only pursuit that enhanced her understanding of the human body during the months she was in Sweden. She took a formal course in physical therapy. Lucy Heyer's teachings were supported and validated for Marion by the progressive nature of Swedish physical culture work.

> I heard about physical therapy training and went to see the man in charge. He was very sympathetic to my plight and interested in my work with Mrs. Heyer. He said I was welcome to join the class. I spoke very little Swedish so took my notes in German.

About a quarter of the way through the course, my notes became Swedish! He let me graduate with the class and wrote a letter saying I had done so. I knew there were some things he appreciated from my earlier work with Mrs. Heyer. The class was very interesting to me, and that was my first formal physical therapy training.

As part of the program, Marion observed various operations, watching hip replacements, bunionectomies, and vertebral disk and brain surgeries. Thus, in two years' time, under difficult circumstances, Marion had gained exposure to some of the most progressive and important work going on in the field.

Marion received her visa at last, and she decided to take the road not previously taken: to go to New York and work with the woman she had met in her mother's parlor in Nuremberg, Gertrude Lederer and Lederer's colleague, Karen Horney. By that time the Germans had invaded Norway and the only route to America was through Eastern Europe, Russia, and Japan. Her sister's visa did not come through, so Marion sailed alone for the United States from Japan at age twenty-four, landing in San Francisco instead of New York. Marion's sister remained in Sweden, married, and reared a family there.

Settling in the United States

After seeing San Francisco and Berkeley, Marion decided to make her home there. She lived with a German family in Berkeley and did occasional work as a physical therapist. She found the early 1940s atmosphere of Berkeley particularly stimulating and, much like her mother, she began to seek out interesting people who were accomplished in their fields.

A young woman physician who was familiar with Marion's work, along with the woman's husband who was a physicist, felt Marion had the potential to become a physician. They encouraged her to begin a pre-med course at the University of California, Berkeley. Once can only imagine what contemporary students must have thought of the tall young woman with little money and a German accent in the man's world of pre-med studies on the Berkeley campus of 1944. She managed to maintain a B-minus average, not high enough for admission to medical school.

Besides attending school, Marion was working the "swing shift" as a physical therapist at Kaiser Hospital in Richmond, treating injured workers from Kaiser shipyards. After the war there was a tremendous need for physical therapists for the wounded. Marion learned of a tuition-free program at the Mayo Clinic in Minnesota that trained people for the relatively new (in the U.S.) field of physical therapy. She enrolled and because she was an advanced student, was accelerated through the course to graduate in six months.

She returned to Berkeley and resumed work at the Kaiser Hospital in Richmond, California, but found she had little zest for the hospital environment. The staff was overworked and had insufficient time to give to individual patients. She often treated forty patients a day.

Soon, she and her former supervisor at Kaiser formed a partnership and went into private practice in physical therapy, an innovative step for that time. They opened an office in the basement of a physician's office building in Oakland. There Marion continued to treat patients for over thirty years.

Marion was married for a short time, and in 1949 she gave birth to a daughter. Marion's original partner retired soon after. Marion then joined forces with another woman for a short time, and then with her present partner, Gritta Green, who is now semi-retired. Marion's reputation grew slowly but steadily. Her office was near the offices of several orthopedists whose patients often required long-term physical therapy. Physicians making referrals to Marion soon learned the value of her opinion and treatment. Many patients were sent with the simple orders, "Do what you think is best."

In her daughter, Marion found herself with a living laboratory for observation of the development of the human body and psyche. Marion's strong opinions about the effects of child rearing practices upon the free and natural movement of the body stem from her own experiences as a parent.

Patients who came to her with problems with physical origins taught Marion the potential of the body to heal itself. They taught her a great deal about the nature of the will to be well as a factor in maintaining body movement and health. She noticed that patients who talked to her about the events of their lives at the time of their accident or injury were the ones who recovered most quickly. She became convinced of the connection between mind and body and became increasingly successful in treating patients with psychosomatic illnesses—those with origins in emotional stress and withholding.

Marion continued developing her techniques and theories in this setting for thirty-five years. Despite her expertise, and with an ever-widening reputation and roster of successes, she herself lacked the conviction that she had developed any special process. She knew only that she was a caring physical therapist and also a very busy single parent at a time where there was far less support for that role than there is today.

Some of Marion's friends came to her occasionally for the treatment of tight muscles or tension-related aches and pains. One of them asked Marion for something to do to prevent the aches and pains. From this simple request Marion began her movement classes in 1957. She used the range of motion tests she used in physical therapy as exercises, set them to music, and had the women do them once a week to keep their joints lubricated and the muscles moving freely and fully.

She held her first class in the living room of one of her students. The original five students were soon joined by others, making it necessary to move to a larger space. As attendance and interest increased, a second class was started. These two classes, taught by Marion, have remained in continuous operation, with several of the original students still in attendance.

As her daughter matured, Marion found more time to consider the achievement of her life's work. A patient brought her the key to an important life change. A woman whom Marion had been treating with little result appeared upon her therapy table in a suddenly much improved condition. Marion asked what had brought about the change. The woman told her that she had just taken a weekend course with Werner Erhard called "Mind Dynamics." Marion had never heard of the training but sought it out, so impressed was she with the change in her patient.

Marion credits the Erhard seminar with giving her the confidence and perspective to seek new opportunities in her life and to take credit for work well done. In her words:

> I had become aware of knowing really much more than I had ever let out. So I began to say things to my patients, and it seemed to make a great difference. This is how I reawakened an interest in the verbal part of my work and really when it began in earnest.

As Marion began to open up to the possibilities of discussing patients' conditions with them, she began to realize that she did indeed have something to teach and so began her training of students by apprenticeship.

At present, Marion is actively involved in guiding her students in Berkeley and abroad. She has come to accept the role of leader, a difficult one for her. She remains a student as well. Marion continually seeks to understand more fully the mystery of the mind-body relationship and to support the value of self-knowledge and self-acceptance.

Chapter 2: Theoretical Basis

> If you do not let yourself be the way you are, your body cannot function. The same is true for the emotions. The only way you can be who you are is through surrender and self-acceptance.

The Rosen Method flows directly from the practice of physical therapy. It evolved through years of clinical practice of physical therapy apart from other intellectual, academic, and philosophical influences. Until the establishment of the Rosen Institute, little effort was made to describe systematically the operating principles and ideas underlying the method. It was fiercely pragmatic and relied solely on the evidence of clinical experience.

Only after Marion Rosen accepted the challenge of teaching did she have to transform her accumulated knowledge to a more literal and transmissible one.

Part of the difficulty of discussing the philosophy of the Rosen Method is its very simplicity. When asked to explain the philosophical basis of her bodywork, Marion replied:

Naturally, as we come into this world, we are not beings that hold back; we are beings that are open. When we are born, when we start getting up and we start moving, we move according to very elementary mechanical and physiological rules. The body works when you move and behaves according to these rules. No effort to it. But we put something in the body that makes it more difficult to move, and then we freeze in this position. Why does this happen? There is always something that seems to necessitate a certain way of non-movement, non-living in a certain way. And every time something stimulates it again, we hold again. We hold a little bit more. And we have forgotten that this is what we do. These elements are partly in the physical body and partly in our emotional being. And in the end, probably in our spiritual attainment.

The underlying concerns of the approach are transpersonal and transcending, based on our common experience as embodied beings. The method is based on the premise that a natural and optimal state of human physical and psychic strength exists. The Rosen Method aims at obtaining or regaining this optimal state where the full range of possibilities for expression and authentic, spontaneous behavior exist. As such, Rosen Method is a pathway to self-awareness and self-acceptance.

Rosen Method treats mind and body as an interactive unit. The body does not have meaning as an object in the way it does, say, for a surgeon. Body is imbued with mind, and mind is embodied. The Rosen practitioner acknowledges the potential power of all psychic elements of which some knowledge exists—the unconscious, the parapsychological, and so on—but places particular emphasis on the role of the emotions, because it is the emotions that have emerged, again and again, in her work. All her technique is similarly rooted in her client's experiences. Her methods are those that have proved to have practical application for her clients.

Because mind and body are inextricably linked, Rosen practitioners reach for each through the other. Their particular talent is affecting the mind and body by contact with the body. The point of entry to the system is through the body.

In bodywork, it is easy to assume that some manipulation is being done *to* the client. The Rosen Method practitioner is a facilitator of awareness and change, not the creator of it. The practitioner observes the places in the client's body where chronic tension is held and where free movement of the breath is not allowed. Through contact with the tight muscles, often called barriers, the practitioner meets the holding at its own level, as though reminding the muscle that it is holding, and that it has the inherent possibility of relaxing. The client's awareness follows the practitioner's hands, and relaxation becomes an option.

When the practitioner contacts a client's tight muscles, and his awareness makes it possible for them to relax, the experience of the earlier event is often felt. From this insight, the tension pattern that the client developed can be assessed and the client brought closer to his authentic or true self. This information is never new to the client. What one learns as true in life is that which one has already experienced but not accepted, has not acknowledged, or has forgotten. There is no new knowledge, simply a new knowing.

The Rosen Method practitioner pays close attention to the breath and breathing. A change in the mind/body relationship will occur or can be detected via the breath. In Rosen Method the breath is the indicator of change in the mind/body and is the intersection between conscious and unconscious processes.

The diaphragm, the major muscle involved in breathing, is innervated by both the voluntary and the autonomic nervous systems. Because of this dual innervation, attention can be, and is, paid to the "unconscious" or "natural" breath. When a client relaxes and stops performing or "doing" his breathing, the practitioner watches this breath for changes. She looks for changes in the natural or unperformed breath that indicate has made a connection with repressed emotion linked to tension in the muscle being touched. When the practitioner observes this change from her external perspective, she can verbalize her observation and give the client an opportunity to connect this change with his inner experience.

The breath is the intersection between mind and body. The breath is the most readily available channel for tuning in to the mind/body dialogue. The breath is doubly interesting and valuable because it is both a voluntary and involuntary action. Voluntary breathing is linked to conscious activity, involuntary breathing to unconscious activity.

Marion Rosen's apprenticeship with Lucy Heyer initiated her concern and interest in the breath. Heyer had studied with Elsa Gindler, and both were in agreement that breathing, although not completely understood, was an important area of investigation for bodywork theory and practice. This interest and conviction has become central to the Rosen Method.

When the diaphragm is tight, the body does not function at its best. As the major muscle of breathing, the diaphragm is essential to a state of well-being. Its free, full movement can only be allowed; it cannot be performed. Holding in the diaphragm represents a state of "doingness" in the body, a state with an emotional counterpart.

The client's unconscious processes shape the body. In the socialization process most people adopt roles, play games, wear masks, put up facades, and put barriers in the form of muscular tension between themselves and others. They feel or believe that their genuine or authentic self is unacceptable. The roles, games, masks, barriers, and facades develop subtly in response to unspoken demands and pressures from the child's caretakers, become structured in the body, and require muscular tension to maintain.

Our bodies and our characters are shaped by the social forces at work as we mature. The attitudes taken on as a result of socialization are carried and expressed in the body, forming habit patterns that are embodied as rigidity and restricted movement.

For example, a baby has no trouble at all expressing feelings spontaneously, usually by crying. As the baby grows, he or she gets the message that crying is not permitted or valued as a means of expression. When the tears come, the child stops crying by tightening the muscles of the neck and chest. When the urge to cry comes on again, the child tightens the neck and chest and refrains from crying.

Later on, the tightening of the neck and chest muscles becomes habitual, and the child no longer feels the feelings that would make him or her cry. Repression in complete, and the child grows into an adult with a chronic stiff neck and non-movable chest and shoulders.

This pattern of tension often makes a body top-heavy with a thick neck and flushed face, a form frequently seen in men who grew up being told, "Big boys don't cry."

One may have a chronically tense body without becoming severely disabled. The most damaging long-term effect of unregarded bodily tensions is the capping of the individual's potential for self-actualization. Self-actualization can result from allowing chronic tension or habitual holding to soften, with a resulting shift towards the authentic expression of emotions as they occur. Rosen Method practitioners can feel, see, and trace the movement of the client's breath into formerly held areas.

No value or importance is placed by the Rosen practitioner on the trauma in one's life that made it necessary at the time to create a barrier or chronic muscle tension. A barrier is a barrier. It doesn't matter if it was formed because the child didn't get a jelly sandwich or because of a major loss. The practitioner meets the barrier, not the experience itself. But the client may become aware of the emotional content of the barrier and thereby gain access to a new way of behaving.

The content of the barrier or holding is unimportant to the practice of the method. What is important is to acknowledge the need to repress in the first place, the chronic muscular tension required to maintain the pattern, and the examination of whether that need still exists.

When the client experiences the content of the barrier, he invariably finds it interesting. Sometimes, however, the relaxation happens without the content or story coming into consciousness. Even if the content does not surface, the client still experiences relaxation and the possibility for choice. If, however, a story is available along with the relaxation of the muscle, the client should be helped to say what it is. The event become real if it can be shared, and the original need to repress it loses its impact. As the habit of repression is thereby challenged, future repression is less likely.

Ilse Middendorf

Ilse Middendorf was born September 21, 1910, in Frankenberg, Germany. Between 1932–36 she studied breath therapy, nerve massage, and gymnastics at various institutes in Germany. From 1936–41 she studied graphology. Her subsequent education included lay analysis and a seven-year study of psychology. Professor Middendorf's work today is known throughout Germany, Switzerland, and Holland, particularly among dancers, musicians, actors, and psychotherapists. In 1965 she founded the Institute for Breath Therapy in Berlin, where she engages in private practice and offers extensive training in breath therapy. She is married and has one son.

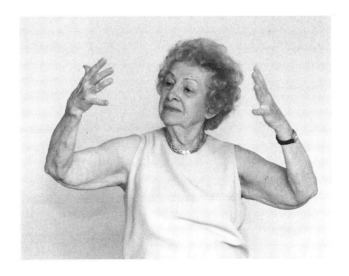

Interview with Ilse Middendorf

Elizabeth Beringer

Beringer: I know you have more than fifty years of experience working with breathing. How did that start? What is your background?

Middendorf: I was born in a little town in Saxony, Germany, called Frankenberg. My childhood was very happy. I used to spend a lot of time outside in the garden—to look after it, but also just to spend time there. One day, when I was in the garden, a voice called to me saying, "You have to breathe." I was very astonished. I sat on a bench for two hours, just thinking about the meaning of this. Then I went to my mother, who said, "Just let it go. I don't know what it is. Don't bother about it."

Beringer: How old were you?

Middendorf: Eleven, maybe twelve. I don't remember exactly. I was always introverted. At the age of five, I played the piano and loved to dance. Then I heard this voice, this sentence, which I forgot about for a time, but it came back later, and I remembered it strongly. I was exposed to gymnastics from the time I was very young; and when I became older, I wanted to study more.

Beringer: Would you speak about this further? You mean something different from what we do with the word "gymnastics."

Middendorf: I studied the Menzler Method which is based on very good internal sensing and movement. I began this when I was about five years old and continued throughout my schooling.

Elizabeth Beringer. "Interview with Ilse Middendorf." *Somatics* Autumn/Winter 1988–89. 15–17

Beringer: Was this part of the German school system at that time?

Middendorf: No, it was not common; it was just one of many kinds of training, but I had the opportunity to do this. There were other methods like Kallmayer, Menzendieck.

Beringer: These were offered in the schools?

Middendorf: It was a special opportunity to be taught by a student of these teachers. I had such an opportunity to study with a teacher trained by Dora Menzler. It was not usual—something that was more for the upper classes. But it suited me totally. When I was older, I studied "gymnastics" with Gunther and Trumpy (two women). I had to pay for this training myself. I was short of money; it was difficult, but I knew that was what I wanted. I was about twenty years old then.

Beringer: So you had training in this type of work all along. When did you start really focusing on breathing?

Middendorf: Directly after my training, I taught breathing. While in training, I began to feel that breathing was not stressed enough and that the movements they taught were against the natural movement of breath. I felt that the "breath movement" had a different shape. Then I had a lot of fights with my teacher. During this time, I also went to study with a teacher out of the Mastanang movement. This is a kind of work where body state and mind are interrelated on Tibetan movements. They had seven specific breath exercises. Later, I began teaching this system as well.

Beringer: Some people in the workshop mentioned that your work reminded them of chi kung, or other types of Oriental systems they had studied, but that it was more personal. I wondered if you'd had any contact with those systems.

Middendorf: I was in China and noticed that they often worked with breathing in a guided way, by will. The Tibetan system was the same. The most important difference between those kinds of methods and ours is the feeling that we want to follow the law of breathing. We are into this law—not above or beside it. We want to know: What does *breathing* mean? That is a very important differentiation. These other systems I studied may have suggested some directions, but my work comes entirely from my own explorations. When I was teaching the Mastanang work, I did my own daily explorations between five and seven in the morning before I went to work. I wrote notes, but I never read them again because it wasn't necessary. Once you have had an experience, you don't have to read about it anymore.

Beringer: Did that go on for many years?

Middendorf: Yes, I still do this two hours every day. Here in San Francisco, I get up at five and still work two hours. But, back then, I had no one else to confirm the rightness of what I was exploring. I gave lessons in the Mastanang Method for six years—while I was doing my own explorations every morning. Then I met Cornelius Veening, and this was a revelation. He came from the same roots. He was a master teacher. He had only a few students, ten or fifteen, whom he chose. He had no institute, and he completely refused to write anything, He hated to see anyone teaching from notes. He had connections to Jung and Heier, a pupil of Jung's. He made it possible for me to teach my own work. He confirmed the work I was doing privately; and, all at once, it opened like a flower. I needed that confirmation. I worked with him for almost thirty years. Once or twice a year, I would go to work with him for ten days. He died three years ago.

Beringer: Did he live in Berlin?

Middendorf: Yes. He was in Berlin until the 1950s, and then he moved to Holland. I don't know exactly when. He was Dutch.

Beringer: Could you speak more about Jung's ideas in relation to your work?

Middendorf: Jung's importance was his focus on self-reliance, and his work was with images and dreams. My work is on breathing.

Beringer: You see them as having similar goals with similar paths?

Middendorf: Yes. If a person finds his way based on the experience of his breathing, he finds his own power and creativity.

Beringer: You talked a great deal about people not being complete and that we are always creating ourselves. Is that the same idea?

Middendorf: Yes. It's a process. Every person has his own way of processing: through the experience of his breathing, he finds his way, his path. One person goes inside, senses the breath moving, and his experience of breathing is based on that. Another one goes outside to experience the breath moving there, and comes back slowly. . . . And the one who first went inside goes outside the next time to experience breathing there. A person with restricted breathing has to experience first his own rhythm and to experience how it widens. Those parts which are too narrow straighten up. They have to find a way into the wideness, and those parts which are too wide have to find the way back. The work to find balance is very important. You have to find the balance that is changing again and again and all the time.

There is only one rule: It is centering breathing. Whenever you sense that you are centered and breathing, there is also sensing of being centered. That's the whole thing. Out of that you make your own start, and you find your own process, but it is all based on that: Sensing, Centering, Breathing.

Beringer: Could you describe what kinds of things you would do in a class to facilitate this kind of process?

Middendorf: It's very hard to talk about his. This is the point where it gets difficult. I can say that we start with stretching. When you stretch, you can say where the stretching is; it brings you inhalation, and so on, but this goes right to the head. That is not what we want in this work. We work with different processes which we call stretching, pressure points, vowel-space breathing, cave breathing, and movement out of the breathing. I cannot really describe them here in words because it would not do the work justice.

Beringer: In what context do the teachers of your work practice?

Middendorf: Many practice in their own offices, or schools, or sanitariums; others practice health counseling. There are many different types of situations.

Beringer: When did you found the Institute and begin to teach others?

Middendorf: I started the Institute for Breathing Therapy in 1935, and I began to train other teachers in 1965.

Beringer: In your work you have both group classes and private sessions. How do you decide what someone needs?

Middendorf: It is individually based on what this person needs at any movement—either only private sessions or classes or the two mixed together, to match their process. What we look out for is: What does this person want? We don't say, "You must take ..." We say, "Look, we offer this and this. What would you like?" And sometimes when people come and ask for private lessons, I ask, "Is this really necessary for you?" I don't open the door and say, "Come in, come in." I say, "Really, look at yourself."

Beringer: Many people do various kinds of yogic breathing. What is your impression of that work and how is that different from yours?

Middendorf: All the yoga ways of breathing come out of the male way. The Eastern way of thinking is to find god in one direction, in a male way. "The way is directed. I go there and I have to go; I must go." This way needs will; that is also the reason why, in this case, breathing is connected. It has something to do with will. This male way of being needs will. When this is the basis, the breathing is under the law of the will.

We are the opposite of the male way. In our work we can grow spatiality, a breathing place. This space is a power you can experience in reality; it is a real thing. Out of this, we have direction. But to get this space I have first to be centered, to sense, and to breathe. For instance, you have a kind of power from the armpit, you have the power from the middle center, you have the power of the lower space, and so on. And in this way, I'm inside a big whole which includes everything, like an egg.

Beringer: I like very much the image you used in the workshop—that your work is not a ladder, but that one can approach it from any side, as if it were a sphere.

Middendorf: In this work you can experience so much power that it has to go out. It looks for a way to go out, for a direction that's "me," myself. In fact, this is Tao. It has nothing to do with ego. The male way of being grows out of the female. In the next decade, we have to experience the balance between those two things: male/female, yin/yang, whatever you call it. It has to come, this balance.

Beringer: When you mention the centers, does this relate to the chakra system?

Middendorf: No. We don't have chakras. We have some centers which manifest themselves during the experience; they have similarities, similar experiences, but they can change every time. You can sense a center [of energy] wherever you are wide and narrow. During the same experience, many are centered in the *hara* [the center of the body]; others, in the middle of the heart or throat—but it's not necessarily fixed.

Beringer: That's interesting because, in fact, different chakra systems do not agree on the number and placement of their chakras! So you do not think in this system?

Middendorf: We think in the system of experience. I am sure that the chakras are important and that we are in relation to them in this work, but we do not work directly with that idea. It can happen that the movement of the breath can match experiences from other systems. Many people who do T'ai Chi say there's a similarity that shows up in the movement. If you see someone do T'ai Chi, you might say that it is similar to a person who is moving out from his own breathing, as we do. The difference is that T'ai Chi is 3,000 or 4,000 years old, and it is now a pattern that a person puts on. We let all these forms grow up new every time out of our experience. T'ai Chi comes from the outside, and our work grows from the inside.

Beringer: When I had a private session with you, I was able to feel my breathing much more clearly, and the pattern of my breathing had changed. What role does the individual's physical awareness of the process have in your work?

Middendorf: Put your hands here (indicates my lower ribs) as you sit upright. We sense the breath movement and wait until the new inhalation comes of its own accord.

Sensory awareness grows and begins to have its place more and more in a person's daily life. You feel all the time; you sense your feet, everything. It is in your sensory awareness. When you do this, your breathing movement is conscious because you sense all the time. Your sensory awareness is such that you are aware of your breathing movement at all times. It is hard to put into words.

Beringer: That's clear. This would be hard to put into words, even if we were all speaking the same language.

Middendorf: Because of this power of sensory awareness, we can experience, say, illness at its inception—not only when it appears. We can feel when something is not in good balance with respect to illness. Then we will probably change something. For instance, I can feel a coldness in the bronchial system, and I act on it at that time. I take a hot bath or I drink a glass of wine or I breathe. My breathing is reacting automatically to some change. I don't wait. I'm aware, and I don't go on for days and suddenly get a cold. When I talk about breathing, I mean one's whole being: body, mind, and spirit.

Beringer: In the workshop, you talked about different psychological or spiritual states associated with different parts of the body. In your work, do you make practical use of this concept, or is it more theoretical?

Middendorf: I'm working with that concept, but I don't label it. I have people experience their bodies in the deepest way I can. Out of that very personal experience comes, eventually, an enlightenment about how one's bodily state reflects one's psychological state.

Beringer: Is there anything else you'd like to add?

Middendorf: I'm very happy still to be growing in the process of building up this work. There are processes I discovered only two years ago, and others I found forty years ago. I'm finding new things all the time. It is never completed; it is always growing.

The Perceptible Breath:
A Breathing Science (Preface)

Ilse Middendorf

In this book, I want to explain, what I have experienced in almost fifty years of work with breathing. It is meant not only for everyone who has worked with me, but also for those who are able to open themselves and get to know and to experience the breath, not only by "doing" it, but also by "letting" it happen. I also want to direct myself to those who believe that one should not experience one's breath "consciously"(here I mean: feeling it consciously), since it can easily be disrupted, so that it should remain exclusively unconscious.

This book is not meant to be a scientific explanation in the ordinary sense, but it is based on experiences that certainly are scientifically precise. Developments and laws in the sphere of breathing will be discovered that are not only the mind's control, but also the ability to feel. This can only be achieved by a constant ability to feel together with an undisturbed composure. I am aware of the difficulties putting an experience into words, so I shall try to describe it as I have perceived it. Thus "focusing-perceiving-breathing" will be the basis of it.

The body was ignored for various reasons, amongst them religious ones. It is used to serve as an instrument, a means to an end of the spiritual-mental life. At best it was to provide "enjoyment of the pleasures of life" and in this way was accepted or banished, but more often ignored as "dull nature." During the last hundred years or so, a change has been taking place, allowing the "packhorse body" become more conscious. Today the human body as a whole or its part are a matter of popular interest from many different points of view. It became inter-

Paderborn, Germany: Junferman Verlag, 1990. 9–15

esting, because of people's existential helplessness, in which it is hopelessly involved and which it cannot resolve. The human body is often "discovered" by subjecting it to specific physical exertions, in the hope of revealing its secrets by these clumsy external means. The body is sought by supposed "methods of research" that in the end do not take the body into consideration at all.

The all round nature of the human existence, however, continually allows and requires new ways of approaching physical existence. We can see nearly every day, how new "methods" originate, but their values must be dubious for lack of balance as we had seen, for example: the mechanization of our movements, the achievement-oriented way of life, use of the body as a vehicle to achieve certain mental or spiritual states.

The reasons why there are so many different keys to corporality, are because the body "carries everything in itself," since life and soul, mind and body form a whole. How strong has our discernment to grow, until we are able to realize what this marvel, "the body" is, and judge it in terms of its overall importance! How often, even in our own times, is the body looked upon and judged as an object. But how could reality develop in human life, in the Now, without the reality of the body?

German and Indo-European linguistic history allows us to distinguish between the Körper (corpus) and Leib (body).

The history of the New High German word Körper (corpus) starts with its Middle High German borrowing from the Latin word corpus, body flesh, corpse, shadow (of a dead person), trunk, belly, person, nature, and others, and leads over the years to the latest form. This borrowing was encouraged by the Christian church (communion and worship of the corpse) and through the art of healing. In meaningful contrast was the development of the German word "Leib" (body) originating in the Germanic word for "life."

Thus:

Old High German:	Lib:	Leben (life)
Middle High German:	Lip/Lib:	Leben, Körper (life/body)
Anglo-Saxon:	Lif:	Leben (life)
Old Norse:	Lif:	Leben

In the English word "life" we can recognize phonetically the German word "Leib" (body). German is the only Germanic language since the middle ages which has transferred the word meaning "life" to the body itself (Lip, Leib=body).

So Lip = Leib (body) means life and concentrates on its entity, whereas corpus = body, seems to express more substance—a circumstance which the breathing person can easily be aware of and experience.

In Germany, Jahn, the father of gymnastics, opened the first door of the prison of "bodily unconsciousness." According to the tradition of the western world it was started from the "outside." Soon, though, deeper layers were also presaged within the physical.

Then Hede Kallmeyer began her expedition of discovery into the world of movement of gymnastics. Her work is based on that of the American G. Stebbins, whose great model was Delsarte. In her excellent book *Heilkraft durch Bewegung* (Haug Verlag), Hede Kallmeyer attributes the dawning of body consciousness to Delsarte (1811/1871) which develops until nowadays. Wars and political turmoil have been unable to hold up its subsequent development without interruption by such famous names as Kallmeyer, Gindler, Mensendieck, Gode, and Medau in gymnastics, and Duncan, Laban, Mary Wigman and Palucca in dance. The field of gymnastics and acrobatics covers "physical exercise," athletics and competitive sport, but despite its variety, this awakened consciousness of the body still lacked something. Leaving aside that even in antiquity, in Egypt, Greece and in the civilizations breath was thought to maintain the contact with divinity and to be a carrier of vitality; when at the beginning of the century there were at first only few and then increasingly more and gifted people who recognized the essential importance of the breath and who opened the way to an entire feeling and experiencing of the breath: Clara Schlaffhorst and Hedwig Andersen (1928) whose work even today lives on in the training of teachers of breathing, speech and vocal training.

The psychological root of the world of breath was mentioned by C.G. Jung and emphasized by Gustav Heyer. Cornelius Veening and Margarethe Mhe elaborated their original intuitions into a "breathing-psychological" path and made clear what the deep contact of the breath with the essential meant.

Karlfried Graf Dürckheim must also be mentioned here as the breath is embedded in his existentialist teachings. And in Lowen's bioenergetic teachings you can find Wilhelm Reich's *Wissen vom Atem*. Ludwig Schmitt (1956) was the first to bring the medical side of breathing home to us. While his first work *Das Hohelied vom Atem* shows quite clearly his consternation about the significance of breath, his second work *Atemheilkunst* (1960) forms an important basis of medical breath therapy.

This short review is meant to show the roots of the germinal body-consciousness, which we owe to those who worked with the breath in earlier times and which is developing to become a vital empirical science. Those who have published fundamental works on the subject "breath" are: Volkmar Glaser (1980), Udo Derbowsky (19878), Horst Coblenzer (1976). There is no space here to quote all those who have created developments in breathing; I want to emphasize that a group of people who devoted themselves to working with the breath, who are searching and understanding can open up a core of vital breathing conscience in all its range of possibilities. Body-soul and spirit can now be lived and experienced as a unity. The breath is an energetic core that may influence all kinds of aspects of human life: it influences movement, art, medicine, psychology and religion. Here we may consider work with the breath as an autonomous discipline with its own special laws.

Breath is a connecting force. It creates a bodily equilibrium and balance and helps us to make inner and outer impressions interchangeable. It connects the human being with the outside world and the outside world with his inner world. Breathing is an original unceasing movement and therefore actual life. The ineffable has given nature various autonomous laws which have still to come to fruition. Experiencing the breath means to start to live in a new way. Breathing became my "guide rope" that enables me to lead the body and with it the spiritual and mental into a new "opening" to life where meaning is, to achieve a wider consciousness and greater expansion in the inner and outer spaces.

In a time of impatience during earlier attempts, when I wanted to make more and quicker discoveries in the field of exercising with breathing, I had a dream, which I should like to describe in broad outline: I stood right on the bank of a river with a very strong current. One the other side there was a broad, sunny landscape, woody and light green in color, with an impressive farmhouse in the foreground, crowded with animals and friendly people at work. I knew that I had to cross the river to get to the other bank and that they expected me there, gut there was no bridge leading across the nearly torrential stream. Instead, there was a strong rope connecting the two banks floating partly on, partly in the water. I gave way to an impulse, jumped into the water, grasped the rope first with my right hand, then with my left, and so moved, hand over hand, along the rope over the river towards the other side. That was very difficult and sometimes it seemed impossible to reach the goal. But finally I made it and was welcomed by the people on the other bank and woke up.

It became clear to me that I had to continue patiently the "guiderope of breath" until the clarity of consciousness could develop out of "understanding the unconscious." I still like using the metaphor of the "guiderope of the breathing," because it always leads us on to something new, as long as we entrust ourselves to it.

It was that, which I had experienced with the breath that made me follow the path which I mentioned in the book. When I was eleven years old, I had similar experiences which grew into a steadily increasing body of experience accompanying my professional life.

The success I had as a gymnastic teacher was not enough for me while I was young. I searched for an essence in the movements and for a medium to achieve or to create one. The transformations or changes which the people who worked with me underwent, seemed to me far too superficial and not intense enough. I was looking for something more direct and more involved with human reality. Full of presentiment I kept turning to the breath, but shied away from the particularly single-minded methods. While it seemed for me that some training methods placed too much emphasis on will power leaving no room for breathing and creating reality. So I was grateful to have found an extraordinary teacher, who brought home to me the unity of our human appearance by means of movement, breathing, and meditation: Ewe Warren, a dancer with great human maturity. To her I owe the preparation which enabled me to experience the breath later on. Many thanks to her!

Then I met my second teacher, Cornelius Veening. With him something opened up inside me that had not been able to free itself before: The break-through to the essence in the breath and immersion in its creative and inspiring nature. In the years of working with the breath he made me conscious of and clarified the so far unknown powers, encourage, criticized and supported me until I started to become independent and acquired the power of creativity, I needed to go my own way. I owe a great deal to this great master, but especially my opening up to my own development and, above all the liberty I found in myself.

C.G. Jung's psychology is also very close to working with the breath. For decades I have turned to his work and he has given me many important insights and clarified things inside me of great importance to me and my work. Intensive talks with Charles F. Herreshoff (Charlottesville, USA) made clear to me that the world of pictures is not identical with the world that opens up the ability to feel and experience in oneself, which is what this book is about. I should like to thank Herreshoff very much for his extensive collaboration during its preparation, his advice on certain psychological basis, and their relation to the perceptible breath.

Finally I should like to add that this book is based on experiences at times difficult to "understand." Patience is the key to your understanding and experiencing: patience in repeated reading and practice to reach eventual clarity and understanding.

2.

Structural Wisdom

F.M. Alexander

F. *Matthias Alexander (1869–1955) is perhaps the oldest significant influence on Americans in this area of embodiment. His method is widely practiced by schools of acting. John Dewey was his pupil for twenty years, and Pragmatism and Progressive Education bear the marks of his work. The Alexander Technique, a one-on-one teacher-student method, involves learning how to inhibit one's automatic reactions to the simplest stimuli—beginning to speak, getting up out of a chair, taking up oars to row a boat. Out of the experience of inhibiting the rush to do these activities, one learns how to move with more grace and ease, how to be more fully present in this movement. The lessons generally take place by way of very subtle verbal instructions, and sometimes a very light touch.*

A Conversation with Marjory Barlow

Joan Schirle

*Marjory Barlow is a Master Teacher of the Alexander Technique. The niece
of F.M. Alexander, she began lessons in her teens and has been teaching for
fifty-four years. In this conversation with Joan Schirle, she talks about Alexander himself, the nature of his work, and the demands of being a teacher. It
was taped on August 12, 1986, during the First International Alexander
Teachers' Congress in Stony Brook, New York.*

Schirle: Would you say that F.M. Alexander was an extraordinarily
patient man to have experimented with himself in this way—to come
up with this?

Barlow: I simply can't believe it—it's the most fantastic story! I think
that he was a very passionate, very tempestuous man, and in his initial state very quick-tempered. My mother said that if he saw someone ill-treating an animal or something like that, he literally saw red;
they were afraid he was going to murder somebody one day! He was
really so quick, and this is his initial endowment, really. Before I started
going to Ashley Place to have lessons, my mother warned me; she
said, "You'll be in tears every day." Only once—but it wasn't F.M.
who did it. (laughs) And this was the fantastic change, you see—and,
of course, it was very important to him to apply the work to these ter-
rifically quick, deep emotional responses. In a way that was why the
work appealed to me when I first read *Constructive Conscious Control*:
that it was possible (a) to become more aware, to reach perhaps a level
of awareness that was a little bit better than the one I'd got, and (b)
not to be so subject to these emotional swings. I was like a pendulum.

Somatics Spring/Summer 1987. 22–25

Schirle: Was it difficult for F.M. to be patient with beginners?

Barlow: It *had* been, obviously—from what mother told me about how cross he was going to get with me—but by the time I landed up there, it was 1932, and he was never impatient with me or with anybody I saw him teaching. He realized, you see . . . he really knew and remembered how difficult it was. He used to say to me sometimes: "People who come here are the salt of the earth; but if they knew what they were going to have to undergo, they wouldn't come." Then he added: "But where else can they go?"

Schirle: How would you talk about what Alexander called "Direction"?

Barlow: I would say that every time an idea comes to you to do anything at all, messages are sent from your brain through your nervous system to the rest of you—I'm not a scientist, I'm an Alexander teacher, and this is the way I see it, very simply, really—and the movement is then carried out. Before we have lessons, all this is totally automatic. Habits are built up, and they are built up in the nervous system. It is not the old muscles and bones—it is the direct connection. There is no division between your brain and the rest of your nervous system, and it is that immediacy that is so wonderful; when you send a message, a conscious message, it is there before you know it. And if anything gets into the work that is interposed—for example, a lot of people have "images," or all that sort of nonsense—that is all unnecessary.

Schirle: So when you speak of how we interfere with ourselves, you are speaking of that neuro-response that takes place between the brain and the rest of the body, and how we interfere with the purity or the directness of it?

Barlow: Yes. When the stimulus comes—I mean, this really brings us back to inhibition, doesn't it? *This* is the keystone of the whole Alexander Technique. You see, he could not get anywhere. He tried going up every avenue that he could think of, and it was not until he realized that every time that the stimulus came to speak, back went his head. And he tried *everything*, from putting it [the head] forward to ... everything. One day he saw that it was his response—his automatic habitual response to a stimulus—that was the trouble: It was so quick. He realized that his first work—when the stimulus came—was to say "No!" Not to say "No!" to the stimulus—and this is very important—but to say "no!" to the *first* reaction to that idea. What happened at first was a habitual thing. If you say "No!" there is the stimulus , there is the response. But if you do not say "No!" it is like that—it is habitual, it is perpetual motion—just like an automaton. We are a lot of robots really. But if you do not allow that response to happen when the stimulus comes, there's a little bit of space between the two, a little bit of freedom there—and the only freedom we'll ever have in this world, I think. People talk about freedom in a big way. But if you can refuse to respond to the stimulus, you have three choices: You can allow your habitual response to happen, because it is the most appropriate for the situation you are in; or you can decide to make a conscious new response; or, best of all, you can decide to do nothing—if that is appropriate. It gives you the chance to respond appropriately to this moment.

Schirle: You are one of the few teachers whose writings talk about the emotions and the spirit relative to the ideas of conscious control. Does that come from your own personality, or was Alexander himself interested in these areas and we just do not hear so much about that aspect of his work?

Barlow: I'm glad you've asked me that, because it is very difficult to define what a religious person is. One thing he was *not*, was dogmatic. He was asked about religion, because people loved to pin F.M. down—to get his opinion on this, that, or the other. And they would ask him direct questions; for example, "What do you believe, F.M.?" He would reply: "I believe everything and I believe nothing."

He would not pontificate on subjects that were not his special province. He had his own way, his own beliefs, his own relationship with the universe—it sounds a bit silly, really—but he had a sense I'm sure, of the universe being a rather intelligent place. He had a great sense of purpose in his whole life, for he had had a very strict religious upbringing. Church on Sundays, three times a day, Sunday School in the afternoon, all the children—my mother told me this, of course. He was a very religious boy and a young man. He had a younger brother who got meningitis and screamed; because they were very far from doctors, nobody could do anything. F.M. prayed and prayed, but the baby died. And this made him think again; this really brought him up short. To me, he was the most religious person, in the real sense, of anybody I have ever met. And he was so inspiring. He really could lift you if you were in a bad state: Just by talking to him, somehow, and talking about the work ... suddenly you were up *there*— you know, rather like Bach's music—and it sort of all made sense....

Schirle: In your own work and studies you have made connections between his work and some very practical Eastern spiritual philosophies. There are some teachers who consider that this work applies only to the body and mind, but the spirit and emotions can be affected as well.

Barlow: Of course. It is the whole person, isn't it? And I think, rather like F.M., that I had a very strong religious sense from the beginning— from wherever one gets it—and have gone down quite a number of paths. You see, you have criteria ... since I started doing the work, I would explore these various avenues. When I came up against a contradiction with the Technique, it was the other thing that went. I have that lovely guide with me in everything, really; and if it conflicts with what I know about the Technique, I can't be interested any longer. But there are certain things which do not conflict at all. I do not allow these things that I pursue for my own personal development to come into my teaching, except indirectly, of course—one cannot help saying what one believes. But I certainly would not approve of any kind of admixture ... I do think the battle is to keep the Alexander teaching pure. By that I do not mean that people cannot develop their own ideas: but when it comes to a bit of T'ai Chi and a bit of yoga and a bit of this and bit of that, there isn't time in a training course for that— there really isn't time.

Schirle: Do you think there is a lot of that going on in the teaching now?

Barlow: Well, there is, isn't there? I know that it is inevitable with any teaching, when you look back through history. With time, it becomes diluted, it becomes changed, it becomes adulterated, if you like; and we all have to bring to it what we are. This is really what we are talking about, isn't it? What the person *is*. The extraordinary thing about F.M. was that he had no school. He was entirely himself . . . he was absolutely original.

Schirle: What have you found to be the most difficult thing for a teacher-trainee to learn about Alexander's work?

Barlow: The whole idea of the training course to me is teaching people to know how to work on themselves—to get those experiences which cannot come from wonderful teachers' hands—of actually making your own new experiences with what happens when you work on yourself. Otherwise, they haven't got anything to teach their pupils about how to work on themselves. So a lot of the time is spent working on yourself, just as it was in F.M.'s class.

Schirle: How important do you think good hands are to a teacher?

Barlow: I think they are very, *very* important. And if the person has really worked very hard on himself, that delicate . . . "craftsmanship"— I think that is the word—is terribly important, because you can put people awfully wrong by giving them a wrong stimulus. But I do not think it is the main thing. The main thing in teaching is really insisting that the person himself *works*. You see, this is not something you get from the outside. I always go back to F.M.—what happened with him. There he was with a problem. What did he do? What was the method he used to get from(a) where his problem was to(b) the solution? He used to say, "Anybody can do what I do, *if* they will do what I did." None of you want anything to do with that—nobody wants to use this.

There are many important things about the hands. It is very important how you put your hands on. You've got to be watching yourself all the time: That is the important thing. And another thing that is frightfully important is how you take them off. It is almost as important—how you take your hands off. You are giving somebody the direction; then you get an idea you are going to go somewhere else in the body, and the whole nervous system jars.

Schirle: How do you retain your sense of freedom and excitement about the technique after these many years of teaching? How do you keep from getting fixed about the work?

Barlow: Well, it is such an exciting thing . . . you see, it is always *new*. I have been terribly lucky. I find it more exciting the longer I do it. You are always having new experiences, and I learn from my pupils, all the time—really, I ought to be paying *them!* No, truly, I feel this . . . the whole thing is such an exciting adventure. If you are working on yourself, you are making new experiences, so that it is never the same, even with the same pupil, and that is very interesting. F.M. used to say, "The ideal is—if you can—to approach your pupils every time you give them a lesson as if you had never seen them before and to see them as they are today." You do not bring to this encounter all you know about them—how they have been in the past. "Give them a chance," he said, " to be what they are today." And this is a very important idea. If one could treat one's nearest and dearest this way and not bring—when you see them in the morning—every thing that has happened in the past forty-six years. [laughs]

Schirle: Do you look forward to further developments in this work, either in your work or that of your students? Where do you see the Alexander Technique headed?

Barlow: I look forward to it developing in many, many different ways. F.M. used to say that we are only on the fringe of this thing, only on the fringe. We've got so much more to learn, and it will develop in all sorts of directions and be applied to all sorts of different things. But the danger is that the real basis of it will get lost. He continually said to us: "Stick to principle. If you stick to principle, if you use the basic thing that I used to get from where I was to where I wanted to be, you can't go wrong." People have so many different talents and gifts and directions in which they want to go that, given basic fidelity to that thing, you cannot go wrong. It is when they throw away the baby with the bath water—this is what worries me about the Technique in certain developments. I always go back to F.M.: What did he do? I say to my students, "If you are in doubt, go back to what he did." That is what we've got to do.

Schirle: What do you think has been your major contribution to the technique through your training of teachers or your writings or your work generally?

Barlow: I never thought about it . . . I have had such fun doing it, but it has never come into my head, really. You know, Bill is the writer; Bill is the one who lectures and gives interviews. All I have ever wanted is to be left alone, in peace—not to be interfered with. To work quietly with someone who is prepared to come and spend half an hour with me in my room—that is all I have ever asked of life since I started the Technique. But it is not quite like that, is it? [laughing] The great thing is that it has enabled me to live my life, I hope, in improving what I am interested in; what I have *always* been interested in is knowing what I am doing. Thinking. Think about that for a minute—thinking what you are doing. These come and go; they are in the language. We never think about what they mean . . . "thinking" what you are doing. I like to say "how" you are doing; that is the other one. But "thinking in activity" was such an important idea to F.M.; he used to call it a means of learning to control human reaction. And his idea was that you could bring the body and the mind—in all, the whole organism, the whole *person*—into a unity.

Schirle: This "thinking in activity"—is this different from what we normally associate with the word "thinking"?

Barlow: Oh, yes. It is a very special quality, isn't it? words are so difficult, aren't they? As F.M. would say, "any word I use has got barnacles on it." Everybody brings his past experience of that word. F.M. said to me, "I really need to invent a new language; but if I had, nobody would have understood a word we said." There you are. No, it is very hard to put it into words what "ordering" or giving messages is. It is a very . . . *attentive* process. You've got to pay attention. This is something we all find extremely difficult—our attention span is about a second and a half. Talking about ordering, F.M. said, "Any fool can think of one thing at a time and go on thinking of it; but when you have to go on thinking one thing, and add two, and go on thinking of one, and add two, and add *three*, that is about as much as most of are capable in a lifetime's learning." But he did give us examples of a long sequence of orders . . . in the monkey and going into the monkey and going on the back of the chair with the hands on the chair, because you've got to give the whole sequence.

Schirle: What you have just been discussing is why I think so many performing artists are tuned in to Alexander's work—because they have to be thinking of so many things at once and this is such a wonderful practice for that.

Barlow: That's right. Paying attention to more than one thing is *life*. He used to say that if we hadn't got that capacity, none of us would be here . . . we would not have survived. He was very keen on being attentive to what was going on around you. When you're talking to someone, you've got to be attentive to them, to be *with* them.

Schirle: Did he talk about concentration?

Barlow: Oh, did he not! It was a forbidden word! Verboten! Absolutely F.M. explained that concentration means bringing everything to a point. But what we need is a kind of awareness which is as wide as possible, taking into account as many factors as we are capable of. The reason *why* musicians and people like that are so . . . in the same world . . . is because they have to spend hour after hour after hour [practicing]. When I go to a concert, I look at those instrumentalists and I think, "My goodness! How many hours of solitary disciplined work have gone into the fact that they are sitting here tonight, playing their violin or whatever?" That is what the work is. And unless you do that, especially if you are a teacher and training people; unless you are doing that work *every* day, like playing your scales—F.M. used to say, "*Every* day! Go back to those words."

Joan Schirle is a Senior Teacher of the F.M. Alexander Technique, certified in New York in 1969. She is Director of the Dell'Arte School of Physical Theatre in Blue Lake, California, where she teaches Alexander, movement, mask performance, and self-revelatory theatre.

The Stutterer

F. Matthias Alexander

I WILL TAKE FOR my second illustration the case of man with an impediment in his speech who was sent to me for advice and help. He told me that he had taken lessons from specialists who treated speech defects, and had done his best to carry out their instructions and to practice their exercises. He had always had special difficulty with sounds which called for the use of the tongue and lips, particularly with the consonants T and D, but although he had been more or less successful in doing the exercises themselves, his stutter was as bad as ever in ordinary conversation, especially when he was hurried or excited.

As is my custom with a new pupil, I noted specially the way he walked into my room and sat down in a chair, and it was obvious to me that his general use of himself was more than usually harmful. When he spoke, I also noticed a wrong use of his tongue and lips and certain defects in the use of his head and neck, involving undue depression of the larynx and undue tension of the face and neck muscles. I then pointed out to him that his stutter was not an isolated symptom of wrong use confined to the organs of speech, but that it was associated with other symptoms of wrong use and functioning in other parts of his organism.

As he doubted this, I went on to explain that I had been able to demonstrate to every stutterer who had come to me for help that he "stuttered" with many other different parts of his body besides his tongue and lips. "Usually," I said, "these other defects remain unobserved or ignored until they reach the point where the wrong functioning manifests itself in some form of so-called "physical" or

---

The Use of the Self: Its Conscious Direction in Relation to Diagnosis, Function, and the Control of Reaction (New York: Dutton, 1932), 69–88.

"mental" disorder. In your case, your stutter interferes with your work and hinders intercourse with your fellows, and so you have not been able to ignore it, but this may well turn out to be a blessing in disguise if it is the means of making you aware, before too late, of the other more serious defects which I have pointed out to you, and which will tend, as time goes on, to become more and more exaggerated." I assured him that my long years of practical experience in dealing with the difficulties and idiosyncrasies of people who stutter had convinced me that stuttering was one of the most interesting specific symptoms of a general cause, namely, misdirection of the use of the psycho-physical mechanisms, and I did not wish to take him as a pupil, unless he was prepared to work with me on the basis of correcting this misdirection of use generally, as the primary step in remedying his defects in speech. I could promise him, however, that if he decided to come to me and I was successful in making certain changes for the better in his manner of using his mechanisms, a change for the better would also come about in the functioning of his organism, and his stuttering would tend to disappear in the process. He saw the point and decided to take lessons.

Now in my experience stuttering, like the golfer's tendency to take his eyes off the ball, is due to habitual misdirection of the use of the mechanisms, so that the remedying of the defect in both cases presents fundamentally the same problem. Like the golfer, the stutterer needs to have this habitual misdirection of his use changed to a more satisfactory direction, and the new and improved use, associated with this change in direction, has to be built up and sufficiently stabilized in him before he will be able to employ it practically as a means of overcoming his particular difficulties in speaking.

In the case of this pupil, therefore, I began by pointing out to him various outstanding symptoms of his wrong habitual use, one of the most marked of these being the undue amount of muscle tension that he was in the habit of employing throughout his organism whenever he tried to speak. This extreme muscle tension was an impeding factor in the functioning of his mechanisms generally, and rendered impossible a satisfactory use of his tongue and lips, and the more he tried by any special effort of "will" to speak without stuttering, the more certain he was to increase the already undue muscle tension and so to defeat his own end.

The reason for this, I explained to him, was that he did not start to speak until he had brought about the amount of tension which was associated with his habitual use and which caused him to *feel that he could speak;* i.e., he would decide that the moment had come for him to speak only when his *feeling* told him that he was using his mechanisms to the best advantage, and this moment, in the last analysis, was when his sensory appreciation (the only guide he had as to the amount of muscle tension necessary) registered to him as "right" the amount of tension which he habitually employed in speaking and which was therefore familiar to him.

Unfortunately, the familiar amount of tension that "felt right" to him was the unnecessary amount associated with the wrong habitual use of his mechanisms of which his stuttering was a symptom, and I therefore urged him to recognize from the beginning that the "feeling," upon which he was relying to tell him when his use was right for speaking, was untrustworthy as a register of muscle tension, and that he must not depend upon it for guidance in his attempts to speak. How, I asked him, could he expect to judge by his feeling the amount of tension he should employ in speaking, when he was unfamiliar with the sensory experience of speaking with the due amount? Obviously, he could not "know" a sensation he had never experienced, and as sensory experience cannot be conveyed by the spoken word, no amount of telling on my part could convey to him the unfamiliar sensory experience of speaking with less tension and without stuttering. The only way to convince him that he could speak with a less amount of muscle tension would be to give him this unfamiliar experience.

To this end I adopted a procedure based upon the same principle as the procedure employed to the end of giving the golfer the experience of keeping his eyes on the ball, my aim being to give my pupil, first, the experience of employing a conscious direction of a new and improved use of his mechanisms generally, and, secondly, the experience of *continuing to employ this conscious direction whilst using* the mechanisms concerned with the act of speaking in the manner best suited for the purpose.

I began by giving him:

1. the directions for the inhibition of the wrong habitual use of his mechanisms associated with the excessive muscle tension;
2. the directions for the employment of the primary control leading to a new and improved use which would be associated with a due amount of muscle tension.

I then asked him to project these directions whilst I with my hands gave him the new sensory experiences of use corresponding to these directions, in order that the trustworthiness of his sensory appreciation in relation to the use of his mechanism might be gradually restored, and that by this means he might in time acquire a register of the due amount of tension required for speaking, as distinct from the undue amount of tension associated with his stuttering.

I continued this procedure, until I had repeated for him the new sensory experiences of use often enough to justify me in allowing him to attempt to employ his new "means-whereby" for speaking and for saying the words and consonants that caused him special difficulty.

It is impossible in the space at my command to put down all the details of the variations of the teacher's art that were employed to bring my pupil to this point, for a teacher's technique naturally varies in detail according to the particular needs and difficulties of each pupil. Those of my readers, however, who have followed the account of the difficulties I encountered when I attempted to employ the new "means-whereby" in my reciting, will be able to realize the kind of difficulty we were faced with all along, when I say that my pupil was a confirmed "end-gainer."

At the beginning of this new stage in our work together I reminded him how his progress up to this point had been hampered by his habit of end-gaining and of "trying to be right," and I warned him that unless he succeeded in side-stepping it, he would have little chance of applying his new "means-whereby" to his difficulties in speaking, for if, at the critical moment of starting to say a difficult word, he still went directly for his end and tried to say the word in the way that "felt right" to him, he would be bound to revert to his old habitual use in speaking and so to stutter.

Events proved how difficult it was for my pupil to take practical heed of this warning. I would repeatedly urge him, whenever I gave him a sound or word to pronounce, always to inhibit his old habitual response to my request by refusing to attempt to pronounce the sound or word until he had taken time to think out and employ the new directions for the use which he had decided upon as best for his purpose. He would agree to do this, but as soon as I asked him to pronounce some sound or word, he would fail to inhibit his response to the stimulus of my voice, and forgetting all about the new directions he had been asked to employ, he would immediately try to repeat the sound, with the result that he was at once dominated by his old habits of use associated with the extreme muscle tension that *felt right* to him, and so stuttered as badly as ever.[1] In short, his very desire to "be right in gaining his end" defeated the end.

In every stutterer of whom I have had experience, this habit of reacting too quickly to stimuli is always associated with sensory untrustworthiness, undue muscle tension and misdirection of energy, but in this pupil's case the habit of going directly for his end, and of trying to "feel right" in doing it, had been positively cultivated in him by the methods employed by his previous teachers in trying to "cure" his stutter.

It would appear that the "end-gaining" principle underlies every one of the exercises given by teachers who, whether by orthodox or unorthodox methods, deal with stuttering as a specific defect, and I will take as an example the exercises that had been given to my pupil to meet his special difficulty in pronouncing works beginning with T or D.

His former teachers had recognized that the use of his tongue and lips was unsatisfactory for the purpose of pronouncing these consonants, and in order to overcome the difficulty had instructed him to practice certain exercises involving the use of these specific parts in saying T or D.

Now this procedure could only aggravate the difficulty, for the idea of trying to say T or D acted as an incentive to the pupil to employ the habitual use of himself associated with the wrong use of his tongue and lips. As long as this wrong habitual use remained unchanged, this association persisted and he had little chance of getting rid of this incentive, so that to ask him under these conditions to practice saying T and D as a remedy for his stuttering was tantamount to giving him an added incentive to stutter.

This was borne out by what I observed when he showed me how he had been practicing his exercises. I watched him closely and saw that as soon as he started to do them, he at once made an undue amount of tension generally, continued to increase the tension of the muscles of the lips, cheeks and tongue, and tried to say T or D before his tongue had taken up the best position for the purpose. This attempt was as bound to result in failure as would the attempt of a motorist to change gears before the clutch has done its work in getting the cogs into the position in which they will mesh. It was evident that he had been trying in all his practice in the past to gain his end without being in command of the means whereby this end could be successfully gained, and the fact that the majority of these attempts had been unsuccessful had brought him to a state of lack of confidence in himself, which added considerably to the difficulty of breaking his "end-gaining" habit.

As far as I am aware, all methods of "curing" stuttering, however they may differ in detail, are all based on the same "end-gaining" principle. The adviser will select some symptom or symptoms as the cause of his pupil's stuttering and will give him specific instructions or exercises to help him.

I am well aware that it has proved possible by such methods to stop people from stuttering, but I would question the common assumption that because this is so, a genuine "cure" has been effected. For in cases where it is claimed that a stutter has been "cured," there is usually something peculiar or hesitating about the manner of speaking, and those concerned do not seem in the least perturbed that the harmful conditions of undue muscle tension, misdirection of energy and untrustworthiness of sensory appreciation, present in the case when the "cure" was begun, are still in evidence now that what is considered a successful "cure" has been brought about.

No method of "cure" can be accepted as effective or scientific, if, in the process of removing certain selected symptoms, other symptoms have been left untouched and if new, unwished-for symptoms have appeared.[2] If this test is applied to a stutterer after he has been "cured" by such methods, it will be found too often that the original defects of undue muscular tension, misdirection of energy and untrustworthiness of sensory appreciation have been increased in the process of the "cure."[3]

I admit that these defects may not bring about a recurrence of the stutter, but even so, they are almost certain to lead to the further development of other undesirable symptoms which constantly remain unrecognized. This invariably happens when defects and diseases are "cured" by specific methods, and explains why, in spite of the immense number of "cures" recorded, the troubles in the human organism would seem to be increasing and calling for more and more "cures."

It is important to remember that there is a working balance in the use of all the parts of the organism, and that for this reason the use of the specific part (or parts) in any activity can influence the use of the other parts, and vice versa. Under instinctive direction this working balance becomes habitual and "feels right," and the point at which the influence of the use of any part will make itself felt will vary and the influence of the particular use be strong or weak according to the nature of the stimulus of the end activity desired. If a defect is recognized in the use of a part, and an attempt is made to correct this defect by changing the use of the part without bringing about at the same time a corresponding change in the use of the other parts, the habitual working balance in the use of the whole will be disturbed. Unless, therefore, the person attempting to make a change in the use of a specific part has an understanding of what is required to bring about at the same time a corresponding change in the use of the other parts which will make for a satisfactory working balance and therefore be complementary to the new use that he is trying to bring about at one point, one of two things is bound to happen, either

1. the stimulus of the desire to gain his end, by means of the old use associated with the habitual working balance which "feels right," will be so strong that it will dominate the stimulus to cultivate a new and improved use of a certain part associated with an unfamiliar working balance which "feels wrong"; or,
2. if the change in the use of a part is made in the face of imped-

ing factors in the use of the other parts (as happens in any specific method of treatment employed to correct a defect in a part), the working balance between the use of that part and the use of all the other parts will be adversely affected in their turn, and new defects in the use of these parts developed.

After my pupil had shown me the exercises he had been told to do, I explained to him that in practicing them he had been indulging in his old wrong habits of general use of himself, and thereby actually *cultivating* the wrong habits of use of his tongue and lips which had made him stutter. I impressed upon him once more that if he wished ever to be confident of saying T and D and words in which these consonants occur without stuttering, *he must refuse to respond to any stimulus either from within or without to say T or D;* in other words, whenever the idea of saying T or D came to him, he must inhibit his desire to try and say it correctly, until he had learned what use of his tongue and lips was required in his case for saying T or D without stuttering, and until he could put into practice the necessary directions for this new use of his tongue and lips *whilst continuing to give the directions for the primary control of the new and improved use of himself generally.*

He understood the reason for this, but his attempts at cooperating with me proved more or less unsuccessful for some time. Over and over again I got him to the point where the use of his tongue and lips in association with his general use was such that I knew he could pronounce T and D without the undue muscle tension that made him stutter, but when at this point I asked him to repeat one of the sounds, he would either

1. forget to inhibit his old response, change back to his old conditions of use and increase the tension to the point when he *felt* that he could say T or D, try to say it in this way and stutter, or
2. on the occasions when he remembered to inhibit his old response and to employ the new "means-whereby" for saying T and D without stuttering, he would make no attempt to repeat the sound.

In both these cases he was actuated by the same motive. He associated the act of speaking, especially the pronunciation of consonants that were difficult for him, with a given amount of muscle tension, and as I have already shown, he had come to believe that it was impossible for him to speak until he *felt* this undue amount of tension. This explains why he made no attempt to speak until he had deliberately brought about the familiar but excessive tension which caused him to stutter. In this way he simply reinforced the old sensory experiences of undue muscle tension already associated with his habitual use, and with his habit of trying to *feel right* in gaining his end.

To deal with this difficulty I made a point of giving my pupil day after day the experience of receiving a stimulus to gain a certain end and of remembering to refuse to gain that end, since this refusal meant that at one fell swoop he inhibited all the wrong habits of use associated with his habitual way of gaining that end. In proportion as he was successful in inhibiting his immediate response to any stimulus, he became able to defeat his desire to gain his ends in the way that felt right to him, and *as long as he continued this inhibition,* I on my side was able to repeat for him, until they became familiar, the new sensory experiences associated with an improved general use of his mechanisms, including the right use of his tongue and lips. By continuing to cooperate with me on these lines, he gradually acquired sufficient experience in the direction of this new use to be able to employ it successfully as the "means-whereby" of pronouncing the consonants which had caused him special difficulty.

But, more important than this, my pupil in the course of this procedure had learned that if he inhibited his immediate instinctive reaction to any stimulus to "do," he could prevent the misdirection of his use and the associated undue muscle tension which had been the marked feature of all his reactions to stimuli, and which had hampered him no only in his speaking but in all his activities, both "physical" and "mental," and if he chose to apply this principle to his activities in other spheres, he would have at his command a means of controlling the nature of his reaction to stimuli, that is, of acquiring a control of what is called "conscious behavior."[4]

Certain features of this pupil's case occur with practically every pupil.

During the earlier stages of a pupil's lessons when the use of his mechanisms is still unsatisfactory, I have constantly found that he fails to inhibit the old instinctive direction of his use, with the result that his directions for the new use do not become operative. Before I can get a chance to help him, he proceeds to gain his end in accordance with his habitual wrong use, and it is practically impossible under these circumstances to stop him from gaining his end in this way.

On the other hand, when he has learned at a later stage in his lessons to inhibit the instinctive direction of his use and the directions for the new use have become operative, so that I am enabled to give him the corresponding sensory experiences, I have found that although he now has at his command the best conditions possible for gaining his end, he will not make any attempt to gain it. He cannot believe that the end can be gained with these improved conditions present; they "feel so wrong," as he puts it, that he instinctively refuses to employ them.

When this difficulty arises, it is necessary for me to give him the actual experience of gaining his end by what he feels is a wrong use of his mechanisms, and when I have succeeded in doing this, he invariably remarks how much easier this new way is than the old way, and how much less effort it requires. Yet in spite of this admission, the actual experience of gaining his end in this new way has be repeated for him again and again before the improved use "feels right" to him, and before he gains the necessary confidence in employing it.

The lesson to be learned from all this is that since our particular way of reacting to stimuli is in accordance with our familiar habits of use, the incentive to try to gain any given end is inextricably bound up with this familiar use. This explains why, if a pupil's familiar use is changed to one that is unfamiliar and therefore unassociated with his habitual way of reacting to stimuli, he has little or no incentive to gain a given end by the familiar wrong use appears to be almost irresistible, but when these conditions have been changed to conditions which are best for the purpose of gaining the end, there seems to be practically no incentive to gain it.

This is not surprising, for when a person's sensory appreciation of his use is wrong and his belief as to what he can or cannot do is based on what he feels, gaining an end by a use that is unfamiliar means for him taking a plunge in the dark. Even when I have explained to a pupil why this difficulty has arisen in his case, and he understands the reason for it "intellectually," he will need, more often than not, considerable encouragement and practical assistance in order to be enabled to make the experience of gaining a given end by means of a use that is new and unfamiliar to him. Once this has been done for him, however, he becomes conscious of a new experience that he is desirous to repeat, and repetition of this experience in time convinces him that his previous beliefs and judgments in this connection were wrong. As a result there gradually develops in him an incentive to employ the new use, and this becomes at last far stronger that the incentive to employ the old use, for its development is the outcome of a reasoned procedure which he finds he can consciously direct and control with a confidence he has never before experienced.

One of the most remarkable of man's characteristics is his capacity for becoming used to conditions of almost any kind, whether good or bad, both in the self and in the environment, and once he has become used to such conditions they seem to him both right and natural. This capacity is a boon when it enables him to adapt himself to conditions which are desirable, but it may prove a great danger when the conditions are undesirable. When his sensory appreciation is so untrustworthy, it is possible for him to become so familiar with seriously harmful conditions of misuse of himself that these malconditions will feel right and comfortable.

My teaching experience has shown me that the worse these conditions are in a pupil and the longer they have been in existence, the more familiar and right they feel to him and the harder it is to teach him how to overcome them, no matter how much he may wish to do so. In other words, his ability to learn a new and more satisfactory use of himself is, as a rule, in inverse ratio to the degree of misuse present in his organism and the duration of these harmful conditions.

This point must be understood and taken into the practical consideration by anyone forming a plan of procedure for improving the use and functioning of the mechanisms throughout the organism as a means of eradicating defects, peculiarities and bad habits.

Towards the end of his lessons my pupil asked me why it should be so much more difficult to overcome the habit of stuttering than the habit of over-smoking. He then went on to tell me that at one time he had been an inveterate smoker, but realizing that the habit was getting too much of a hold on him, he had decided he must give it up. He had first tried the plan of reducing the number of cigarettes he smoked per day, but as he found that he could not keep within the prescribed limit, he had decided that the only way for him to succeed in breaking his habit was to give up smoking altogether. He put this decision into practice and had become a non-smoker. He now wanted to know why his efforts to overcome his stuttering had not been equally successful.

I pointed out to him that the two habits presented very different problems.

The smoker can abstain from smoking without interrupting the necessary activities of his daily life, and as the temptation to smoke to excess results, as every chain-smoker knows, from the fact that each pipe, cigar, or cigarette smoked acts as a stimulus to the smoking of another, every time he abstains from smoking he is breaking a link in the chain.

The stutterer, on the other hand, cannot abstain from speaking because his daily intercourse with his fellows depends on it. Every time he speaks, therefore, he is thrown into the way of temptation to indulge in his familiar wrong habits of use of his vocal organs, tongue and lips, and so to stutter. The stimulus to speak is one that he cannot evade in the way a smoker can evade the stimulus to smoke if he so wills it, so that the habit of stuttering calls for a much more fundamental form of control.

Satisfactory control of the act of speaking demands a satisfactory standard of the general use of the mechanisms, since the satisfactory use of the tongue and lips and the required standard of control of the respiratory and vocal organs depend upon this satisfactory general use. This being so, the unsatisfactory general use of the mechanisms which, as we have seen, is present in every stutterer, constitutes a formidable obstacle in the way of mastering his habit.

The situation is very different for the smoker, for the act of smoking does not demand any such high standard of use of the mechanisms, and although unsatisfactory conditions of use are frequently present in his case, the influence which they exercise in preventing him from overcoming his particular habit is small in comparison.

Still another element enters into the case. The habit which the smoker is trying to overcome is one which he has himself developed in the process of satisfying a desire. The stutterer, on the other hand, is dealing with a habit which has not been developed in the process of satisfying a desire, but which has gradually grown to become a part of the use of the mechanisms which he habitually employs for all the activities of his daily life. This explains why the smoking habit is relatively superficial in this degree to overcome, and why my pupil had been able *by himself* to solve the problem of his over-smoking, but had not been able to deal with his habit of stuttering without the help of a teacher who understood how to give him the means whereby he could *himself* command that satisfactory use of his mechanisms generally which includes the correct use of the tongue, lips and vocal organs for the act of speaking.

I would emphasize here that the process of eradicating any such defect as stuttering by these means makes the greatest demands on the time, patience and skill of both teacher and pupil, since, as we have seen, it calls for

1. the inhibition of the instinctive direction of energy associated with familiar sensory experiences of wrong habitual use, and
2. the building up in its place of a conscious direction of energy through the repetition of unfamiliar sensory experiences associated with new and satisfactory use.

This process of directing energy out of familiar into new and unfamiliar paths, as a means of changing the manner of reacting to stimuli, implies of necessity an ever-increasing ability on the part of both teacher and pupil to "pass from the known to the unknown";[5] it is therefore a process which is true to the principle involved in all human growth and development.

Since this chapter was written, I have received a letter from this pupil, and with his permission I am quoting the following extracts from it, as they are of interest in relation to the development of sensory awareness of an improvement in use:

I hope that you have not construed my prolonged silence to mean that I have lost interest in you or in your work. Quite the contrary is the case. I am interested in little else.... I feel quite sanguine about the possibility of making considerable progress if I can come this year. I am optimistic enough to believe that I am almost ripe for some real new experiences.... I have now come to the point that when I feel my back working I also feel my jaws relax. I really believe that I have been using my jaw muscles to keep myself erect! I am really beginning to appreciate how little I have used my tongue and lips in speech, in fact, I have scarcely used them at all. It is this great improvement in my sensory appreciation that gives me such hope for the future.

Notes

1. In order that the reader should not think this difficulty was peculiar to this pupil, I wish to state that I have had similar experiences with all my pupils. How could it be otherwise when "end-gaining" is a universal habit?

2. As Dr. Dewey writes in his Introduction to *Constructive Conscious Control of the Individual*, "the essence of scientific method does not consist in taking consequences in gross; it consists precisely in the means by which consequences are followed up in detail. It consists in the processes by which the causes that are used to explain the consequences or effects, can be concretely followed up to show that they actually produce these consequences and no other."

3. As an example of this, I will quote a statement made to me by an intending pupil at his preliminary interview. He told me, among other things, that he had cured himself of stammering and I asked him how he had done it. He replied that he had been a very bad stammerer, but that one day he was forced to run to the top of a long flight of stairs to deliver an important message, and found to his surprise that after this experience he was able to speak without stammering, and he had continued to be able to do so. Most people, of course, would look upon this as a "cure," but I could not, because I saw that his use of himself generally was still very bad, and which, in my opinion, amounted to "stuttering" in other parts of his organism. The fact is, the experience to which he attributed his freedom from stammering had not changed his unsatisfactory condition of use to those satisfactory conditions which are not found in association with stammering. Consequently, similar experience was just as liable to cause a recurrence at any time of the vocal stammering,

and as his unsatisfactory manner of use was still present, he had a predisposition to develop other troubles.

4. The following is of interest in this connection. One of my pupils has just told me that before he came to me for lessons he used to have uncontrollable fits of temper, but that since having the work he has no trouble in that way, and that all his family notice the change. He asked me to explain how it was that what he looked upon as a "nervous" or "mental" symptom could be affected by the kind of work I was doing with him. In reply I asked him how other people knew when he had lost his tempter, and he answered that they would know by the tone of his voice, the expression of his face, the look in his eyes, or by his gestures and excited manner generally. I then asked him how these reactions could be possible except through the use of what he thought of as his "physical" self. For instance, the voice must be used if we are to judge its tone, there must be use of the eyes if they are to flash, of the muscles of the face for change of expression, and, for excitability to be manifested the whole of the mechanisms of use must be stimulated into undue activity and muscle tension.

Change the manner of use and you change the conditions throughout the organism; the old reaction associated with the old manner of use and the old conditions cannot therefore take place, for the means are no longer there. In other words, the old habitual reflex activity has been changed and will not recur. If loss of control can be manifested only by means of the use of ourselves, it follows that a conscious direction of an improving use will bring us for the first time within striking distance of a conscious control of human reaction or behavior.

5. The late Mr. Joseph Rowntree after one of his lessons described my work as "reasoning from the known to the unknown, the known being the wrong and the unknown being the right."

Moshe Feldenkrais

A breathtaking work of genius, the Feldenkrais methods—one
("Functional Integration") hands-on with an individual teacher;
the other ("Awareness Through Movement"), group movements directed
by a teacher—teach a person how to liberate oneself from the narrow
range of stereotypical movement patterns that we learn in our culture
and to find a wider range of moving, and being. These works have had
an enormous impact on the medical practice of physical therapy, since
restricted movement patterns are associated with trauma, and freeing
them produces significant relief of pain.

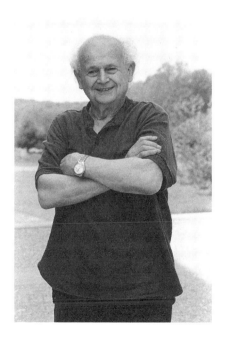

Interview with Mia Segal

Thomas Hanna

Mia Segal is one of the principal heirs of the teachings of Moshe Feldenkrais (1904–1984). Her years of having worked closely with him, including assisting him in developing his public trainings, give her a unique authority in articulating his work. She trains practitioners in Israel.

Somatics: When you were quite young, you did some research and writing on the Israeli underground. Did your parents want you to be a writer?

Segal: I had the background for it. My father was the managing editor of *Davar*, the labor newspaper in Israel and, at that time, the largest. I was brought up to take pride in knowing literature, poetry, and the Bible. To be able to express yourself beautifully in writing was very important in my family.

My mother, who was born in Jerusalem, taught Hebrew there at a time when other languages were taught in the schools, and Yiddish was spoken at home. My mother had joined other teachers to bring about a revolutionary change—to teach Hebrew in the schools. She took pride in using the language correctly and poetically, with the correct pronunciation.

Somatics: Was your father a writer or, actually, a scholar?

Segal: I would say—both. When Israel was established as a state in 1948, there was no Israeli law. My father was asked to be responsible for the drafting of the laws, and he left the newspaper to do this.

Somatics: He was not a lawyer?

Somatics Autumn/Winter 1985–86. 8–20

Segal: As a child in Russia, my father attended two of the most famous religious schools. He was considered an *ilui,* a child genius, and was qualified as a Rabbi.

He came to Israel with the "second immigration," as did the builders of our State. Palestine at that time was governed by the Turks; my father, among others, was drafted to serve in the Turkish Army during World War I. As a result he spoke Turkish fluently. After the war, we were under a British Mandate. My father then studied law. Having acquired a thorough knowledge of Jewish, Turkish, and British law, he was later qualified to compile and draft the new Israeli laws. The Israeli State also had a language problem because the old Biblical vocabulary did not suffice for all the new concepts; so the Academy of the Hebrew Language was founded, and my father was one of its distinguished members. His library, books, and manuscripts are now at the Academy in a special place dedicated to him.

Somatics: You were in the Army, weren't you?

Segal: Yes, I was.

Somatics: Did you work for the newspaper?

Segal: I never worked for the newspaper. I assisted in collecting, writing, and editing the history of the Haganah, the Israeli underground defense. My line was in the area of writing—not in bodily activities.

Somatics: When did you first do anything which involved any kind of bodily skills?

Segal: After I married. One day Maurice had an attack and could not breathe. I had never seen anything like that before. It was a terrible shock—I thought he was dying. Maurice said that he had had it before: It was asthma. He called a doctor who gave him his medication, and he seemed to be O.K. again. However, a week later, he had another attack, and I couldn't understand it, being most inexperienced in the field of sickness and health.

In 1952, Maurice, who had been injured in an air crash, had to go to England for a series of leg operations. I remember thinking: "I know the leg will eventually heal. I am going to find out about asthma." I was still so scared, and I was determined to find out. In England, I asked everyone I met: "What do you know about asthma?" Eventually, I met a medical student from South Africa who said, "Oh, yes, I know about asthma. If you want someone to help your husband, take him to see Charles Neal. He practices the Alexander Method."

I went to see Charles Neal who told me he could help. Since Maurice was permitted to leave the hospital between operations, I took him in for a consultation. Charles said, "You don't know how to breathe properly. You have bad breathing habits." This was a revelation! After two or three sessions with Charles, Maurice was much better; he learned a way of coping during an attack, and the fear of losing control disappeared. I asked Charles if I could learn how to help Maurice in the future—when we were back in Israel. He said, "I don't train anyone officially, but you can stay here and observe what I do." Charles had been a star student of F. Mathias Alexander.

Somatics: Were both the Alexander brothers living then?

Segal: I don't know. I understood that Charles and Alexander had had an argument. Charles then went on his own, taking with him some of Alexander's pupils. He was sponsored by Isabel Cripps, wife of the Minister for the Colonies, and opened the Isabel Cripps Center.

I enjoyed my work at the Center. Although I wasn't officially a student, Charles required me to take a course in anatomy on my own. He also gave me a list of the things he wanted me to study. This was my first contact with the human body. After two years, Charles said, "I think I'll give you a room here, and you can start to work with people." At that time, only a few others were working at the Center: Charles, of course, Eric de Peyer, Mrs. Gibson, and Lois Kaink. That's how I started.

Somatics: Were they official instructors or outside the field?

Segal: I know of no other Alexander teachers at that time, although there are many now.

Somatics: Did Charles Neal give you some sort of permission to be a practitioner?

Segal: Charles gave me a letter saying I could teach, but he didn't mention pupils—no official pupils. But I did have his permission to go ahead and work, and I felt I was effective in my efforts. I did this for two years. Then we returned to Israel.

I stopped working when my children were born. Then Charles Neal wrote that he was coming to Israel to see his old friend, Moshe Feldenkrais. I was delighted, of course.

Somatics: You didn't know Feldenkrais at the time?

Segal: No, but I'd heard of him. He was well-known. I did know he was working with Ben-Gurion. At the time, Moshe was actually looking for someone to assist him in his work, and Charles recommended me.

Somatics: What was the relationship between Neal and Feldenkrais?

Segal: They thought highly of each other and were good friends.

Somatics: And with Alexander?

Segal: I heard that while living in England and writing *Body and Mature Behavior,* Moshe met Alexander. Moshe used to say that Alexander had the best hands he had ever felt. If I remember correctly, Moshe showed him *Body and Mature Behavior,* and Alexander said, "Actually, you copied it from my book!" This, I suppose, ended the relationship.

As I understand it, Alexander was strict about his work: The placement of the head, back, and the body was exactly specified; everything had to be just so, and no variations were permitted. I understand now those who follow the Alexander Technique have become more flexible.

Charles Neal, on the other hand, had slightly broadened the scope of work, though he too was restrictive: only the head, neck, and back. He was very open and organized in every way. He was remarkably agile: He could walk into a room and jump upon the table without any obvious preparation—just as he walked. From him I learned how important sensitivity of touch can be.

Somatics: When did you decide to assist Moshe Feldenkrais?

Segal: It's interesting how that came about, because I had said to Moshe, "Look, I can't work with you now. I have children; my son is four months old; I am too busy." He replied, "Why don't you just come and see what I am doing?"

I went the next day. Moshe had a small apartment on Nachmani Street. I entered a small room where an old lady (she was in her late eighties then) was sitting cross-legged on a bed doing embroidery.

"I've come to see Moshe," I said.

"Sit down," she replied. Continuing to do embroidery, she suddenly said, "I've lost my needle. Young woman, come help me look for it." We searched everywhere but could not find the needle.

I said, "Maybe you'll find it tomorrow."

"Tomorrow!" she exclaimed. "Do you know what I'd be if I had said, 'tomorrow'?"

"What?" I asked.

"A virgin!" she replied. This was an amazing statement for a Jewish woman of her age and tradition. That's how I met Moshe's mother.

Moshe came in and said, "I'm glad you're here. Will you come to my workroom?" I'll never forget that day. I even remember the details of the room: the color of the bed cover, the desk, and the chairs. The "pupil" was lying on the bed. Moshe sat down and just took up her head with his two hands. Although I had been working with people for two years or more, I had never seen that quality of work before. It was very similar to what I had seen Charles Neal do and what I myself had learned. However, there was a difference in quality—perhaps it was the sense of purpose and the integrity of his approach which were new. I realized how much I did not know. After that I came there daily, and all I wanted to do was just to observe and learn. This all began in 1956.

Moshe was a wonderful teacher. After every lesson, he would ask whether I had any questions. If I had, he would push aside the papers and books on his table, take a piece of paper, and explain what he had just finished doing. His explanations were excellent, his reasons for what he was doing were very clear, and he was most generous with his time. Sometimes he would keep people waiting in order to explain something that puzzled me. He was a remarkable teacher.

Years later, Moshe commented, "You know, I made you into the most wonderful pupil."

And I replied, "That's nothing, Moshe. I made *you* into a wonderful master!" And he really was.

Somatics: Did you begin working very soon after that?

Segal: I really don't know when I began working. Moshe had a special way of teaching and building up my confidence. One day I found myself working on someone; and, suddenly, I realized I didn't know when I had started to work there.

Somatics: Did he always use a bed?

Segal: No, that was the amazing part—there seemed to be no end to his inventions: bed, chair, on rollers, sitting, kneeling.... It was O.K. to use any device or position imaginable. He was so ingenious and free in his approach.

I also kept up my correspondence with Charles Neal, describing my insights and experiences. Charles wrote: "Learn from him, and one day I'll come and work with him too. He does things I cannot do."

By this time, Moshe had become a member of the family—a "brother" to Maurice and me and a "father" to my children; and my parents got to know him very well and enjoyed his talks and stories. He usually spent the weekends with us and seemed to enjoy himself immensely. He knew all our friends and was involved in the upbringing of our children. At times, he would get all of us to lie on the floor, and we would do "exercises."

Somatics: Was Moshe known because he was connected with the Israeli government or for his work in electronics?

Segal: He became known mostly because of his work with Ben-Gurion. By word-of-mouth, people soon discovered that he could help them in remarkable ways, and they began coming for various problems— pain, malfunctioning, and the like. Some came in desperation after medical treatments had failed; others came for self-development or to learn how to be better at sports, dance, or gymnastics.

Long before I started working with Moshe, he had classes of what we now call ATM (Awareness Through Movement). Some of the people had been coming regularly for thirty or forty years. I knew nothing about the "exercising" side of his work. My experience was in Functional Integration (although it was not called that then). I remember Moshe saying to me, "If you want to work with me, I suggest that you experience ATM." I was surprised and wondered, "What is to be learned there?" It turned out to be a remarkable experience, for I gained a better understanding of my own self and everything I had done. For a long time, I had the strangest feeling that it was magic. I'd say to Moshe, "How do you prepare your new lessons?" He did not seem to need any preparation. I'd come to work, and he would say, "it's four o'clock, and we've got to start the classes." He was never late for a class in the fifteen years I was there, nor did he ever miss one. He was very loyal to his pupils and his work.

Somatics: Are you suggesting he improvised?

Segal: Yes. Once I asked him what "exercise" lesson he had planned for that day—just as we left for class, and he said, "While we drive to class, I'll figure it out."

Somatics: Did he ever explain how he started planning that way.

Segal: Yes. When he came to visit, we would often sit and discuss how he did his preparation for a lesson, and then he would demonstrate. He'd say, "Look, I'm thinking: 'How do I move to do this?'" Then he would show me how he went through the process in his own body. In other words, he would do what was necessary in order to discover how to do a movement more efficiently; what the connections were; what changes in breathing occurred; what was going on in his neck or back. He would say, "This is what is happening to my breathing and going on in my neck ..." He would explore his body for hours at a time in order to discover the process and its connections. I'd often come home and find Moshe lying on the floor with his legs up and head down, working something out. He never cared whether he was alone or among our friends—he did his own thing. Sometimes, he would say "Oh!" and lie down on the carpet, and our friends got used to seeing him do this. He drew his lessons from his own internal observations: By noticing what movements occurred in his body and then analyzing the process—by observing what happened within and how it occurred.

I once joked, "Moshe, what are you going to teach them today?"

He replied, "You do not understand. Actually, I am always teaching the same movement—only with a different sauce."

Somatics: What do you think he meant?

Segal: Whatever you do, the initial origination of the movement, or motivation, is the same; however, there are many different ways one can go about it. The difference lies in how it is done.

How do you initiate an activity? What Moshe did, I think, was to discover how to execute a movement and what is the most direct, efficient and precise way: How to behave so congruently that when you move in one direction, every part of your body should participate; or, that even your little toe should know what the head is doing and enhance that activity. Even if you cannot see the movement of the little toe, there should be no interference from it. Those parts of you which are unaware that there is movement are interfering with your movement—not assisting it. How do you keep the various parts from interfering? By becoming aware that you have these areas. That is where his genius lies: in the discovery and differentiation of this process.

Somatics: Part of Moshe's genius was his tremendous self-awareness. Did you see that in him? Did he make it clear how self-awareness and movement—the "awareness through movement" that came out of that—flows into the functional integration work?

Segal: As I worked with my hands, I became more and more aware of my own body; and as I did his ATM class, I discovered more about how to work with others. He did not have me make conscious connections between movement and self-awareness. In this way, he was a master-teacher in the Japanese tradition. Moshe was like a Japanese master in that he let you have the experience first before he would discuss it. He would watch and wait until he thought I was ready. He had a clever way of using his hands. (It is the way we work in Functional Integration now.) You bring a person to feel a certain organization of his body. When you ascertain that he had this awareness, only then do you point it out verbally. He taught me the same way: When I eventually understood what I was doing, we would walk about it.

Somatics: So then, you have worked with Charles Neal and with Moshe. What other sources have taught you important things about the body?

Segal: Maybe through judo. Moshe had told wonderful stories about his experiences in judo. He was a great story teller, and he had had so many amazing experiences. When he told you about some of the things he had done—he had come to Israel as a pioneer and fought the Arabs—you knew he had lived those experiences. Even though he no longer practiced judo, he loved to talk about it. He was then either fifty or sixty years old—at least, he claimed to be sixty years old.

"But, Moshe," I said, "your mother says you are fifty."

He answered, "She wants me to get married, so she makes me younger than I am."

To this, his mother would retort, "He doesn't know—he wasn't there. *I* remember when he was born!"

So there was a ten-year gap. Anyway, whether he was fifty or sixty, he had not been active in judo for some time. But he never lost his ability to walk like a judo master—that special way of walking with a certain balance and lightness.

One day, my family watched Moshe do a rolling breakfall all around our big lawn without stopping. We were very impressed.

I began to study judo by getting a copy of Moshe's book on judo. A very good friend of mine from Australia was also interested in the martial arts; and, together, on the living room carpet, we followed the exercises laid out sequentially in Moshe's book. The next day, I could not walk, nor could my friend, who commented, "My whole back is split near the tailbone." Of course, I was in equal agony.

Later, I said to Moshe, "Your book and your teaching—just look what happened!"

He retorted, "You must be stupid to think you can learn judo that way. You need a proper mat and the right teacher."

So, with many stories and after much thought and discussion, my husband and I decided to take the children and go to Japan. At this point, I had worked with Moshe for fifteen years. When I told him that we were leaving for Japan, it was a difficult time for all of us: I was his only assistant at that time, and we were his family—especially on weekends. However, it was the only time Maurice and I could go, for the children would have to return to Israel in three or four years to finish school and subsequently go into the Army.

We arrived in Japan in 1969. It proved to be a fantastic experience. I studied judo every day, including Sunday. We all learned Japanese and lived the way the Japanese do, and we enjoyed doing so. My son and daughter practiced nearly every day. Maurice was working in architecture, so he would join us when he could find the time.

At that time, working with other people in the Feldenkrais way was pushed into the background, and I became a student again. However, the Japanese master's traditional style of teaching was new to me. For example, I found out immediately not to ask questions—that I was to copy ... copy ... just copy.... You had to get the feeling of the whole thing yourself. If you asked a master how to do a certain movement, he would reply, "I do not know. One minute ... "; and then he would do the movement in order to demonstrate it. He never explained; he just did the movement, saying, "It's like this ... and like this...." It was similar to the way Moshe taught me: You felt it; you knew it—except that Moshe would then discuss it.

I found all kinds of judo masters, some of whom were excellent. Two were outstanding; one was Hiroset who was a seventh degree black belt. I think of him as being a modern *samurai*. He devoted his Sunday mornings to our family. We would all go there for three hours of instruction. He would say things like this: "Now father strangles son and mother strangles daughter." He later came to visit us in Israel.

Somatics: How did you become interested in Japanese theater?

Segal: My interest in Japanese theater was aroused when I heard a European girl singing. The quality of her voice was fantastic—a tonal quality I had never heard before. I asked her where she had learned to sing that way. "I'm studying with a Japanese master of theater," she replied. When I expressed a desire to study with him, she gave me his name and address. I had never had singing lessons, but her voice was so special in quality that I wanted to learn how to sing that way. I decided to go and see this man—but the next day I broke my leg while practicing judo.

That's an interesting story. In judo, when you plan to throw someone, you first take your opponent off balance and then follow through by "sweeping" the feet out from under him, so that he falls. Although I was being taught by someone who was very experienced, strangely enough, he was being playful; instead of taking me off balance, he just kicked. I heard a crunch, looked down, and saw my left leg at a different angle from normal, broken at the calf. Since it had just happened, I felt no pain. Everyone in the room heard the noise. My teacher, a lady teacher, came over and said, "You broke your leg." All the others continued practicing. The master teacher was in charge; and, as most judo masters, she was a professional *honetsugi,* or "bonesetter." Very expertly she set the bones of the left leg, including the many small bones of the ankle, which were also pushed out by the break. She set the leg so skillfully. Using two pieces of bamboo as splints, she bandaged the leg. Then she said (laughing), "Come back tomorrow, but do not drink any sake." I agreed. Amazingly, there was still no pain.

Arriving home, I said to Maurice, "I broke my leg." He phoned my teacher to say that he was taking me to the doctor.

"If you take her to the doctor, I will never touch Mia again," she replied.

"But the doctor can X-ray the leg," Maurice insisted.

"My fingers X-rayed the leg, and she is coming to see me tomorrow," she replied.

That night, my leg became swollen, black, and dreadfully painful. The next day, I could not walk and had to be carried in to see her. She looked at me and laughed, "You did not sleep last night." Then she took off the bandage and checked the leg. She reset the leg and bandaged it, as before. I had to come back every day. On the third day, she asked, "Why aren't you walking?" So I started walking. After all, I had another leg, and there was nothing wrong with the rest of my body. Six weeks later, I was in full judo practice.

About the same time, a man from Greece had suffered a similar injury. He insisted on being taken to the hospital, which meant a loss of at least fifteen minutes while he was in transit. It was another ten minutes before a doctor set the leg, and he was in agony. I had resumed practicing judo when I happened to see him in the doorway, his leg still in a plaster cast.

As soon as I could walk, I went to see Ohkura, the master of theater. He considered himself the carrier of the tradition of Kyogen which was started by his family twenty-three generations earlier. His first son was named Mototsguo, "the Continuer"; his second son was Motogushi, "the Helper"; and they were trained from birth to carry on the family tradition.

Ohkura was an extraordinary man. You will recall I described Moshe as walking like a judo master or tiger. This man could walk like the wind. You were not aware that he was moving—until you felt the breeze. I told him I had come to study singing and that I did not wish to act or go on the stage. he agreed and told me to come "anytime, on Friday." What I did not know at the time was that you do not give conditions to Japanese masters; and as for the time for the lesson, you come and wait for your turn.

On the Friday I joined his group of students, we waited on one side of his small room. Ohkura would call a student who then would bow and sit opposite him. The master would start singing, and the student repeated the same sounds. There were no instruments—only a leather-covered, wooden block and two sticks on which he beat the rhythm. I listened and thought I'd have no problem because they seemed to be talking rather than singing—that's what I thought until it was my turn to sing, and I could not repeat the sound. I couldn't believe it: It was not a lesson in singing so much as how to use your abdomen. The master had said to one opera star, "I'm not interested in your notes. Repeat after me." He never explained what was to be repeated. He would make a sound, and you were expected to repeat it. What I learned, I had to discover for myself, for he never explained.

I had to copy him exactly. There was one instance when I seemed to be copying him exactly, yet it wasn't the same sound. He said, "Yes, so listen again." When I finally realized that my master's end did not "die at the end," he confirmed my discovery. But I had to work it out for myself. Even now, when I practice singing, I feel wonderful, and my voice becomes strong. Breathing this way gives you a sense of power, and you do not need a microphone to be heard.

In Tokyo, performances were usually given on a stage. While Moshe was in Japan, I had to perform in an open-air shrine where only a strong voice could be heard in that large space.

The teacher later taught me a song which I had to practice at home. A dance was connected with it, which I also had to learn, although I wondered why. It was danced with a fan. I had to copy his movements exactly, but I really did not know what I was doing. I was to have another lesson the next Friday.

Two weeks later, the master asked me whether I would like to see a Noh play. I was quite interested and agreed to be at a particular shrine at ten o'clock in the morning. Maurice went with me. Mototsugo was waiting for us outside the theater. "Come in quickly," he said. "You have to change your clothes." I though that this must be a very traditional theater since traditional clothing was required in order to attend a performance. When I was dressed, I was taken to a small door where my teacher and his two brothers, who worked with him, were waiting. The door opened, and he said, "Go in." I bent down to enter, certain I was to be seated with the other members of the audience, only to find myself on stage!

I stood frozen. Then I heard my master say, "Walk to the center of the stage and kneel." I did so—like a robot. "Open the fan and start singing," he directed. By now, my master and his brothers, who were to be in the choir, were also on stage, sitting behind me, as is customary in Japanese theater. I started singing, and I was supported by the choir behind me. Subsequently directed to dance, I got up and don't know what I did—it must have been a kind of dancing. All this time, the choir was singing behind me. I saw the crowd and my husband's amazed face. It was a terrible experience: All I wanted to do was go home to Israel: no judo! no Kyogen! no singing! no Japan! I just wanted to go home.

Finally, the performance was over. I went back to starting position and bowed to the crowd, holding the fan in the customary way, just as I had been taught to do after a lesson in the master's home: You bow to the teacher and acknowledge that he has taught you and to show gratefulness for the instruction you received. However, I was informed later that the performer is the "master" on stage and does not bow to the audience. To my surprise, there was applause—more than I ever got later on. I suppose they know all about novice-actors. I went back through the small doorway.

I had barely entered the adjoining room when I saw my master on the floor in front of me—in a deep bow, with his head near my feet. I was going to protest; but whenever I opened my mouth to do so, there he was, thanking me again. Then he got up, as light as the breeze; and, saying that the next performance would take place in two weeks, he disappeared.

This was the beginning of my "acting career," and, more importantly, of a close friendship with the master and his family. My children called the master and his wife "father" and "mother," and their children did the same with us. We spent a great deal of time and many holidays with them. Their children often stayed overnight at our house, or our children at theirs. Eventually, the master had our children learn traditional plays which they performed—very likely the only European children to act in a traditional Japanese theater.

This went on for two years. When Moshe came to spend a month in Japan, I took him to the master's house for a lesson. I have a photograph of the two of us sitting and singing. Moshe was most impressed with the *sensei* and often talked about him. Because of our friendship with the master, Moshe had the opportunity to experience Kyogen as well as judo. We went with the master to Isse, a famous shrine. We had rooms at the same inn, and Moshe took a bath with the master. He talked about that bathing experience many times thereafter. Moshe also came to watch the performance at the shrine the next day, and we all had a wonderful time.

Moshe was treated as a master by the Japanese who revere age and experience. They saw the light in his face. I had often talked about my great master, Moshe, before he came to the Kodokan. He met people there who remembered his previous connections with judo, and Mr. Kotani gave Moshe a badge which delighted him no end.

Somatics: When did this take place? In the late '60s?

Segal: We were in Japan in 1969, 1970, and 1971, so it was during the third year we were there.

Our own private teacher was Shimizu, an extraordinarily fine judo master who was in charge of judo training at the largest sports university in Japan. He also took a special interest in us, since it is most unusual in Japan to have a European family—father, mother, and two children—all in judo. He used to say, "Sixty years old, everything is sixty years old ... my legs, my arms—but I'm twenty!" A wonderful man!

Shimizu invited Moshe to teach in his place, introducing him to all his students as a great judo master from whom they could learn a great deal. This made Moshe very happy. I took photographs of the event, but something happened to the film, and I don't think Moshe ever forgave me. "Of what use are you?" he said. I, of course, was so sorry.

Somatics: Moshe often spoke of someone he had met in Japan who was a special kind of healer. Who was he?

Segal: That was Dr. Noguchi, an amazing man. I heard about him from a viola player, a Bostonian who was a member of the Tokyo Philharmonic. At the time, I wondered whether he would turn out to be another "bluffer" who was into healing. Although I had no intention of going to see him, I made a note of his name and address. Shortly thereafter, when I was in Tokyo, I decided to go and see this healer after all. Then the taxicab arrived at the address, I could not believe my eyes: There were fine cars parked outside and people wearing festive kimonos were coming out from a house that looked like a shrine. There was a large garden in front—a rarity in Tokyo. The house itself was among trees and had built on a hill—almost a "mountain" by Tokyo's standards. In the garage, there were two cars, both made by Rolls-Royce!

I decided to go in, even though I was simply dressed. I entered a downstairs room and met two people. After I ascertained that this was indeed Dr. Noguchi's residence, I asked why there were so many cars and people there and was told that one of the staff was getting married and the celebration was being held upstairs. So I went upstairs and entered into a huge hall. All the sliding windows, so typical of Japanese houses, were open, and the effect was that of living in the trees.

I asked a guest, "Where is Dr. Noguchi?" It was as though I had asked, "Where is God?" He pointed to a short man, no more than four feet tall, who was dressed in the Japanese style—a man's kimono, like a dress. The brandy glass he was holding was huge. By this time, I was wondering what I was doing there anyway and was thinking of leaving, when Dr. Noguchi looked straight at me. I realized Dr. Noguchi and two men were coming toward me. As he approached, he said to the two men: "See this lady. She works on people, just like I do; and she makes them better, just like I do."

Somatics: Did Dr. Noguchi expect you?

Segal: No! He didn't know anything about me. I was so surprised. I looked at him and said, "I don't think I do what you do, but I would like to come and learn from you."

He retorted, "What do you mean by 'I don't do what you do?'"

I collected my wits and said, "But I have had a master in Israel who does what you do."

He evidently wanted to know more about Moshe, for then he asked, "Does he treat the body or the spirit?"

I could only reply, "How can you separate them?"

Dr. Noguchi turned to the two men and said, "See, I told you!"

From that moment on, I knew I had to learn from Dr. Noguchi. He wanted to know whether I worked with groups or individuals. "The latter," I replied, "but my Israeli master works with groups, sometimes as many as forty people at a time." Dr. Noguchi said that he also worked that way and that I could come and see for myself on Friday at the university, which turned out to be located close to where we used to live.

This particular group assembled in a basketball stadium where the Olympic Games had been held. There was this short man standing and speaking in the center of that immense space, surrounded by at least six thousand people (I arrived at that figure by counting the seats). Dr. Noguchi spoke in traditional Japanese which I found difficult to understand. (He did write books, but not much is available in English.) At one point, he said, "O.K., now come do your exercises." The people got up from their seats and went down to the center of the stadium—waves of people, all exercising on the stadium floor. They did what he called *katsu-gen-undo,* a vitalizing movement wherein people move in any way that the body makes them move. It is supposed to become an unconscious way of moving, and it gains a certain momentum. It was a strange happening to see.

Somatics: Did he tell them what to do, giving specific directions?

Segal: He would tell them to start exercising. They would begin to move, and their body movements would get bigger and bigger. Some would continue moving in this way. Others would be jumping up and down, crawling, sitting, standing—whatever they wanted to do. When they were told to stop, all went back to their seats. After a while, I decided to go home—I just could not watch it any longer. Before I could escape, Dr. Noguchi was at the door inquiring why I was leaving. Instead of answering his question, I asked if I could come again. He then invited me to come and observe his private lessons on the several days he worked with individuals. The time "From morning till evening," he advised.

So I went to see how he gave private lessons. The waiting room was the same beautiful room used for the wedding reception, and people were quietly waiting their turn. Classical music—Beethoven, Brahms, anyone you can think of—played nonstop all day long. The person to be treated would go behind the screen, lie on the floor, and Dr. Noguchi would use his hands to treat the problem. That is how he did the healing.

I was waiting outside with the others. Then he saw me through the door and invited me to come in. "Sit here and watch," he ordered. That was a fantastic experience for me.

Five men were waiting behind the screen. When Dr. Noguchi pointed to one of them, the man would bow low and lie on the floor next to the master. Dr. Noguchi would run his fingers along the spine— as if he were playing the piano. Then he would move the vertebrae deftly; pull a little here and there—and that is all he did. He would move the legs and do something very fast. he worked quickly; all five of those waiting were treated in about twenty minutes. After five sessions, he would take a break and go to a small adjoining room to have a drink of brandy.

I once asked, "Dr. Noguchi, don't you ever get drunk?"

He laughed, "Yes, but there's this vertebra in my back. When I do this (demonstrating), I become sober!"

Dr. Noguchi spoke only Japanese. In my limited Japanese, I asked him why only classical music was played. "You must understand," he said, "that classical music revitalizes your energy. Anyone who wants to get his energy back should have a background of European classical movement."

Somatics: What was his background? Was he religious or part of a cult? You said he laid hands ...

Segal: The story is that he was a man of the middle class who was a great healer and that he had married a princess who was a cousin of the Emperor. The house he lived in had been her family's palace, moved to Tokyo piece by piece.

This is how I learned what he did: He asked me how I worked, and I offered to show him. He said, "If you will wait until I finish at seven tonight, you can work on me and show me what you do. Then I will work on you to show you what I do." So that is what happened. I gave him a Feldenkrais lesson which he found interesting. Then it was his turn. I found what he did equally as interesting, for his hands were as skilled as Moshe's. That is all I can say about it. It was just a quick adjustment of my body, and I know that most people seemed to get very powerful results.

He scheduled the instructor's classes so that he'd work days ending in the number *two* one month and in the number *three* the next month, each unit lasting for three days and three nights. I was invited to join about two or three hundred students who came from all over Japan.

Somatics: Was he out of a tradition of healing?

Segal: He taught that everyone had the power to heal. He himself had discovered that he had the power when he was a young child. I believe a horse had fallen and broken a leg; when he touched it while it was lying there in the street, the horse got better. This is how he discovered he had the power to transfer vital energy from his hands to another living creature. It was like electricity—or whatever you wish to call it. That is what he was teaching his pupils to do. He lectured and demonstrated the technique of passing electricity to another person. He was known as a great expert; and many students voluntarily worked for him.

My limited knowledge of the Japanese language prevented me from understanding everything he said. Every three hours, he would take a break and head for his room, inviting me to go along. There he'd take a drink and ask me if I had any questions. I had so many questions I couldn't even begin to ask them. I used to watch him intently to see what he was doing. I had a very disconcerting experience. I would look at him and think, "His face is so crooked on the left side." After a few hours, I'd think it was the right side of the face that was crooked—not the left. After a while, still undecided, I wrote my observation down on a piece of paper: It's the *right* side. But then a few hours later, it was the *left* side. His mouth was twisted, his eye closed, and his body seemed to have shrunk. Finally, I found the courage to ask him about my impressions.

"Excuse me, but you seemed to be a little crooked, once on one side and then on the other," I said.

"How do you think I can teach for two days and for two nights without sleeping?" he replied. "Every time, half my brain is asleep."

I'll never know whether or not he was pulling my leg. I later wrote to Moshe about my experiences with Dr. Noguchi.

As soon as he arrived in Japan, Moshe wanted to meet Dr. Noguchi. I still have photographs taken at the time Dr. Noguchi invited Moshe to teach his pupils, and Moshe did—all three hundred of them. With

Dr. Noguchi looking on nearby, Moshe gave a demonstration of Functional Integration and also of ATM. Moshe had them work on one side and then told them to imagine the movement on the other side. After the demonstration, we went to Dr. Noguchi's room. Moshe wanted to know Dr. Noguchi's reaction to the ATM demonstration. Dr. Noguchi stated, "It was interesting, especially the part where you told them to imagine the movement on the other side. That was new to me. As for Functional Integration, there is no difference between what you do and what I do, except that I give them the food and leave it next to them; you feed them and digest it for them." That was a most revealing insight. As I said earlier, his lessons were very short, and his pupils had to assume responsibility for further improvement.

On the twentieth of the month, Dr. Noguchi would give a big party to which he invited "the cream of the Japanese culture." It was held in his magnificent private home (not in his work place). There would be an elaborate buffet, followed by a cultural event: poetry or a musical performance held in a special room (auditorium) and recorded by expert sound technicians. Only European music was played. For someone who had never been exposed to European culture to be so devoted to its music was surprising and unusual. On one occasion, there was an exceptionally fine performance of Schubert's *Arpeggione Sonata* by a famous cellist, accompanied by his sister, a pianist. After the performance, Dr. Noguchi said to the cellist, "Hold your bow like this (demonstrating). Isn't that better?"

The London Symphony came to Tokyo. Some of the musicians were old friends who had played quartets in our home in Israel. When I asked Dr. Noguchi if he would like to hear them play, he was delighted and arranged to have them come to his home on a special evening. Afterwards, Dr. Noguchi made similar comments to them.

Every concert was recorded and added to his huge collection. There were thousands of records on shelves from floor to ceiling and sound equipment ranging from the earliest Gramophone to the latest recording apparatus. I once asked him about a certain record, only to have him climb to the top shelf, quickly find the record, climb down and give it to me. His movements were unique. Compared to my singing teacher who seemed to float like the wind with no visible movement or change in the body, or Moshe's graceful tiger walk, or my judo teacher's leopard walk, Dr. Noguchi walked like an animal that can turn spontaneously and effortlessly in any direction at any speed.

Somatics: He was an expert in movement. Did you learn anything from him that you have used?

Segal: Yes, I continued to go to all his classes. When the day's work was finished, we would exchange lessons. I was considered to be more than an acquaintance, yet I never formally studied with Dr. Noguchi. I did not learn much about his technique because I do not do that kind of work. I was influence by his attitude and philosophy, perhaps, because you absorb whatever makes an impression. His comment to Moshe about "feeding students and digesting the food for them" had quite an impact on me. I decided not "to digest" in the future but to have student ponder about the unexplained parts of a lesson. I did cut my lessons shorter after that.

Moshe himself may have been influenced by Dr. Noguchi's observation. He even cut short one of our trips around Japan in order to return and see Dr. Noguchi again.

At one point, Dr. Noguchi had Moshe and me hold hands with some of his students to pass electricity. I asked Moshe later if we did pass electricity. "I don't know," he replied.

Dr. Noguchi also gave a party for Moshe. We arrived in time to see the pupils standing in a corner of the room. They pointed to a plant with a flower bud and said that they were planning to use electricity, or a vital power, to make a bud open into a flower. I said to Moshe, "You can't tell me you can influence a plant!" But they stood about two feet away from the plant and pointed to it, like this (gesture). The bloody plant's bud opened before our eyes. They claimed it was the heat from their hands that made the bud open into a flower.

"Well, Moshe?" I asked.

"I can't explain it," he replied.

Somatics: Did you learn about acupuncture points in Japan?

Segal: Yes. A lady who did Kyogen with us told me that she was having acupuncture treatments. I went to see Dr. Sato. Here's another instance of a great Japanese master: He did not want publicity and lived so privately you could hardly find his house: a simple, beautiful, peaceful place. He was startled to see me, a European. First, I asked to be taught acupuncture, but he said that he was not a teacher. So, I asked him to be my doctor. "What is wrong with you?" he asked. His treatments were extraordinary. Afterwards, I felt divine. He had the lightest hand in using needles. I would also bring my husband and my children for treatment, and they too came to love it.

One day, Dr. Sato said, "If you come next week, I will teach you." Then he wanted to know whether I had studied European medicine. What to tell him? I wanted to say that I was a qualified medical doctor—how could he find out I wasn't? I was about to say, "Yes," but, to my amazement, I heard myself answering, "No." Dr. Sato said, "Yes, I will teach you. But if you had studied medicine, I would not do so, because doctors have closed minds." I was to bring my daughter to serve as a model and my son to interpret Dr. Sato's instructions; my son understood Japanese better than the rest of us. My family was delighted to learn that Dr. Sato was going to teach me acupuncture— and then I told them they were to be part of it.

I bought a special copybook, and off we went to Dr. Sato's home for our first lesson. "Come in," he said, "and let's have tea." We were sitting there, and I began wondering when the lesson would begin. "I want to show you my teacups. Look at this . . . it's beautiful. . . ." Dr. Sato went on and on. "Which tea would you like—this one or that on?" My children were wondering if I had misunderstood Dr. Sato when he said that he was going to give lessons. I was also wondering if I had understood him correctly. Eventually, I decided I had misunderstood Dr. Sato's intention, so I put down my notebook and pen. Then I heard him say, "In this spirit, we can start learning." Wasn't that wonderful!

From then on, we came for an hour twice a week. This busy professional set aside time for us, even though his waiting room was always full of people waiting to see him. He refused to accept payment for the lesson, insisting that he was not a teacher. To show my appreciation, I decided to give him an exquisite ceramic piece made by a famous artist. I gave him the gift. "Thank you very much," he said, as he put it down. At the end of the next lesson, he handed me a box. It was a present—a much more expensive one. Then I understood that he really did not want to be paid, even though he gave me two hours a week for a year.

Dr. Sato also treated Moshe's knee. Moshe and Dr. Sato liked each other immensely. Dr. Sato is the one who said of Moshe, "There's a lot of life and wisdom in his face."

Somatics: You had a wonderful time in Japan. How long were you there?

Segal: Just over three years. It was quite an experience. Among those people I often felt I was an ignorant child. They had a certain wisdom.

Somatics: You changed your way of working because of Dr. Noguchi. Did judo, acupuncture, or the other experiences you had every change your work in other ways?

Segal: Acupuncture had very little influence on my work. Just before I left, I asked Dr. Sato, "When do you think I will know acupuncture?" He replied, "I have been doing this for forty years, and only now have I started to understand a little." Some of the things he taught me, I could do. I am not really an expert, far from it. For a while, I did not do any at all. I still have the needles and *moxa*; and I might use needles on a member of the family if it's a complaint I can handle.

Acupuncture is more like medicine than teaching: It is doing something to a person. I once thought of combining acupuncture with teaching; for example, being able to relieve a student's acute pain, thus facilitating learning. But I did not know enough about acupuncture to use it that way.

Somatics: Philosophy does have a lot to do with it. The Japanese and the Chinese are more sensitive to the broader philosophical—in some sense, the religious—issues in their approach to medicine.

Segal: That's right, but I think their philosophy is the same as Moshe's; that is, in the way both consider the whole body as a unit. Their philosophy lets you look at the whole person instead of the particular part; for example, if a patient has a pain in the kidney, the ear may get the treatment. If I learned anything from acupuncture, it was to look at the body as a unit, as a pattern, rather than divided into parts.

Somatics: Moshe always had an interest in that aspect of acupuncture, for example, treating the kidney through the ear. His fascination probably had something to do with types of reflexes—skin reflex areas that lead to the brain; in fact, it was like a detective mystery to him.

Segal: It is a very different approach.

Somatics: You have talked about many significant things in your life.

Segal: To sum it up, even after all the masters I have had, I am doing Moshe's kind of work: You could say that he incorporated all the other things I learned. He used his knowledge of methods in the most practical and economical way, and he was able to teach very clearly and explicitly. He gave his many pupils all the necessary elements.

Somatics: It is as though his knowledge of judo and ju-jitsu through the years and the relationship of his own body to these disciplines enabled him to see through to the wisdom of the Japanese tradition: That hidden wisdom you said was in the culture. There is something profoundly Japanese about Moshe's insights.

Segal: Yes. Definitely Eastern. He had absorbed their spirit or essence to which he added his fantastic European way of thinking and the sharpness of scholarly, logical mind. Moshe had a certain fire, really. His eyes were brown but became black when he was excited about something. Very strange, piercing, wonderful eyes!

Somatics: He would be working on someone, and it was deeply impressive to see his eyes as he looked up whenever something unusual was happening as he was manipulating the body. Did you experience that?

Segal: Yes. It was fascinating to watch him working. That is how I learned for many years. After a time, Moshe was photographed and videotaped as he worked. I got a terrible shock when I saw the first videotapes: His head, eyes, shoulders, chest, and breathing were not shown. I did not know what I was watching. I suddenly realized that the last thing I watched were his hands. In the videotapes the camera cut off part of Moshe's body and focused on his technique—how he moved a toe.... When I worked with Moshe, I would look at him— rarely the way his fingers were manipulating a body. I found nothing at all in those videotapes.

Somatics: You get back to a spirit, a way of being. You sit around a watch the master. There is no explanation. That is typically Japanese.

Segal: You can't take out the details and think that you have the substance: The details are not the substance. I loved to watch his wonderful hands, but it really was not what I had been watching for years.

Somatics: That is where his students so often got lost. They considered what he was doing an engineering technique, so their eyes focused on the hands alone—watching which bone he was pushing as if that there the secret of it all. What was important, as he often stressed, was the *how,* not the *what.*

We have talked about various things, from Israel through Japan. What about the U.S.A.? I believe you've had some acquaintance with the psychotherapist and hypnotist, Milton Erickson. Were you impressed by Erickson? Has it made a difference to you?

Segal: Yes, I was impressed. However, I don't think I know enough about what Erickson and his students do to say I was affected in any way. In some ways, what Erickson does explains much of the mystery of Moshe's intuitive understanding of the psychology of the person. It has nothing to do with the hands. When I would ask Moshe to explain how Erickson knew certain things, Moshe would say that it was because of his "experience in life." Although both of them had a lot of experience, it was the way they looked at life and their understanding or inner wisdom.

Somatics: Some people say it is intuitive; others say that it is psychic. There are all sorts of names for it. Moshe would never use "psychic" or "intuitive." Do you agree that he'd say it is *experience?*

Segal: Yes, Moshe was so down-to-earth. He was centered in everything he did, and he was always balanced. That was Moshe: never a flag flying in the wind, but always closely tied to the earth! So how could he talk about the psychic? His center of gravity was close to the ground, and his work and teaching were down-to-earth and logical. He didn't use words without meaning—real meaning. That, too, was his greatness.

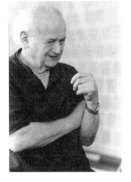

The Elusive Obvious
(Introduction)

Moshe Feldenkrais

I AM KNOWN FOR the beneficial effects of what I call "Functional Integration" and "Awareness through Movement." In both these techniques I use everything I have learned to improve the health, mood, and ability to overcome difficulties, pain, and anxiety of the people who turn to me for help.

In my twenties, while playing left back in soccer, I badly injured my left knee and could not walk properly for several months. In those days knee surgery was not the simple intervention that it is today. It was learning to function with a knee like mine which impressed upon me the urgency of doing something more. Our knowledge will undoubtedly improve in the future, but with good theory much of what we know now can be useful and applicable.

I have tried to write only what is necessary for you to understand *how* my techniques work. I have deliberately avoided answering the *whys*. I know how to live and how to use electricity, but I encounter enormous difficulties if I attempt to answer why I live and why there is electricity. In interpersonal affairs *why* and *how* are not so sharply divided and are used indiscriminately. In science, we really only know how.

I was born in the small Russian town of Baranovitz, and at the time of the Balfour Declaration, when I was fourteen, I went all by myself to the British mandatory territory of Palestine. There I worked for several years as a pioneer, largely in a manual capacity. At the age of twenty-three I matriculated; I had studied mathematics and then served for five hears in the surveying department doing mathemat-

Capitola, CA: Meta Publications, 1981. 1–12

ics for producing maps. I saved sufficient money to travel to Paris where I took an engineering degree in mechanics and electricity, and proceeded to the Sorbonne to read for a doctorate. While at the Sorbonne I was attached to the laboratory of Joliot-Curie who later, of course, received the Nobel Prize. At the same time I met Professor Kano, the creator of Judo, and with help from him and his pupils Yotazo Sigimura (6th Dan) the Japanese ambassador, and Kawaishi I gained my Judo Black Belt. I formed the first Judo Club in France, which today has nearly a million members. After the German invasion of France in the Second World War I escaped to England, and worked there as a scientific officer in the antisubmarine establishment of Scientific and Technical Pools of the British Admiralty until the end of the war. I participated in Budokwai in London before finally returning to Israel to be the first director of the Electronic Department of the Defense Forces of Israel.

At the age of fifty or so, after writing *Body and Mature Behaviour,* first published in England in 1949 by Routledge and Kegan Paul, I encountered many people who thought I had some extraordinary knowledge which could perhaps help them. That book was an exposition of the up-to-date scientific knowledge of the time which had led me to my practical applications. My views on anxiety and falling, and the importance of the vestibular branch of the eighth cranial nerve are now almost universally accepted. As a result of the needs of others, I gradually developed Functional Integration and Awareness through Movement which I have subsequently taught in a dozen or so countries of the world. During this process of helping and teaching, I have been privileged to examine, by touching and moving, more human heads than I dare to say. They have come from all walks of life and from many races, cultures, religions, and all ages. The youngest was a five-week-old baby whose neck was injured at birth by forceps, and the oldest was a ninety-seven-year-old Canadian who had been electrocuted and was paralyzed for over thirty years.

I have also handled many workers from a very wide range of activities. These details are of little importance other than to demonstrate that the primary and real object of my learning is the practical effectiveness of my actions. I am still learning, reading, and annotating several books a month in spite of my multiple obligations and travels. Some of the authors I would advise you also to read, many of them are priceless: Jacques Monod, Schrödinger, J.Z. Young, Konrad Lorenz, Milton Erickson. They all discuss philosophy, semantics, and evolution, and they show an insight and knowledge of the psychophysical world which is edifying as well as interesting.

I touch with my hands and this I do to many thousands, be they white, mongolian, black, or of whatever human races exist. This touching, handling, manipulating of living human bodies enables me to see in the books of these superb writers and turn into practice the science they teach. Probably they themselves do not know, how useful their knowledge is already when translated into the nonverbal language of the hands, i.e. Functional Integration and the verbal Awareness through Movement.

I suggest, and I believe that I am right, that sensory stimuli are closer to our unconscious, subconscious, or autonomous functioning than to any of our conscious understanding. On the sensory level communication is more direct with the unconscious, and is therefore more effective and less distorted than at the verbal level. Words, as somebody said, are more to hide our intentions than to express them. But, I have never met anybody, man or animal, who cannot tell a friendly touch from an evil one. Touching, if unfriendly even in thought, will make the touched stiff, anxious, expecting the worst, and therefore unreceptive to your touch. Through touch, two persons, the toucher and the touched, can become a new ensemble; two bodies when connected by two arms and hands are a new entity. These hands sense at the same time as they direct. Both the touched and the toucher feel what they sense through connecting hands, even if they do not understand and do not know what is being done. The touched person becomes aware of what the touching person feels and, without understanding, alters his configuration to conform to what he senses is wanted from him. When touching I seek nothing from the person I touch; I only feel what the touched person needs, whether he knows it or not, and what I can do at that moment to make the person feel better.

It is essential to understand what I mean by "better" and "more human." These apparently simple words do not mean the same thing to all of us. The things a handicapped person cannot do have a different meaning to him than to a healthy person. I remember a boy of thirteen brought to me by his mother. He came into the world with his right arm first, and not his head as is customary. He had no luck, and an inexperienced doctor, or whoever it was, pulled him out by his protruding arm. The right clavicle was broken, which is not a serious matter at that age, but a brachial plexus was damaged. The arm became flaccid, hanging helplessly, in spite of the fact that his mother had taken him to see every specialist who might have been able to help. I may tell you later how he learned to drive a car, become a father of healthy children, and a professor of mechanics.

When the boy became one with me he told me, with tears running down his cheeks, something you will never guess—anyway, I was surprised: he complained nobody had ever hit him at school, in spite of all his provocations. Whatever he did his schoolmates would not touch him, as teachers and parents had all impressed upon them that he was not to be hurt. He was miserable because he had never had the pleasure of being beaten up. Think, now, what "better" and "more human" meant to this boy. His mother did not know what was needed, and neither did anybody else. When I touched him he felt as one with me, and he sensed that I knew he was miserable and that I had no pity. At that point he could tell me what it was impossible for him to utter to anyone else. It was a nonverbal situation as I had asked nothing. What happened that enabled him to cry and then talk to me?

A girl with cerebral palsy, aged fifteen, was brought to me from Paris. Her mother was the principal of a lycée and could not leave, so her father brought her, and her grandmother stayed with her in Tel-Aviv. She also surprised me, for she wanted to be a dancer, this when she had never been able to put her heels on the floor and could not bend her knees, which knocked into each other at every step. If you have ever seen a person severely affected with cerebral palsy you may be able to imagine her arms, spine, and gait. Nobody with common sense could think that she was so unaware of her condition as to have such an idea about herself. My job, nothing more or less, was to help her to be what she wanted, and she did, several years later, join a dancing class in Paris. I would like you to think about what was "better" and "more human" for this girl. She was a bright girl at the top of her class until the time she went to the university, and I promise myself to look her up the next time I am in Paris.

I hope you will not jump to the conclusion that I am concerned only with cripples. To me they are all just people who seek help to be better and more human. Many doctors, actors, orchestral conductors, athletes, engineers, psychiatrists, architects, housewives—the whole range of what we can be—all sense that it would be better to be better and more human one way or another.

In fact, if normal intelligent people had more wisdom, I would give them all my attention. Their growth would make a difference to life in general. When I first began to work with people as such it was with Professor J.D. Bernal, a man of universal culture; Lord Boyd-Orr, Professor of Medicine and First President of the World Health Organization; Professor Aaron Katzir, Director of the Weitzman Institute; and David Ben-Gurion, founder of the State of Israel—all of them extraordinary human beings, famous, successful, and socially integrated. J.G. Crowther who was then the Secretary of the British Council, on hearing Bernal praise my work exclaimed, "There are probably only another three brains like his so you will not reach many more." As it turns out, socially successful, very clever, important, creative people may devote no time to their personal growth. They find their whole life is their work, ignoring themselves far too often. Such people listen to me seriously only when they are incapacitated one way or another. Even so, I have reached by now thousands of them through their misfortunes. It is sad to admit that it was only by attending to the crippled that I was able to learn how to help normal people as well. This is a generalization which, fortunately, was not always true.

I believe that this is as important for me to share some of my thoughts and experiences with you as it is for you to improve your life experiences, as they helped me. You may learn to make your life more as you wish it to be; your dreams could become more precise, and, who knows, they may even come true.

While writing, I am aware of only some parts of my body and also some of my activity. You, while reading, are equally aware of only some parts of yourself and of parts of your activity. Immense activity goes on in both of us, far greater than we appreciate or are aware of. This activity is related to what we have *learned* during our whole life from inception to this moment. Our actions largely depend on our heredity, on what we have been through in our lives, on the image we have formed of ourselves, on the physical, cultural, and social environments in which he have grown and the ones in which we now function. The activity in us which makes me write and you read is mostly autonomous, some of which can be said to be unconscious and some intentional. While writing, my conscious intentional activity seems to be the only one that concerns me. I have only occasionally to pay attention to my spelling or the flow of words "autonomous," "unconscious," or "conscious" is what I intend to convey for you.

For many years I have been involved in working with people who have turned to me for help. Some complain of physical pain, others of mental anguish, and only a few ever speak of emotional troubles. I have some difficulty in explaining to my followers that I am not a therapist and that my touching a person with my hands has not therapeutic or healing value, though people improve through it. I think that what happens to them is *learning,* but few agree with this. What I am doing does not resemble teaching as understood at present. The accent is on the learning process, rather than on the teaching technique. After each session my pupils have a new sense of well-being: they feel taller, lighter, and breathe more freely. They often rub their eyes as if they have just woken from a sound and refreshing sleep. More often than not they say that they have become relaxed. The pain is always abated and often it is gone altogether. In addition, face wrinkles nearly always disappear, the eyes become brighter and larger, and the voice deeper and more resonant. The pupil becomes youthful again.

How can such changes in mood and attitude be brought about just by touching, however cleverly, another person's body? My pupils try to convince me that I possess the healing touch. I have taught students to do what I do in Israel, the United States, and elsewhere, so that they all now have "healing hands." They were not specially chosen, but they were selected for their academic education and their wish and capacity to learn. At the beginning, in order to explain to my students what happens between me and my clients—I say "clients" reluctantly in order not to confuse you, although they are in fact pupils but not students—I tell them this story. Imagine a dancing party attended by a man who never dances, for reasons best known to himself. He always declines all invitations to participate saying that he does not know how. One woman, however, likes the man sufficiently to persuade him to take the floor. Moving herself, she somehow manages to make him move too. The dance is not very complicated, and after a few awkward moments when his ear tells him that the music has something to do with it, he becomes conscious that her movements are rhythmical. Nevertheless, he is relieved when the dance stops and he can return to his seat and breathe again. At the end of the evening he finds he can follow her movements and steps more easily, and can even avoid bumping into her feet. Half thinking, he feels that perhaps he has not performed so badly, although he knows that he still cannot dance.

After going to a second party, he makes sufficient progress to shake his conviction that dancing is not for him. At the next party, finding a woman left sitting alone like himself, he asks her to dance, still protesting that he is not very good. Ever since then he has danced, forgetting to begin with an apology.

Consider the woman who could dance, and how she made a pupil or client dance also, without teaching musical rhythms, dancing steps, and all the rest of it. Her friendly attitude and her experience made him learn without any formal teaching. A certain kind of knowledge can pass from one person to another without a healing touch. However, the man must have learned to use his legs, hands, and the rest of him before a friendly touch could help him to use his experience and learn to dance so easily. He learned notwithstanding his ignorance of his latent ability.

In saying that I work with people I mean that I am "dancing" with them. I bring about a state in which they learn to do something without my teaching them, any more than the woman taught the dancer. We shall see later in a more detailed fashion that, in general we do much without knowing consciously how we do it. We speak and we do not know how we do it. We swallow and ignore how we do it. Try to explain to a Martian how we swallow and you will realize what I mean by knowing. Some very common everyday acts, like sitting or getting up from a chair, seem easier to know. But, are you really sure of what we do when getting up from the sitting position? Which part of our body initiates the movement? Is it the pelvis, the legs, or the head? Do we contract our abdominal muscles first or the extensors of the back? We can do the movement just by intending to perform it and not knowing how we do it. Do you think that we really do not need to know? Suppose that somebody cannot get up for some reason (and there more reasons for that than meet the eye), and asks you for help. You can show him that you can get up, but then he knew that. So it seems you can do it but cannot explain how you do it. Suppose you are in need of the explanation, for how can we be sure that without knowing how we do something it is being done as well as our potential capacity will allow? Certainly most of the simple actions we do are good enough to meet our needs. Even so, every one of us feels that some actions are not as good as we would wish them to be. We organize our life around that which we can do to our satisfaction, and avoid those acts where we feel we are inept. We decide that the activities that involve our ineptitudes are not congenial to our character, are uninteresting, and we usually have more important things to do.

I did not draw in my early life for there were no drawing lessons in the schools in those good old days. One had, instead, to prepare for an active and socially useful life. When my book *Body and Mature Behavior* was published after the Second World War I did not realize that I had changed my future in direction it was to take me. One morning a medical doctor in London telephoned me, and said he had read my book, and asked when I had studied with Heinrich Jacoby. He had recognized in my book some of the things he had received from this great teacher. He had difficulty in believing that it was the first time I had heard that name mentioned. To come to the point, he suggested that he should arrange for me to meet Heinrich Jacoby for our mutual benefit. Heinrich Jacoby lived at that time in Zurich and was much senior to me, not only in age; I felt clearly when I learned that what I had believed to be my personal discovery was in a way the kind of thing he had been teaching for years to a distinguished group of disciples comprising scientists, doctors, artists, and the like.

A few months later, when I could avail myself of my annual leave from the laboratory where I worked at the time as a research physicist, I went to meet Jacoby at the date he had fixed for me. I would very much like to tell you what happened during the three weeks I stayed with him and of all our conversations and mutual teaching, which often meant we saw the sun rise before we went to sleep. A book would be rather long if I were to relate all the important things I learned and those he said he learned from me. I will, however, tell you of my first overwhelming experience in drawing which I had with him, as it concerns the kind of learning we are dealing with.

I was an athlete of some repute and of strong build. Jacoby was a tiny, fragile little man who had learned to walk, he told me, when he was seven years old. He looked like, and was a hunchback, but moved gracefully. Even so, my first impression was that the man was no match for me. I felt that, way in the back of my consciousness, although I was certain that I had done the right thing to visit him. After a few minutes, when he explained that I was being recorded on tape and photographed by his cinecamera, he offered me a sheet of drawing paper, charcoal, and a piece of soft bread to be used as an eraser. He then asked me to draw as best I could the lamp on the piano in front of me. I told him that I had never drawn anything before except for the technical drawings I had to do for my engineering degree before reading physics at the Sorbonne, which brought me later to the Joliot-Curie Laboratory, my doctorate, and all the rest. He replied that he knew all that but I should nevertheless have a try, as he had something else in mind other than just to see me draw. I drew a vertical cylinder with a truncated cone at the upper end and a kind of ellipse at the bottom for a stand. It looked to me to be a lampstand as good as I thought a lampstand drawn by me could be. He looked at the drawing and said it was the thought of a lamp and not the lamp, and I realized then that I had drawn the abstract notion of the word "lamp." All the same, I retorted, only a painter could do what he expected of me, and I was no painter, as I had said before I started.

He insisted that I should try again and draw only what I saw, and not what I thought I saw. I just did not know how one draws what one sees. In my, and it may be also your, way of thinking he asked me to be a painter when I was not a painter. "Tell me what do you see?" "A lamp," I said, "do you see any of the outlines which you have drawn?" I had to admit that I could not identify in my drawing a single line of the real lamp, except that the proportions were more or less those of the lamp in front of me. "Do you see lines?" Again I had to admit that none of the lines on my drawing were actually to be seen. "If you do not see lines, then what do you see when looking at this lamp? What do your eyes see in general? They see light. Then why do you not draw the lighter and darker patches which you see. You have charcoal in your hand, and if you put too much of it on the paper then you have the bread to remove the superfluous and obtain some grading of the patches so that they become more as you see them."

I took another sheet of paper and this time started with dark patches of charcoal where there was no light, then it dawned on me that nowhere were there brighter patches than where I put no charcoal on the paper. The stand was no cylinder, the shade on the top was no truncated cone, and the bottom was no ellipse. I had extraordinary feelings when I looked at the assembly of charcoal rubbings and the parts removed with the bread kneaded with my fingers. This drawing was not mine, but one which I thought only a painter could do. I had not even tried to think that way before because it had felt to me to be like cheating, pretending to be what I was not.

I believe you are understanding for yourself the extraordinary transformation that was occurring in me. I am not a painter, but then who is? When I do or act painter, the result is what only a painter can do. Am I being changed, am I losing my identity? I did not really think in those terms at that moment, but I felt unsafe because of the change which operated in me under Jacoby's questioning. He did not show me how to do it. Remember the dancer with his girlfriend? Can you see anything in common in the two cases of learning in two such different circumstances? I can.

When I left Jacoby and went to my room I saw there on the table a glass jug half filled with water. I felt an inner challenge—no, an inner conviction—which expressed itself in an urge to reproduce the jug on paper. Childishly, I also thought that I could show Jacoby that I was not so really so inept as I appeared to him. I did not draw any lines at all but used instead minor touches, and the rest was blobs of light and dark. When it was finished you could see the level of water, the play of light in the water as distinct from the light on the glass, although both were transparent. I felt that I had produced a master-piece and I believed that I had grown taller by six inches at least.

It turned out that there is no limit to the quality of being a painter, and I have to make an effort not to tell you how I became a real painter during the few weeks when I danced with Jacoby, who never taught or showed me how to paint or draw. With his tongue in his cheek he asked me why I did not follow my own teaching when I drew.

Ida Rolf

Ida Rolf (1896–1979) developed a method of deep manipulation of body structure, "Rolfing," based on a brilliant synthesis of classical osteopathy, tantric yoga, and a host of other body practices which she explored throughout the world until the end of her life in 1978 at eighty-three years old. Two assumptions characterized her method: the radical plasticity of the body, and the healing effects of moving bodily structure into alignment with the pull of gravity. She taught practitioners how to use their hands to capitalize on the inherent mobility of the bodily tissues, and how to move these tissues in directions that produce more balance in a person's life.

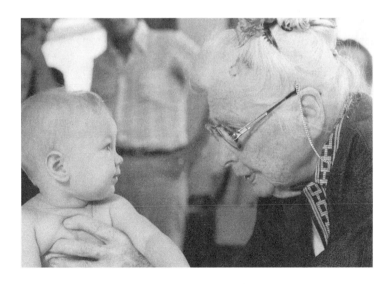

Ida Rolf Talks about Rolfing
and Physical Reality (Introduction)
Rosemary Feitis

Introduction

I first met Ida Rolf at Esalen ten years ago. What is now called "human-istic psychology" or the "human potential movement" was then just beginning to hit its stride. People like Will Schutz, Abe Maslow, and Fritz Perls had been doing their own work for years, but when they got to Esalen it was as though they had been handed a megaphone. Showing your work at Esalen could either make your reputation or break it—Esalen was always a turning point. This was equally true for Rolfing. Ida Rolf had been working for twenty-five years in New York; she had been teaching all across the United States and in Canada and England since the 1950s. Yet it was only after she began at Esalen that Rolfing became widely known, the subject of much notice and some controversy.

The people who came to Esalen for workshops stayed to get Rolfed. Some wanted to be trained to do Rolfing, and soon there were classes in Big Sur every summer. Eventually, like so many other new things that were cradled there, Rolfing outgrew Esalen and moved out into the world. In these ten years, 180 Rolfers have been trained; there is now a Rolf Institute,[1] with a home in Boulder, Colorado, and a group of teachers, and the beginnings of research; any number of articles have been written and books are coming into being.

I was one of the people who trained as a Rolfer. And, after I learned Rolfing, I worked with IPR[2] a few years longer—as secretary, orga-nizer, friend, chief-cook-and-bottle-washer, associate, and assistant in

New York: Harper & Row, 1978; 1–28, 33 ff.

writing. The outcome of that time was a book: *Rolfing: The Integration of Human Structures,* by Ida Rolf. It is a big, complex book full of illustrations and intricately put together. It was a formal exposition of the nature of the human body as understood by the principles of Rolfing.[3] It was quite literally an education for me to work on that book with IPR, and work on it we did for five years.

As we wrote, rewrote, and edited, I realized that I would like to see another book, one that was less formal, one that could capture the everyday feeling. Spending a day with IPR, working together, was so often a matter of moments that could shed light on a whole landscape. She was generous with her responses, unguarded and quick to let you know what she thought. This is the feeling that I've tried to capture here. My hope is that the serious student of Rolfing will read this book in conjunction with the formal exposition, the person who was just Rolfed may read it to get some amplification of his or her experience, and others may find in it some wisdom from a pioneering, original mind.

People like to ask about the origins of Rolfing—even to speculate and invent. Dr. Rolf tends to be reticent. On one occasion, a friend and I tried a trick. We made up a plausible lie for an article to be published in the *Bulletin of Structural Integration,*[4] saying that she had started her career in an ashram in Bombay. We hoped to the get the real information as she edited the piece; she changed it to read "an ashram in the Bronx" and let it go at that. Finally, years later, IPR and I spent a pleasant afternoon taping an interview about her early days. I found out that the "ashram in the Bronx" wasn't so very far from the truth.

IPR was born in New York in 1896 and grew up in the Bronx. She attended Barnard College, graduating in 1916 in the middle of World War I. At the time, with young men fighting in Europe, the supply of qualified technical personnel in so many fields was pre-empted, and so she was given a unique opportunity for a woman in that time. She was hired by Rockefeller Institute (now Rockefeller University) in New York City, and allowed to continue her education while working there. She received a Ph.D. in biological chemistry from the College of Physicians and Surgeons of Columbia University and continued at Rockefeller, eventually attaining the rank of associate. In the late

1920s, family business, including the management of her father's estate, forced her to leave.

Dr. Rolf started to work with people almost accidentally. As she tells the story:[5]

During the early war years, a friend of ours one day brought his wife to call; it must have been around 1940. I was talking about the fact that I had been visiting schools. I used to come into New York once a week and visit some of the experimental schools, trying to make up my mind what kind of school I wanted to send my kids to. I think the school I was talking about was the Ethical Culture School; at any rate it was somewhere they did unusual work with music. We were talking about this work and that I admired it, and so forth—just afternoon-tea conversation. And she said, "It sounds like the work my sister Ethel does." I said I'd like to meet her sister, Ethel, but she said, "There's no use meeting her because she's been through an accident and she can't teach music any more. She can't play the piano, she can't use her hands, she can't even comb her own hair."

And I said, "Well, I'd like to meet your sister Ethel anyhow." So the day came when Ethel came up the front lawn. She'd fallen on a hole in the pavement in New York and she had very badly injured one hand and arm, and the other wasn't that good. I looked at her and I said, "I bet I can fix that. Do you trust me to try? You can't be worse off." (She had just sued the City of New York and lost the suit, and she had paid all kinds of money in doctors' bills and so forth—$20,000 anyway. So she was feeling pretty low in her mind.) I said, "I'll make a bargain with you. If I can get you to the place where you can teach music, will you teach my children?" She said yes. And so I started in. I started, really, with yoga exercises, which I myself was using at that point. After we worked together about four times, she was in good enough shape to start teaching music. So we had a small class for four kids in Manhasset at my house. And that's where Rolfing really started. Because, of course, Ethel had a friend who hadn't been able to get help, and this friend had a friend, and so forth. And from then on my doorstep was pretty much filled with people who hadn't gotten help elsewhere. This was the beginning of the war, by the way, and Ethel was accepted as a WAC in a year or two, so you could call that a successful undertaking.

This story contains a number of the elements of IPR's personality that brought Rolfing into being. She had always investigated what was new and was never afraid to take what she learned and use it. She already knew a fair amount about yoga and osteopathy and had done considerable reading in homeopathy. All of these she investigated out of concern for her own health, because she was one of the people who hadn't been able to get help elsewhere. She told me:

> As a young woman, I had been struck by a horse's hoof on a trip to Colorado. As a result of that I had some symptoms that looked like pneumonia. The accident occurred the day before I was leaving for Yellowstone. It was a horrible trip. I had a temperature of about 104 degrees and was stranded alone in a cabin that was heated only by a stove and had no hot water. Eventually I landed in a hospital in Montana. The doctor there wasn't satisfied with my progress and so he said, I'm going to send an osteopath in. So a young man came and after his ministrations I could breathe again. When I got well enough to "walk home" so to speak (there was railroad strike in those parts at the time, I could barely get across the country. Eventually I did get across, and my mother took me to a blind osteopath in Port Jefferson, Dr. Thomas Morrison. (He was very highly regarded by his confreres: shortly before his death, they planned to build an osteopathic hospital or center on Long Island and wanted to call it the Morrison Center.) It was unusual to go to an osteopath at the time; there was still a great deal of controversy going on between the medics and the osteopaths and they were not accepted at all. I got to be friends with Morrison, and I became interested in the theory of osteopathy—that structure determines function.

Osteopathic treatment changes the way the bones of the body relate to each other, freeing obstructions between joints and thereby improving well-being. This is easy to understand in an injury caused by a traumatic impact such as Ida's kick from a horse: in that case the simple mechanics of the situation dictate that if a rib is out of place, breathing will be difficult. When the rib is put in its proper position, breathing will be easier. Osteopaths work directly with the bony structure throughout the body.

Similarly, Rolfing seeks to enhance function by changing structure, but it differs from osteopathy in two important respects. As Rolfers, we see that bones are held in place by soft tissue—muscles, ligaments, tendons, etc. If a muscle is chronically short, it will pull the attached bone out of balance. Repositioning the bone is not enough; the individual muscle and allied tissue must be lengthened if the change is to be permanent. In addition, when one part is in trouble, the body as a whole gets out of balance. This is easy to understand in a static structure, such as a house. If, for example, a door doesn't swing true or close properly, it really isn't enough to rehang the door. Probably the house has settled; in order to balance the door permanently, it would be better to look to the symmetry of the foundation. Structures must be balanced as a whole—this is as true of living structures as it is of houses and bridges.

Dr. Rolf learned about homeopathy in the early 1920s when a friend of hers, who was seeing a Dr. Schmidt in Geneva, told her to "go and get what they call a chronic." She remembers:

> I had plenty wrong with me; I was a curvature case but I didn't know it. And I was a prediabetic and didn't know that either. (Hypoglycemia hadn't been invented in those days.) I went to Switzerland on a leave of absence from the Rockefeller Institute. I studied in Zurich during the week and on weekends I went over to Geneva and got hold of the homeopathic *Materia Medica*. I read all Saturday night and all Sunday night and I went back to my physics classes in Zurich on Monday morning.

Homeopathy is a branch of medicine not frequently practiced in the United States, where allopathic medicine is more popular. The difference between the two types of healing lies principally in the choice of remedy. The allopathic physician will use whatever works to alleviate a given symptom. The homeopathic physician, on the other hand, will endeavor to arouse his patient's healing powers by giving him something that produces a temporary increase in his symptoms and then leads to what is known as a healing crisis. (This is, in some respects, similar to the ideas underlying vaccination.) One of the central theories of homeopathic medicine has to do with chronic complaints. A "chronic" is usually seen as an accumulation over time of different diseases imperfectly resolved, which then gather together and express themselves in a form that is long-standing and does not readily yield to treatment. In order to remedy this type of condition, the homeopathic physician must find his way back through the history of the complaint, treating first the most recent symptoms, then the earlier ones, and so on back to the earliest beginning of a the problem. They believe that in this way chronic disease can be permanently dispelled. The sequence of "unraveling" the problem was called by Hahnemann (founder of homeopathy) the "law of cure."

Osteopathy and homeopathy were known to Dr. Rolf, and contributed to her early understanding of the body. But the cornerstone of her thinking was yoga (she called it "yog"). All through the 1920s, she belonged to a group that practiced yoga asanas (positions) and held meetings and lectures and discussions. Her teacher then was an American, Pierre Bernard, who maintained a beautiful center for yoga instruction in Nyack, New York.

His father had been a tantric and he was brought up as a tantric. He had spent most of his childhood in India. In tantric families, boys of seven years of age are taken from their families, put into another home of the same culture grade, and are brought up with the other family. This is part of their educational system, so that the child is taught without the kind of emotional attachment that are inevitable between father and son, etc. In Hindu tantric families, through the centuries, the basis of the boys' education was the Tantras—the five Indian sacred books. These they had to learn by rote, which is something like the mental equivalent of doing five hundred cartwheels.

I'm sure you've heard me tell this story: There was a teacher whose name was Max Müller, an old German working at Oxford. He got very interested in the manuscripts from India that were being brought

West at the time because of the British Raj. He would get these old manuscripts, and a word would be erased or a whole line would be erased or worn through. He had four Hindu high-caste Brahmans from India being trained in Oxford. Now, when this happened, he would send for one after another of them, and say, "How does line so-and-so in verse such-and-such of chapter so-and-so go?" And the kid would spout it—only he wasn't a kid by this time, he was a young man. Müller would put that down, and then he'd send for the next one. He'd repeat the same thing, so Müller knew it was right. That was education in those days. So you can maybe even understand why I feel the way I feel when I listen to some of these fools spouting about how they want to go and do yog training and all that sort of stuff. They haven't got the where-with-all, and this they can't face.

So-called hatha (gathusta) yoga is the yoga of the body; it has as its premise that work with the body will improve not only the physical but the emotional and spiritual life of the individual as well. In physical terms, the principal aim of yoga asana is to increase the space at bony interfaces (joints). That is to say, the assumption of yoga is that bodies need to lengthen, and the means by which this length is achieved are positions in which opposing body parts pull or twist each other.

Yoga aims at developing the superior human being; it is a collection of techniques and teachings developed by its originators in the belief that this would bring out the highest qualities in man and educate and develop them. This is what attracted and held Dr. Rolf's interest, at first in connection with her own development and the education of her children. In those years of practicing yoga and discussing its principles, she was establishing the basis of all her future work; that bodies need to lengthen and be balanced, and that a balanced body will give rise to a better human being. When she was working with Ethel and all the people who came to see her after Ethel, she first worked with the techniques of yoga, instructing through moving. Slowly she realized that the asanas did not achieve length and separation of the joints, that in too many cases there was actual contraction of the joint surfaces. Something else was needed.

While she was teaching, she was also learning, investigating other exercise systems and incorporating what she found useful into her own understanding and work. IPR learned exercises from a Miss Brown, and one day Miss Brown's teacher came to town. The teacher proved to be a great big husky sixty-odd-year-old osteopath whose name was Amy Cochran. She is the one who first taught me the exercises which I've been teaching ever since. She claimed she had them by psychic perception from Dr. Rush—the medic who signed the Declaration of Independence. She had come East for a time and I started observing her teaching and trying to figure out what she was doing.

When Amy Cochran went back to California, IPR followed. This was in the late war years. She traveled by car across the country with her two small boys and a big orange cat. They stayed one night in a motel just outside the Mojave Desert. When they were ready to leave, the cat was lost. They had to leave. In those days there were no air-conditioned cars; the desert could only be crossed at night. When the man at the agricultural inspection station into California asked if they had any plants or pets, the story of the orange cat came out. And when they got to the rather dismal war-shortage housing in San Marino, California, the cat was there to welcome them. It had been found sitting by the side of the road and spotted by an agricultural inspector, and been taken to the business address left at the California border. (Very few cars were traveling across the war-time America, and agricultural inspectors were, evidently, able to take a personal interest in what came their way.)

A year later, IPR barely made it back home to New York; she had trouble explaining to the rationing board why, in a time of gas shortage, she needed to travel across the country twice. But make it home she did, and when she got there, she applied what she had seen—manipulative techniques and exercises—to the people who were still standing on her doorstep. One of them was Grace.

> Grace was a completely crippled woman. When she came to me, she was about forty-five. As a child of eight or so, she had been a great tomboy. She and a boy were diving off a roof of a pavilion. Things were getting "higher and higher"; she went off the roof, not having told the boy that she was going. He got mad and went

after her. He went faster than she and, halfway down, he knocked her against the wall of the pool. She came out of it completely crippled with her back just bent over. Grace always had to have somebody with her. She couldn't do such a thing as reach down and pick up her stockings off the floor or reach out and pull down a shade. So when I got home from Amy's in California, I called up Grace and I said, Grace, we're getting to work and we're going to fix you up. The day I started working with Grace was the day I really got Rolfing going. I would look at her and say, "This is in the wrong place," and I'd say, "Now, Grace, does this feel better this way, or does it feel better in the other direction?" And she'd say, "That way," so we'd organize that corner. This went on for a couple of years, and in the end Grace picked herself up and went to California all by herself. That was when the first principle of Rolfing was really born—moving the soft tissue toward the place where it really belongs.

Grace had worked with Amy Cochran before she worked with IPR, but, IPR said, "Amy Cochran didn't know that bodies had to lengthen." Amy Cochran had the exercises by psychic perception from Dr. Rush, and psychic perception has its disadvantages. It is usually true that any "truth," whether an understanding or a technique, is time- and culture-bound. That is, it is the next step in the processes of its time. Dr. Rush may have been gifted with great insight, he may even have been ahead of his time, but he was necessarily out of joint with the times 150 years later. Not only was new information available, but the tissue quality, the life-styles, the expectations of the people had radically changed. A new therapy was in order.

IPR has a gift of understanding basic principles—new and ancient—and the unique capacity to take them a step farther, so that they evolve to a place of usefulness for her own day and age. She expresses annoyance with people who "never really take an idea apart so they can understand it." IPR is very good at going back to first principles and coming up with a solution to a problem. One of my favorite Ida Rolf stories has to do with the cure of a bad case of poison oak (the West Coast version of poison ivy). I was in the usual state of discomfort and complaining about it; Ida told me to got get a scrub brush and a cake of yellow soap. I was to scrub the soap lather into the rash, being sure to get down to the bottom of the rash. The principle is simple: the irritant in poison oak has an acid base; yellow soap has an alkaline base. The one will neutralize the other if only you have the courage to scrub the blisters open and get acid and alkaline in contact with each other. IPR never lacked courage.

She spent the next years working with people who had heard of her and who wanted to help. As she worked with them she began to see a pattern in her work and how the different principles of yoga, osteopathy, homeopathy, etc., were demonstrated in the changes she saw in her clients. But it wasn't until she started teaching that she felt the need to formulate her work into a technique with principles of her own.

In the meantime, Dr. Rolf continued to explore ideas that interested her. She worked for a short time with a Mrs. Lee, who taught the Alexander technique in Massachusetts. She was also much interested in Korzybski's work, and through this interest she met Sam Fulkerson.

Sam Fulkerson was one of the early angels of Rolfing. he was a great devotee of General Semantics, and was a much older person in that organization than I was—he'd known Korzybski himself, and was devoted to this teaching. I had read *Science and Sanity;* for me it was the first time anybody had applied engineering principles to language. I was very interested, so in about the early fifties, in the middle of winter, I went to a seminar in the foothills of the Berkshires. In that class, I met Sam. He had had a motor accident a couple of years earlier in which he'd broken every rib and knocked out all his teeth, so he was interested in having some Rolfing. He was great big jovial guy. One time, some years after, he said to me, "Ida, you know why there are two pockets in a man's shirt?" And I said no. "Why," he said, "so he can put the top dentures in one pocket and the bottom dentures in the other."

Sam was a smart guy, and he knew that the way to get Rolfing along was to teach it. He was going to see to it that he did his little stint in getting it taught. He was the first man that literally pushed me into teaching. Those early classes weren't the equivalent of the present-day courses. Students were drawn from chiropractors and osteopaths; the classes were set up by leaders in those fields and lasted perhaps a week. And all this was fathered, shall I say, rather than sponsored, by Sam Fulkerson. He started the classes himself, renting quarters in a hotel in Cedar Rapids. He was a distributor in the United States for Professional Foods, and he invited all of the most successful, prominent professionals (chiropractors and osteopaths), who were his customers. He invited them to either the first week or the second week of the course—there must have been one hundred between the two classes.

Another of my favorite stories about Sam happened right in the middle of this first class, during a demonstration. All of a sudden I wanted the plural for pelvis. It had never occurred to me before that I might someday need a plural for pelvis. I didn't know what it was, and I asked a half a dozen of those osteopaths, and they didn't know. So I said, "Hey, Sam, what's the plural for pelvis?" And he stood there and he scratched his head, and he said, "Ah . . . fannies." Until his recent death, he lived in Los Angeles.

In the years that followed, I was teaching all over the country, from Chicago down into Texas and over to Los Angeles. That was what really started Rolfing.

Those chiropractors and osteopaths took the work and they used it as an adjunct to their work, and this I did not particularly like. They wanted to adopt it into chiropractic and osteopathy, and I said no. Rolfing's not chiropractic; it's not osteopathy. I've been saying no to that ever since. But on the other hand, when you start, you start with a couple of broken sticks if that's all you can find. People today don't understand that. When you start from zero, you start from zero, and by God you work. You put your back in it, and your sweat in it, and your head in it, and you don't give any attention to anything else.

Not only did the osteopaths and chiropractors try to include Rolfing as part of their own technique, but even when Dr. Rolf taught what she then called Structural Integration as a separate technique, people tried to take bits and pieces of her work, not understanding that it was an organic whole.

A group of chiropractors in Toronto invited me to come up for a short course, in the role of a graduate teacher. I don't think the course ever came to pass, but at any rate, one incident from that time still raises my—sometimes intolerance and sometimes amusement. I gave a lecture and a demonstration in the auditorium of their school. Needles to say, the demonstration was up on a platform at the front of the auditorium; there were several hundred students in the audience. I did this about six weeks before the course was supposed to be given, as an introduction to the students. When I finally got to Canada six weeks later, I was walking down Bloor street and somebody came up to me from behind and said, "Dr. Rolf, I just wanted to tell you, your system's no good." I said, "Oh really, tell me about it." And he said, "Well, I went home and I tried it on my mother-in-law. She has a heart condition and it didn't do her any good." Frankly, if anybody else told me this story, I wouldn't believe it, but it happened to me.

The whole question of teaching was a thorny one. On the one hand, Fulkerson was right—if Rolfing was to live beyond IPR's lifetime, she would have to teach. But all her early attempts at teaching were unsatisfactory. When she taught osteopaths and chiropractors, they were liable to see her work as a technique rather than a point of view. This kind of cooption was not only an affront to Dr. Rolf's originality, it was also a total misunderstanding of her intention. IPR was not interested in curing symptoms; she was after bigger game. She wanted nothing less than to create new, better human beings. The ills would cure themselves; the symptoms would melt as the organisms became balanced. Curing symptoms let you in for an endless chase around the body. For example, if a man complains of trouble in his shoulder, it's possible to "fix" the shoulder by direct manipulation of the soft tissue locally. Within a week, the man will be back, complaining of trouble in his neck. If you get the trouble out of his neck, he'll be back to tell you about his arm, and then his upper back, and so on.

IPR found in gravity an idiom that could encompass her aims. She shaped her ideas into an article to be published in John Bennett's new journal, *Systematics*. Its title was "Gravity: An Unexplored Factor in a More Human Use of Human Beings."[6] In this article, she pointed to the fact that human bodies exist in gravity; it is the omnipresent, all-powerful, unremitting determinant of their uprightness or lack of it. Humans are no different in their existence in gravity from any other material body. All are subject to the laws of mechanics; one of these laws states that masses must be balanced in order to be stable. Man consists, more or less, of stackable units. The agents of this balance are the bones and soft tissue (myofascia). Bones determine position in space, but bones are held by soft tissue. When the myofascia is repositioned, bones spontaneously reorient. When the tone of the soft tissue is balanced, there is a sensation of lightness in the body. The masses of head, thorax, pelvis, etc., are no longer dragged out of true by their weight; the structure presents less resistance, and gravity can "flow through."

At about the same time she was concentrating her ideas, IPR changed the format of her teaching. What she needed was a sequence of treatment that would apply equally to all bodies. The logic of the body and her own understanding of balance gave her what she needed: she would work to create balances, starting on the surface of the body and gradually working deeper. She established the ten-hour sequence of Rolfing during that time; it has remained fundamentally the same since. IPR first taught her new format in the early 1950s, at a class in Tunbridge Wells, England. Now she met with a new kind of difficulty:

> It was very great disappointment. I was subjected to all kinds of attempts at stealing the work, and so forth. I had asked students from the class to act as assistants later, because there was so much work. When I left England, one of them got together with the woman who had been my secretary, and they got the names and addresses of my clients and tried to build a practice for themselves.

It is never easy to maintain integrity of a new body of work, particularly when it is a manipulative technique. People are so prone to say it's "just like" something else. We all resist the idea that something is new or radical. Then again, it is easier to copy the outer form of a technique than to give thought and understanding to the underlying ideas. It is much easier just to give anyone who walks in the door a couple of stretches here and a push there. It is harder to envision how each individual idiosyncratically pulls and twists away from uprightness, and more demanding still to understand how to unravel the mesh of rigidities and tensions that maintain his shape. But nothing short of this kind of informed seeing was IPR's goal as she taught. She wanted at all costs to avoid the kind of mechanicalness that characterizes, for example, so much of chiropractic work today. Again and again she emphasized in her classes that the early teachers of chiropractic had been brilliant in their field, but the pressures of time and money, dilution of teaching talent, all had eroded their work. She wanted none of this. IPR did her best to protect her brainchild, asking students to sign agreements not to teach until they had practiced for five years. Later, the teaching function came to be administered by the Rolf Institute.

By the time the fifties were over and Dr. Rolf had been teaching and working with people all over the United States, Canada, and England, the form of Rolfing was well-established, and Rolfing was a clear, teachable body of work and a proven therapeutic method, although her students were scattered far afield. It was her good fortune then to meet Fritz Perls and, through him, to come to Esalen. Fulkerson had been her "impresario" through the fifties. Esalen opened up new opportunities.

> There wasn't anything that didn't lead back to Fulkerson, one way or the other, except Fritz Perls and Esalen. How I got together with Fritz was a story. Dorothy Nolte—this was about 1965—went to a lecture Fritz gave on a Gestalt therapy. She saw Fritz in such obvious misery during the talk that when it was over she went up to him and said, "Fritz, if you will come upstairs with me, I think I can make you feel a little better." Fritz had a history of heart trouble, and at that point he was feeling so bad that he didn't argue with her. They went upstairs, she gave him a first hour of Rolfing, and Fritz felt very much better.

Then, typically, Fritz went riding around the country in airplane seats—from California to New York to Florida and back. By the time he got back, he was feeling miserable again. So, once more, he looked up Dorothy and asked her if she would do something for him. But she wouldn't, saying she didn't have the experience to take on a case as serious as his and suggesting that he ask me to come to California. He did ask me, and I thought to myself, Well, what have I got to lose if I go out to Big Sur now, in the month of May, when everything is lovely and sunny and rosy? I decided I had nothing to lose.

I got there Friday afternoon, and Fritz wasn't there, he was down in Carmel, gone to a dentist or something. Finally he came home, and I laid him down, and set to work on him. I worked Friday and Saturday—we worked till the following Friday, every day. I sat in his classes in the meanwhile, and everybody was mad at me because they didn't know why I was there—they thought it a damn shame that here was this woman sitting in his class and she wasn't part of his class, and she wasn't partaking in the class, and who the hell was she anyway?

On that following Friday I gave him the seventh hour, and in the middle of the hour Fritz goes stark unconscious. I had a *very* bad two minutes, and I said to myself, "You bloody fool, taking a man who is dying of a heart failure, putting him through Rolfing, you deserve what you've got. See, the man's dead." And then I looked at him and I said, "Confound it, he's not dead. This is the picture of a man under anesthetic, not a dying heart failure." And so I said, "Well, I'll just wait and see what happens next, and pray to God he doesn't know where he's been."

But God was out to lunch. When Fritz came around, the first thing he said was something that indicated he knew perfectly well that he'd been unconscious. He said that he had once been injured by an anesthetist in surgery. When he had got out of anesthetic he had accused the anesthetist of having injured him; the anesthetist said it was impossible. So you see, when I got into his neck, I began to raise that whole trip. After that he had some minor things which disappeared after a couple of month but he never had another bad heart attack. So I came home, and I went back to Big Sur Christmas of that year to work with him again, and by this time his heart man was saying, "There's nothing wrong with your heart, I can't find anything wrong." He never was accused again after that of being a heart victim. Never.

I tried to get Fritz to commit himself to giving a class together with me. Fritz wouldn't commit himself, but I came out to Big Sur anyway. Never, in the early years that I was in Big Sur, did anybody ever approach me and ask me whether I'd go out there and whether I'd work and would I work under such and such conditions, and so forth. Never. I just picked myself up and I went out there and I paid for accommodations and I put up my shingle and it happened. Fritz, of course, would see this that, and the other one that was really in need, and he'd say, "You know, if you'd go to Ida Rolf, she'd give you some help." And they'd show up down there in the baths, and they'd get something

[Query: You like Fritz's work? You wanted to teach with him?] Well, that doesn't express it particularly. I like having psychological work with these people at the same time that they were having physical work. I had used that method over in England with some psychologists.

So each summer in the mid-sixties, Dr. Rolf would go to Esalen and "hang out her shingle." And the hedonists of Esalen would head for the baths to work with her, wondering a little what they were letting themselves in for. Stories would come up the hill about the receptionist whose back "went out' so that she hadn't been able to straighten up one morning. Ida straightened her out. At first, it was called Structural Integration. Then it was called "getting Rolfed over." Gradually affection took over, and it was called Rolfing.

Esalen in the sixties was a laboratory of new idea, new techniques and often explosive experiments in human change. Physically, Esalen is a collection of buildings located just off Highway 1 in Big Sur, about two-thirds of the way between San Francisco and Los Angeles on the Pacific Coast. Its great treasure is two hot springs, once sacred to the Esalen Indians. These now feed into a bathhouse that looks like a

World War II bunker on a cliff, and has one of the most beautiful views of the Pacific in the world. In the late fifties, three young men one of whom owned the land, decided they would like to attempt something similar to an ashram in the United States. They had at first wanted to use it as a place to learn Eastern techniques, but discovered they had opened Pandora's box on new psycho-active techniques in this country. Within a few years, they were hosting workshops for Abraham Maslow, Rollo May, Will Schutz and many others.

Fritz Perls, father of Gestalt therapy as we know it today, came to Esalen through a Los Angeles psychotherapist, Jim Simkin. Fritz started by giving the usual weekend or five-day workshops, but soon went on to what he called his "circuses." These were weekends when anyone could come; often as many as eighty people would watch him work. He would take all comers, provided they had a dream to work with. In the mid-sixties, a weekend at Esalen might include seeing Fritz working the Lodge, having a massage down near the ocean, learning yoga near the pool, and having a Rolfing session with IPR. It was heady stuff.

Esalen brought IPR a different kind of student, frequently out of sympathy with mainstream cultural values. Some had been successful—a heart specialist turned Esalen dishwasher, a former space engineer; some were pioneers in the field of humanistic psychology; some had refused to find a place in the "system," becoming instead craftsmen, poets, and wanderers. It wasn't always easy to educate this heterogeneous mix, and to make sure they were adequately prepared for Rolfing training in terms of educational, psychological, and physical qualifications. IPR had no time to teach anatomy and physiology, or to qualify her students to deal with emotional and other issues that might come up in a Rolfing session. She had to depend on outside institutions to supply what students didn't already have. It seemed ideal to ask that applicants attend medical or premedical classes, but we soon found out that these focus primarily on pathology, not on the functioning of the healthy body. (One of the most useful general anatomy classes we unearthed was given in an undertaking school in Florida.) The new group processes practiced at Esalen, particularly Gestalt therapy, were excellent training for the necessary emotional insight.

I trained as a Rolfer in 1968, acting as class secretary as well. After that class, I stayed on to work with Dr. Rolf. The first order of business was her book about Rolfing. She had started it the year before, completing three chapters, and was of two minds about whether she would continue. Was it worth the trouble? Would she be able to get her ideas across in writing, or were they better demonstrated through teaching? And, above all, was the right time? She had no consecutive time to devote to writing—she was traveling, teaching, Rolfing, and writing short pieces for journals. "Is the book worth it" became an annual question over the next few years. We gave it one last chance, and as we read it we liked it. It wasn't so bad after all.

Dr. Rolf was trying, in this book, to get across her vision of a balanced body. Clearly, this would entail visual as well as verbal presentation. What was needed was an artist who understood Rolfing. We worked our way through four artists before we were rescued by John Lodge, artist, bon vivant, Rolfing student, and man of infinite patience. He'd work all night long showing how a set of ribs articulated with the vertebral column, only to have IPR say the one in the middle couldn't be at that angle. So he'd correct it, working all night again to make a new drawing, and the next morning he'd find out that the vertebra needed to be moved. The difficulty seemed to be that IPR could move the flesh, so she felt it only reasonable to ask that John move the bone. For John, it meant re-creating the whole drawing each time—flesh is more amenable to movement. On and (mostly) off, the writing the book took the better part of five years; the illustrations took three, and getting it published took another five years. Finally, on IPR's birthday in 1977, she was presented with the first two copies of *Rolfing: The Integration of Human Structures*, hand sewn and hot from the bindery. It looked beautiful to us.

By 1973, the Rolf Institute had come into being and was carrying on its considerable volume of work from an office in Boulder, Colorado. The Institute developed out of the Guild for Structural Integration, which in turn came out of the need for Rolfers to have a center of communication. Earlier, in 1970, the Rolfing office tended to get carted from one class location to the next in the back of a station wagon. In fact, on one occasion a truck sideswiped the station wagon, and the contents of the Rolfing office were strewn over the Berkeley exit of Highway 101, with California Highway Patrol motorcycles (four abreast) slowing traffic so we could retrieve what the wind hadn't taken. It was a windy highway.

The summer of 1970 saw the first meeting of Rolfers, then about forty, at Esalen. We decided to model ourselves on a crafts guild, incorporate as a nonprofit educational institution, and find ways to further Rolfing by supporting Dr. Rolf. There was a pressing need to free her in terms of both money and time, so that she could give her energies to writing and lecturing. Each subsequent annual meeting expressed the same goal, and little by little it was accomplished. Teachers were selected to lighten her teaching load and free her to "bring along" advanced students. A more stable business location and staff took over administrative functions. Eventually, in 1976, the number of Rolfers (180) was sufficiently large to give her substantial financial support out of dues.

What does it mean to say that Rolfing "works"? It's not enough to say that getting Rolfed changes people. In their different measure, so do massage, bio-energetics, clean living, education, vacations, chiropractic, and a new life-style. Nor is it accurate to focus on the emotional release that comes through Rolfing; emotional expressiveness and explosion are more probably a by-product of the process. The main event lies with the individual's use of energy, both his own and the environment's. Human energy is evanescent and invisible; it is difficult to define or measure. Definitions need to be cautiously made. In an introduction to Rolfing written for the *Psychotherapy Handbook*, IPR is succinct and cagey:

> Rolfing is not primarily a psychotherapeutic approach to the problems of humans, but the effect it has had on the human psyche has been so noteworthy that many people insist on so regarding it. Rolfing is an approach to the personality through the myofascial collagen components of the physical body. It integrates and balances the so-called "other bodies" of man, metaphysically described as astral and etheric, now more modernly designated as the psychological, emotional, mental, and spiritual aspects. The amazing

psychological changes that appeared in Rolfed individuals were completely unexpected. They inevitably suggest that behavior on any level reflects directly the physical energy level of the initiating physical structure. The psychological effect is far greater than one would expect to induce in the brief encounter of ten hours of work, which is the normal cycle for Rolfing integration. This effect can be understood if we see it as the emergence of a different behavior pattern resulting from the very much greater competence of physical myofascial organization. Rolfing postulates on the basis of observation that a human is basically an energy field operating in the greater energy of earth; particularly significant is that energy known as the gravitational field. As such, the individual's smaller field can be enhanced or depleted in accordance with the spatial relations of the two fields. It would seem appropriate, at this point in time, to state that following Rolfing a man's greater awareness suggests to him that his energy has been increased. In fact, Rolfing has simply freed his energy, made it more available. His greater structural competence makes it possible to utilize his energy more efficiently.

Dr. Rolf's formal training come to the fore in her writing. The more immediate response, the intuitive flash, the density of her experience are the stuff of the classroom and conversation. She has said, "I don't know *why* it works, I only know *that* it works." In much more explicit and less formal terms, this expresses an important element of what she was saying about Rolfing in the paragraph above. The original impulse for writing the present book was to capture this more elemental talk about IPR's experiences and reflections.

Notes

1. Rolf Institute, Box 1868, Boulder, Colorado 80306.

2. Dr. Rolf, as she likes to be called professionally, didn't think much of the Esalen habit of being on a first-name basis with anyone and everyone. She'd was irritable over the total stranger who would call on the phone and begin with a breezy "Hello, Ida."

3. For a description of Rolfing, see page 212.

4. Dr. Rolf called her system Structural Integration, a name which is

descriptive of the process; Rolfing was a nickname, first coined at Esalen, that has now become the official service mark.

5. This and the following quotations are taken from an interview with Ida Rolf, in July 1976, published in part in the *Bulletin of Structural Integration*.

6. *Systemtics,* Volume 1, Number 1, June 1963.

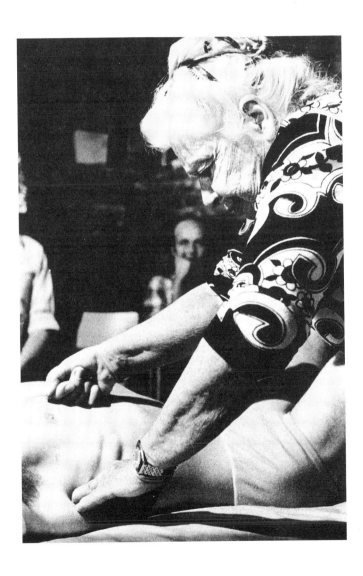

Ida Rolf Talks about Rolfing
and Physical Reality (Excerpts)
Ida Rolf

THIS IS THE gospel of Rolfing: When the body gets working appropriately, the force of gravity can flow through. Then, spontaneously,
the body heals itself.

~•~

Functional disorganization of the body comes as a result of exposure
to the continuous force of gravity. Anybody who builds a house knows
that unless he's building in terms of verticals and horizontals, he's
going to have to understand all about how to reinforce that house
against gravity. If some force lets that house down on one side, he's
going to have to jack it up pretty quickly or he's going to have disorganization throughout the house. The doors and windows won't fit
and cold will come in under the doors, and all that.

We understand about houses. We are used to that idea and we use
it. Even the less informed of us understand enough to look at a door
and see the light under it and say, "You know that wasn't that way
last year, I wonder what has happened." Even the least informed of
us say to a builder, if we value our home, "Do something about this."
If your builder is stupid, he changes the doors. If your builder is smart,
he changes the house. he levels the house, he jacks up something under
the foundation, he puts a new post under a corner. He tries to get the
post to stand on rock because he knows it can't stand solidly on mud.

In your organic house, your body, the same rules apply. The reason they apply is that your organic house, while it may house a spirit
or even be a spirit, is still an aggregate of three-dimensional material
particles in space. Whatever else it is, it is that. As an aggregate of
material particles, it must obey the laws of material particles. A nat-

ural law is a description of how something works under circumstances normal to it.

~ • ~

Nobody can prove what I am about to say, but I think it is so: every energy in which we live is nourishment to us. It is something which is literally contributing food to the individual. If you are living in a field of light, your eyes probably are good; as you deprive yourself of light consistently, the eyes starve and eventually you can't see. If you are living within a field of sound, the same is true of your ears. Now it would be absolutely ridiculous if we lived in a field of gravity and it had no effect on us, yet down through the ages this has been our assumption, that it didn't make any difference. This assumption is still held among a lot of people. They think it doesn't make any difference how you carry yourself because you are a spirit, an immortal and superior something, and it's the superior something which is in charge of the situation. Well, a spirit is in charge of the situation, but not in the way many think. The spirit is in charge to tell the individual that he can so organize his body that he is now in line with a supporting force. He cannot just go on indefinitely striking out indiscriminately against this force that's tearing him down, yet this is what he tries to do. You know average posture: the head way forward, the back way back, the chest almost lacking, the ribs down, no air coming in, etc. His spirit will carry him through? It is an assumption that no longer works; it is the relic of an idea which was universal a hundred years ago.

~ • ~

Old religions used to teach you to sit or kneel and always rock, gently but definitely rock. When you rock, you swing from prevertebral to postvertebral muscles. You'd see the same thing with sailors in the more active days of the war. You'd go down the street and you'd see a man in uniform, but you'd know without checking the uniform whether that man was a seaman or a landman. The landman went down the street boomp boomp boomp; the seaman went down rolling—from the prevertebral to the postvertebral, the prevertebral to the postvertebral. He may not have had a what we would call a really balanced gait, but he did use that alternation which kept the whole body at its peak. And they do this in many religious rituals. So much of ritual, if you look at it in the light of what you know of physiology, can be seen as a form of preventative medicine.

~ • ~

I'm dealing with problems in the body where there is never just one cause. I'd like you to have more reality on the circular processes that do not *act* in the body but that *are* the body. The body process is not linear, it is circular; always it is circular. One thing goes awry, and its effects go on and on and on. A body is a web, connecting everything with everything else.

~ • ~

The Hindu culture discovered many thousands of years ago that if you got a relatively good body, you had a reasonable, mild man. So the way a reasonably good body behaved became for them a the touchstone for morality. When morals are built from the body's behavior, you get a moral structure and behavior which respect the rights and privileges of other individuals. This is a very interesting concept; it has surfaced every once in a while down through the thousands of years that man has been on earth. It went completely out during the more rigid Christian era, when the church began to dictate morals from above rather than morals from within. In doing so, a rigidity came into the concept of morals which people are now rebelling against and have been for the last seventy-five years.

~ • ~

Years ago, I used to have a nice metaphor for how a body is made. I used to say that God felt we didn't have good enough sense to keep our segments together, so He put them into an elastic shopping bag. And then I tell the story of how I went to Macy's. (Those of you who are from New York will get the point of the story.) First of all, I went to get a sweater. But, having bought the sweater and carrying it in a long sweater box, I remembered that I was going to take guests to church on Sunday, and therefore I needed a hat, and now I've got a round box to go with a long box. Well, that was fine. Then I started to catch the Long Island train. To do so I had to cross Seventh Avenue. But to do so I also had to go down through the bakery section and the meat section of Macy's, and as I did this I again remembered I had a whole group of guests coming on Sunday and I needed food for them. So I stopped at the meat shop and I got a shoulder of lamb and a ham, and I had them wrapped.

While they were wrapping those, I lost my heart to some cake at the bakery, and bought a cake. You know what kind of boxes cake comes in; they're very squashable. So they dumped all this stuff at my feet so to speak. I looked at it with despair and I said to the girl at the wrapping desk, "Could you please get it all together?"

I picked it up and gave it to the girl and she got it all together by sliding some cord around it all, and she sent me out. I knew before she sent me out what was going to happen. I got right into the middle of Seventh Avenue between Macy's and the Long Island station, and when the light changed, so did the package.

Now you see this isn't such a funny analogy. You have similar shapes within that shopping bag that the good Lord put around your body to keep things from happening at the corner of 34th and Seventh Avenue. All of these pieces, which are such diverse shapes, are wrapped. Roughly, they're all held together by this elastic shopping bag of the superficial fascia. There is another point to this analogy which is also of interest. That superfascial fascia shopping bag of yours is going to show just where the points of strain are. As those shapes start slipping in the bag it's going to show increased strain here or there, and so it's going to give you clues as to what's going on inside. Now, you see, if that doggone girl, instead of just putting a cord around my packages, has followed the example of Lord and put an elastic shopping bag around, all would have been well.

As I said, I used to use this image ten years ago, but now I'm getting away from it. Nowadays, I insist on thinking in terms of gravity, and my image of a shopping bag has been transformed into a picture of the body as an energy pattern, a structure which lengthens as it gets better tone.

~ ● ~

If you've got to live in a stable world, you'd better quit Rolfing. Your stability lies in appropriate relationships, and that is all.

~ ● ~

Rolfers make a life study of relating bodies and their fields to the earth and its gravity field, and we so organize the body that the gravity field can reinforce the body's energy field. This is our primary concept.

~ ● ~

The message of Gurdjieff, and of Ouspensky who followed him, was that it didn't matter *what* you did as much as *how* you did it. When you come right down to it, this is the message of all teaching of skills in which form is important. That is what form is, whether it be form in performance of any kind: dancing, tennis, or any discipline in which you use your body. Evaluation of form consists in giving points for how the thing is done. We are by far not the first people that understood this. I'm sure the Greeks had a word for it.

Many years ago, in a Sunday supplement, I saw a picture of the Olympic races. Among the first three or four contestants in this picture, the thing that was so outstanding was that the man who won was operating in form and all of the others were operating out of desperation that they had to get there. The front runner was perfectly quiet and easy and could have carried on a conversation all the time he was running. This is form.

~ ● ~

I wish I could be sure I have reached the imagination of every one of you with my conviction that progress will occur in our understanding of this world only to the extent that we can establish something that conforms to the pattern of the real material world. I get so upset when I listen to all the verbal spouting and spouting that goes on all around me. I feel that you are making no progress in understanding your world (or the other guy's) until you stop just passing air in and out of your mouths and start doing something that's tangible and material.

~ • ~

What we want is to go back to an experience and then work out from the event to the first thing that can be inferred—then to the second thing that can be inferred from the first thing, and so on. These are the different levels of abstraction. College courses and business practices tend to jump. They hardly take off their hats and they've jumped to a higher order of abstraction and they say it is reality. But every human being gets experience only as stimuli impinge on nerves—touch impinges on an arm and you feel; sound impinges on an ear and you hear. There are five senses and there are five ways of getting experience into you. Rolfers need to be able to focus on the level that impinges on senses. The sense of taste doesn't really enter into it; the sense of smell sometimes enters into it, but not often. What can be seen is the most important clue; describe what is visible. Typically, we like to think quickly, to think and to infer, to get on with it. But there is too wide a gap between experience and inference. Mistakes get made.

~ • ~

You almost cannot teach Rolfing because you are everlastingly dealing with something that is as uncertain as a water bed. This is the problem, to get secure in an art in which there is no security. Your security comes only from relationships. If any of you think that you're really smart enough to get up and teach Structural Integration as a secure, lecture kind of class, go to it. All kidding aside, if I can get you to a place where you recognize the security of insecurity, you will have made that first step forward. So many people talk as though they really know what Rolfing is all about. But when you turn them loose to work with it, it's a different story. These problems are basically problems of our educational system. Nowhere in our educational system that I know of at the moment (perhaps in some very esoteric order) are there places where they teach you to live on practices which are completely insecure. Part of the goal of present-day education is to get secure ground on which to stand. A Rolfer's only secure ground in a body is to establish a balanced relationship. That is your secure ground, and it is not possible to convert it into something that is solid like a wall.

As Rolfers, the more information about a body you can get quickly through your eyes, the better. As you begin to work with a body, you not only think you're in a morass, you are in a morass. Now how do you deal with a morass? You put on a good wide snowshoe and move. So one of the things I'm trying to tell you is that there is only yourself and what you can learn to see and feel that will give you a certain security. I want to give you the feeling that it's all right to be insecure.

~ ● ~

Fascia is the organ of posture. Nobody ever says this; all the talk is about muscles. Yet this is a very important concept, and because this is so important, we as Rolfers must understand both the anatomy and physiology, but especially the anatomy of fascia. The body is a web of fascia. A spiderweb is in a plane; this web is in a sphere. We can trace the lines of that web to get an understanding of how what we see in a body works. For example, why, when we work with the superficial fascia, does this change the tone of the fascia as a whole?

~ ● ~

This business of living in extrinsics is characteristic of the very young; it is characteristic of the immature. I do not know, it maybe that as long as you preeminently use the extrinsic muscles you are immature. Perhaps maturity occurs as you beg to get intrinsics into the picture and bring both to a balance. That is what it looks like, as you work on kids. Possibly, when this whole thing is threaded out, what you will see is the that there are two different nervous innervations, one for intrinsics (autonomic), one for extrinsics. And it is only as you evoke the activity of both that you get behavior that we call normal (I don't mean average).

~ ● ~

Part of a Rolfer's strategy consists in recognizing that the plasticity of the body has to do with the chemistry of that system of the body which creates and maintains structure—the myofascial system. Realize that this system derives from the mesoderm. Only this system do we manipulate directly, but by virtue of this system we can change the functioning of the entire body. We can change the verticality of the body. So that in this chemical elasticity of the myofascia you have a tool to effect lasting change. In addition, you have the segmentation of the body, which makes the tool usable. Why in heaven's name somebody down through these thousands of years didn't see this long before and use it, I'll never know.

~ • ~

Rolfers are not basically dealing with pathology. A great deal that is labeled pathology is not pathology—it is a perversion of physiology. Organize the structure so the physiology can work without perversion, and it will work that way. If you've got true pathology, it takes a while to change it, but if you've simply got a perverted use of physiological function, you can change it very quickly by changing the structure. At least, that's where I stand—that's where my experience places me.

~ • ~

A friend of mine had a daughter who was twelve or thirteen years old; she had what was basically an emotional problem. He sent that girl from Israel to London to be treated by me because he figured that Rolfing would get the problem out without making conscious the sexual information and emotions concerned. Now he was a smart man. It's easier and faster to change if you get away from the realm of images, into that of material particles, and create new images by creating differently related material particles. It's a very important notion. What I'm trying to do is to create a group who can work back and forth from ideas to substance and understand why and how this is done.

~ • ~

A self exists in a real material body. In order to create a self-image, you have had to put material particles together in a particular way. An image is something which is expressing itself in three-dimensional material. This is a very basic concept, for this is the reality which is restructured in order to change the image. The image is the result. The image may have been the cause from which you started, but at this point the image is the result.

~ • ~

When you're working on the feet, you're not working only on the feet, you're working on the shins as well as the feet. Never divorce in your mind one part from another part. The other end of the ankle is the knee, and so on up.

~ • ~

Rolfing can be like making your bed in the morning. You think you're going to get by without pulling that bed apart, so you pull up this cover and the next cover. When you get all the covers pulled up, you've got nine ridges running across the bed. Now you've got to pull the top covers back again, and you've got to go to a deeper layer and organize the deeper layer, and make your bed on top of that. Then you've got a made bed. Well it's the same with a body: you've got to organize those deeper layers.

~ • ~

I want you to see *structural* organization rather than *physiological* organization. Don't go astray looking for a gleam in an eye. There are so many things that can put a gleam into a young person's eyes (the older ones have more trouble with it). But observe the differences that you see, for example, if you cut off each individual just below the shoulders. Look at the person in terms of his shoulders, the way his neck sits, and the way his cranium sits on his neck. Structure gives you a criterion by which to evaluate people.

~ • ~

I used to say that Rolfers took the safety pins out of the fascia. It's as though you have an overcoat with a safety pin holding the lining. Someone has pinned the lining to your coat, and it doesn't fit anymore. So we are trying to take some of those safety pins of restriction out of the fascial envelope. There are even places where those safety pins went through four times instead of one.

~ ● ~

It's the fascia that crosses joints, not the muscles. Fascial envelopes cross joints. Joints become the red flags; they tell you if and how something is wrong. You have to look for relationship, not only of joints, but within all of the mesodermal tissue. (Fascia and bone both come from mesoderm; fascia is less dense.) This will give you a more inclusive picture of what goes on in a body than if you look only at the muscles.

~ ● ~

There are many ways of doing any movement—nature has a great many alternatives. A child picks one of those alternatives. Nature provides so many options for security that when something goes wrong there is always something else available. A child with a very good body would have several options for any movement and maybe 25 percent of children have many options to begin with. They pick one option that works for them. Why should the change it? Presently it gets to be what is often called a "behavior pattern." I say it's simply a choice of that which is mechanically simplest for them at one period of their lives.

Bonnie Bainbridge Cohen

*B*onnie Bainbridge Cohen, formerly an occupational therapist and a
New York dancer with Erick Hawkins and the founders of Contact
Improvisation, created the School of Body-Mind Centering. Her method
consists of a uniquely sophisticated way of teaching people how to direct
their awareness into experiences of the most intricate recesses of the body:
the thymus gland, the cerebrospinous fluids, peristalsis, etc. The methods involve group work using verbal suggestions and demonstrations,
and hands-on individual work. The effects include remarkable healing of
trauma associated with very specific regions of the body, and dazzling
states of consciousness. Contact The School for Body-Mind Centering,
189 Pondview Drive, Amherst, MA 01002.

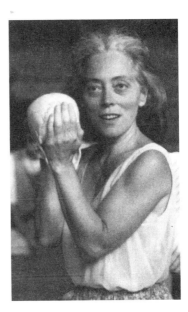

Sensing, Feeling, and Action:
The Experiential Anatomy of Body-Mind Centering (Excerpts)

Bonnie Bainbridge Cohen

The following interview by Nancy Stark Smith, a founder of Contact Improvisation and editor of *Contact Quarterly*, took place in Northampton, Mass., on November 26, 1980.[1]

Smith: You talk of "embodiment" often in your work. Could you say something about it?

Cohen: A good example is a newborn infant. Their hand goes across their face and at first there is only a momentary recognition of something going across their eyes. After a while, as they develop a little further, the hand will go across their eyes and they'll follow it, but there's not the recognition that it's their hand yet. One day, they follow it and they turn their head, and they move their hand back and they turn their head back and you see something in their eyes when they start really manipulating the hand. Another sense opens up that this hand is *me.* And then comes the play between the two hands, and the play of the hands and the eyes.

Embodiment is, in a way, separating out. It's feeling the force that is in this body. But in order to embody ourselves, we need to know what is *not* ourselves. It's a relationship. a child that *only* embodies its hand, for instance, might be considered autistic. If it's carried too far there's self-absorption; there's a certain awareness that this is me, but not an awareness that you're you. If it's just about what's me and what's *not* me, then I don't think it works; there's no counterbalance,

Edited by Nancy Stark Smith (Northhampton, MA: Contact Editions, 1993). 99–100, 114–118.

no definition. What I would call balanced embodiment would include, "this is the end of me; this is the beginning of something else."

Smith: What's the difference between the traditional way of learning/teaching anatomy and the process of embodying it?

Cohen: Generally, when anatomy is taught as I learned it, and as I see it taught elsewhere, you're given visual pictures of it. We have an image of it, but we don't have the kinesthesia of it within ourselves. Maybe we'll even say, "Oh, I have this bone or this muscle *in* me," but it's an intellectual concept, rather than the information coming through viscerally from the proprioceptors of that thing itself. The information is *always* coming in viscerally, but each person is selective in terms of what they choose to acknowledge. The studying that we're doing at the school [School for Body/Mind Centering] is highly selective in terms of receiving input; we go from one system to the other—now we're going into the senses, now we're going to *acknowledge the information* from the skeleton, now from the eye, now from the muscles, now from the organs, from the glands, the brain, the blood, etc. By acknowledging each one, we see that they are channels that can be acknowledged by choice. Once they've been acknowledged *consciously,* we can utilize that information without it remaining primary. One of the things that I think is essential with sensing, is that we reach a point where we become conscious and then we let it go, so that the sensing itself is not a motivation; that our motivation is action, *based on* perception. What often happens is that once we become aware of perception, we forget about the action. The perception becomes the key thing: what am I perceiving. Instead of *eating,* what becomes important is: how does it taste, what is the texture. Instead of just walking it's: how am I walking, what foot's going in front of the other, how are the bones falling. All of that is important, but there is a time to just simply walk, or simply eat for nourishment.

Smith: Then what is the value of embodying? If you can walk anyway, then why bother knowing how it feels in such detail, or getting so involved with it?

Cohen: If we didn't inhibit any natural functioning, there probably wouldn't be any need. In fact, you see that people who don't have a lot of problems, who are fairly well integrated don't spend their time on integrating: they spend their time in some action. Most of us in this work come into it because we have problems; we're inhibited in some way that prevents us from functioning the way we feel we should be able to. By becoming conscious of the processes, we eliminate our unconscious inhibitions, and can function normally. Once we have removed the obstacles and are functioning efficiently, there's no need to keep looking for obstacles. It's not that we're never going to need to be aware again, but there are moments when we can become wholly active, and not have to monitor our activity.

Smith: Another benefit of this kind of work would be that you could perceive and deal with subtle imbalances before they become major problems.

Cohen: Certainly it leads to awareness; it *is* awareness. But I also see that often we, in this work, concentrate so much on the juggling of systems, whatever we happen to be studying, that we end up being sick a lot of the time. I think it has to do with some part of us identifying with the system or the imbalance that we're studying. So in fact we go from one unbalanced state to another. Certainly we become more well or potentially well balancing all these different things, but what I'm exploring now is how we can come to some whole image, a whole state of mind that we would identify with. Then the exploration of each system would be a study, but we wouldn't attach our basic self with the study. Then I think we could become aware of the imbalances without becoming ill.

Smith: How do you see the "whole image" evolving?

Cohen: I see our work going into a transition in the next couple of years. It will go into another kind of approach that will have an overview based on what we've gained from having gone rather innocently into each system. The next stage will be more mind-based, rather than body-based. Both will be there, but just as the mind is in the body area now, the body will be in the mind area.

Smith: What do you mean by "mind-based"?

Cohen: Each individual goes into an area of study with a certain mind, and we usually keep the same mind throughout all of our explorations. What I'm doing now is trying to help people recognize the mind that they're approaching something with, as compared to [the mind of] the material itself. For example, some people might feel things more through the bones, another person more through the muscles, some say they're more into the senses. It's different if you sense something, if you feel it, than if you simply do it. Sensing is related to the nervous system through the perceptions. Feeling and flow are related to the fluid system including the circulatory, lymphatic and cerebralspinal fluids. By approaching everything with the same mind, you are constantly initiating activity from the same place. For example, I think that a lot of people in the Contact work are working with sensing—sensing where they are, feeling weights; they're using their perceptual systems to initiate from, in particular the weight perceptors and the movement perceptors. But there's a funny thing when you do that. The fluids are a counterbalance to the perceptions or the nervous system. So if the perceptual system is always initiating or being the mover, then the fluids are always having to be the support. There becomes a time when you want to reverse that balance, when you want the perceptions to go quiet, to become the support, and let the fluids become the mover. That's when you go into simply moving, without sensing anymore, trusting that the senses have gone unconscious and will support you without them being conscious. When I say forgetting them, I mean letting them go unconscious and letting the fluids become the control.

Take a very large group of people, have them move in a very small space and have them move "sensing." They'll slow up; when people sense, there's this slowing up of the fluids. Then have them drop that and move very quickly in a tight group with no sensing. What you'll find is that you're safer under fast movement with no sensing than you are under the slow sensing. However we've developed, we move best, more automatically, and more efficiently when we move quickly with fluidity—where the sensing goes unconscious and the fluids

188

take the initiative—than when we move slowly with sensing. It happens over and over again. People are surprised that they feel safer under this fast moving than when they are sensing where each person is. And they're less likely to bump into somebody and have an accident. Now if you take a group of people who have never sensed, and have them running quickly, they'd probably be bumping into each other all the time. They'd be running into each other because they don't know where they are.

Smith: So you're using the senses as a support for the fluids and if the senses have never been developed they can't be a very stable support?

Cohen: Then the fluids have never been a support for the senses. It's a balance. It's not to choose one over the other but to have this balance. We have a tendency to get one-sided.

Smith: You said something about "sensing, feeling, and doing." what's the difference between sensing and feeling? Where do we feel from?

Cohen: The fluids. If you're sensing, it's not such an emotional space. But if you're *feeling*, then you get the emotions. A lot of the sensing work is an escape from the emotions. It actually represses emotional integration if it's not balanced. Personally, having been so chaotically emotional at one point, like lava just flowing one way and then the other, not able to handle it, I found sensing was a *haven* from that. And a way to get insight. Through the senses we get insight. But then the emotions got cooled out, and that became an imbalance. Because of the work I'm in and the sensitivity of my systems, I can swing very far from one end to the other, it's not minor changes. So I got into a lot of fluid problems. Then had to go back into the fluids which was for me going back into the emotions. But with *insight* as a balance, as a supporting structure.

Smith: Are the senses able to function more easily as a support for the fluids in a familiar environment rather than in unpredictable surroundings?

Cohen: When you're in an unfamiliar surrounding, the first thing you do is switch to your senses; your perceptions come alive at a point where you don't know what the limits are. You retard the fluids in order to be on the alert. But if you're in an actual moment of danger, if you stop too long to perceive it, you'll be exterminated, you'll die. You simply must act and at that point the perceptions go unconscious. Hopefully you've gained enough perceptual ability as a support that you can survive.

Smith: It's a beautiful distinction you're making between the fluids being the flow, the action, and the brain and nervous system being the perceptions, the senses. Contact Improvisation is interesting in this respect because it seems that you're called upon to act as you're sensing.

Cohen: That's when it's the most beautiful. In terms of *watching* Contact, it gets long and tedious unless you have these moments where someone breaks out and that's when you find your good contacters. You see them break out of sensing, and they simply are acting. It's very exciting and I'm sure you get a rush from doing it. You only see it with people who feel secure, who've sensed enough to know they can let the senses go. Certainly, if you get me out there, in the beginning there's no way I'm just going to respond because I don't know how to respond. I'm going to go very slowly and I'm going to want to feel every little part of my body and where it is and then at some point I'll just go and roll with it. There's no holding back.

Smith: At that point you'd be flipping systems, from sensing to acting? from nervous system to fluids?

Cohen: Things are not seesaw-like, with one end here and one end there. What happens when you go into sensing is that you retard the breathing, respiration, because you're retarding the fluids. The importance of the blood is that it's carrying oxygen to all the cells and taking out the wastes. It's basically about oxygen, which is breathing. So here you have another system coming in, respiration, to be studying in relation to the blood. All of a sudden someone will take a deep breath and you know the fluids have been released. The fluids are the internal respiration as compared to external respiration, the air, which we normally think of as breathing. The external respiration is governed by the blood flowing internally.

Smith: Often in doing sensing work, gravity and relaxation work, at each level of relaxation a deep breath will come, a release of some sort. I've wondered what that was about.

Cohen: By sensing, we release the restriction, whether it's muscular or whatever, which releases the blood. The breath follows. When you feel that deep breath, something has been repatterned into the nervous system.

Smith: Do you feel that in working with one area. such as the eye, that you are also working directly with each of the other systems?

Cohen: I'm trying to do that with the vision class—sensing the skeletal and muscular system of the eye, the nervous system, etc. We do a lot of perceptual work, but what I've been trying to bring out is that vision is not this; that's not how the eye was developed. It was not developed to be perceived, it was developed to have an action. It was developed *to be* active. Perception, when it's working, is an action; it's not a perception, it's not a perceiving of itself. Those of us with visual problems, by sensing, become aware of, say, which muscles are pulling a certain way. That information becomes part of our repertoire. It can go into our unconscious. But when you go to look, don't *try* to move your muscles or your bones, but let the eye respond to the light that's being reflected. We even try to perceive *light;* how do you *perceive* light, how do you become receptive to that phenomenon? Once you become receptive to that phenomenon, let *go* of the reception as your mover or as your purpose and let that become the *support* for seeing.

Evolutionarily, the visual system was developed to *see*, not to be a perceptor of *how* it sees. And if everything was working well, there probably wouldn't be any need for such self-consciousness. However, we have been given problems, and the ability to perceive them, which offers us the opportunity to transform this self-consciousness into self-knowledge. But without action (outer-looking) to balance the inner self-looking, this transformation cannot take place.

Interview with Lisa Nelson and Nancy Stark Smith[2]

Smith: What makes you feel that the first year of life is crucial in the perceptual-motor development of the child?

Cohen: This is when the relation of the perceptual process (the way one sees) and the motor process (the way one moves or acts in the world) is established. This is the baseline for how you will be processing activity, either in receiving or expressing, throughout your life. The importance of working with babies during the first year is that I feel it helps set up a broader baseline, offering more choices in not only how to see events or problems, but how to act on them; it gives them the most multiplicity of direction.

Smith: Why is it important to have a treatment baseline?

Cohen: Well, for example, a lot of adults are limited in how many of the basic perceptual-motor patterns (including developmental movement patterns) they can do. Some are accessible to them and some aren't. Those that aren't accessible are not going to be used in their everyday life—for thinking or for action. Each of the patterns are potentials within us, but until we actually *do* them, they're not accessible to us. Therefore, choices of action and choices of how to see are going to be more limited than if all the patterns developed in their natural progression, at the time that the inner time clock is going off, when the baseline is being established.

Smith: What actually happens if some of the basic patterns aren't developed?

Cohen: In most people that I work with, in fact ultimately everyone, there are developmental underlies to any problem—whether it's social, psychological, or physical. And certainly you can see, for example in the way kids crawl, if they're going to have stress in their knees or back when they're older. When you look at adults, you see those same patterns and how they affect the low back syndrome or sacroiliac problems or knee, ankle, and neck problems. Or, another example might be with babies that aren't transferring their weight through the full foot, you might later get collapsed arches or ankles that are going to be vulnerable to sprains or breaking because they're not supporting their weight properly through them. You can see the things down the line that might become a problem for a baby in the future due to the way it's patterning itself right now. By working on these movement patterns with the baby as it's developing, you can help an infant on a continuum to have stronger, more balanced alignment, action and integration.

Smith: What do you mean by patterns?

Cohen: All natural phenomena fall into patterns. The nervous system is designed to function by patterns. The nervous system has the potential for innumerable patterns, but the patterns are not accessible to us until they are actually stimulated into existence, until we actually do them. Patterns will fall on a continuum between efficiency and inefficiency.

Smith: Could you give an example of a developmental pattern?

Cohen: You could look at the sequence of motor development that we go through from birth to standing and walking, and see four basic patterns—from spinal movement through homologous (both arms together or both legs) to homolateral (left arm and left leg together, right arm and right leg together) to contralateral (left arm and right leg together, right arm and left leg together). The infant lifts its head, it crawls, it sits, it creeps, it stands, it walks. Within each of these phases there are specific patterns, coordinations, that occur (or not). I would call these developmental patterns the neurological organization.

Smith: How are the developmental patterns stimulated?

Cohen: One way is that person just starts doing the movement pattern naturally as that inner time clock determines and the environment call forth or demands it. For example, you don't develop language unless you're talked to. How your parents handle you as an infant also patterns you. Or, later on, the person might be helped more consciously through bodywork or therapy to find access to certain patterns that did not develop during childhood.

Smith: Is it necessary for every infant/individual to go through all of the patterns? It seems that some babies skip a step, like they never creep or crawl but they do end up standing and walking.

Cohen: I think that all babies need to go through them all. They don't need them to survive, but they need them to be fully rounded, to develop this broader baseline that I was talking about.

Smith: If you skip one along the way, is it possible to go back and learn that pattern later?

Cohen: Yes. That's the big key—that you *can* go back as an adult and get the patterns, but it's more difficult.

Smith: What makes it more difficult as an adult?

Cohen: When you do it as an infant, it is unconscious. You don't know how you did or why, but you just have the accessibility, that pattern in the nervous system is opened up without thinking about it. As an adult, if you make the choice to do it, and you have the opportunity, and there's someone around who can guide you through the pattern, they you do with consciousness.

Smith: What is the effect of opening up new patterns for the adult?

Cohen: Well, if the body is the instrument through which the mind is expressed, then one can just play more kinds of melodies, or different kinds of verse, kinds of timbre. As an adult, one's compensatory patterns are also deeply woven into the emotional and thinking patterns, and need to be acknowledged and validated.

Smith: So the patterns can open up different ways of behaving, and thinking, ways of acting, feeling—all of that?

Cohen: Um hm. Whatever would give you quality of mind. We can only express it through the body. The more neurological pathways that are established in the body, and the more basic integration it has, the easier it is to express the multifacetedness, the wider and with more breadth and depth will be the possibilities for expression and understanding.

Sometimes when I'm working with an infant, assisting her through a movement pattern that she is having difficulty with, or missing altogether, a parent will say, "Well, I feel that the child should have the choice to do what they want; they know what's best for them." And that was my feeling too, until, through the years, I've observed, as the children get older, that, in fact, their choice was because of an inhibition in their system and not because they had the insight to know that this was best. The baby is not making the choice from some deep intuitive knowledge, it's making it because it doesn't have any other choice. And because of this inhibition, it is making a choice for a pattern that will give it a less efficient base upon which to grow. Although, if the infant doesn't establish the most efficient pathway of development, that pathway isn't closed—its potential remains for future development.

The Action in Perceiving [3]

Based on an interview with Nancy Stark Smith and Simone Forti, January, 1986. In this article I would like to look at the other side of our Spring/Summer '84 *CQ* article, "Perceiving in Action," to explore the dynamic activeness of perceiving.

Some of the concepts that I would like to share are that movement *is* a perception; that it is the first perception to develop and therefore the most important for survival; that as each experience sets a baseline for future experiences, movement helps to establish the process of how we perceive; and that how we perceive movement becomes an integral part of how we perceive through other senses.

First, we need to differentiate between sensing and perceiving. *Sensing* is the more mechanical aspect, involving the stimulation of the sensory receptors and the sensory nerves. *Perceiving* is about one's personal relationship to the incoming information. We all have sense organs which are similar, but our perceptions are totally unique. Perception is about how we relate to what we are sensing. Perception is about relationship to ourselves, others, the Earth and the universe. And it contains the interweaving of both sensory and motor components.

Traditionally people speak of the sensory-motor or perceptual motor process. In this approach, sensory and perceptual relate to the incoming information and motor relates to the outward relates to the outward movement response to the sensory stimuli.

In this traditional model, after the reception of the information (sensory aspect) there is the perceptual processing, which compares the new information with all previous experiences and interprets the stimuli. Then there is a motor-planning phase, in which one organizes a motor response, and then there is the actual movement response itself. Finally, there is the sensory feedback, which provides information about what happened during the response and then our interpretation and feeling about what took place, i.e., its relationship to us, from our viewpoint. This process is called the sensory-motor loop and its phases can be outlined as follows:

Sensory input – Perceptual interpretation – Motor planning – Motor response – Sensory feedback – Perceptual interpretation

In working with this model for over twenty years, I have found that there are two more phases which are essential for facilitating change by creating the possibility for more choices.

To understand these new phases requires an alternative approach to the traditional concept of perceptual-motor or sensory-motor process. This new approach recognizes that both the input and output aspects of the stimulus/response loop have both motor *and* perceptual activity. This approach also requires an expansion of the traditional list of "the 5 senses": touch, taste, smell, hearing and vision.

It is fascinating and, I must confess, frustrating to me that the sensations of movement and visceral activity have been excluded from this grouping of the major senses. As all sciences are reflections of the socio-politico-religious ideas of their time, it is appropriate that the historical repression of bodily sensation in Western Culture has been transmitted as a matter of scientific fact. Within this view, a phenomenon is usually considered to be "objective scientific fact" if it can be separated from all bodily sensations, i.e., it must be capable of being measured only auditorally and/or visually. If it is measured by bodily sensation, it is considered to be "subjective" and "not scientific."

The *experience* of movement is not considered to be a "scientific study."

In universities throughout this country, in movement science programs, such as Motor Learning and Exercise Physiology, the actual movement has to be separated from all bodily sensation in order to be studied or validated. Most of these programs do not even offer movement classes. Movement is studied via reading and video.

Movement is the First Perception

There are twelve pairs of cranial nerves which process three major types of information:

- special senses of the head—touch to the head, taste, smell, hearing, and vision
- movement of the whole body
- visceral activity

Of all these cranial nerves, the first pair to myelinate (develop a fatty insulating covering) are the Vestibular Nerves.

Nerves myelinate in order of their importance for survival. The Vestibular Nerves being to myelinate in utero by registering the movement of the fetus and its environment (mother). That the Vestibular Nerves myelinate first indicates that they perform the first essential function for survival—before the need for registering touch to the head, taste, smell, hearing and vision.

This indicates that we learn first through a perception of movement. Not only is movement a perception, but as the first perception of learning, it plays an important role in establishing the baseline for our concept or process of perceiving. This original process of perception then becomes incorporated into the development of the other perceptions.

The Vestibular System

The registering of movement is not only the responsibility of the Vestibular Nerves. It is sensed through special receptors located throughout the body. The whole movement or vestibular system is composed of the inner ear, vision, proprioceptive, kinesthetic, and touch receptors located throughout the body, and interoceptors in the organs. To each of these I would add the movement of each cell. More specifically:

- The **vestibular** mechanism located in the inner ear receives information from the proprioceptors, interoceptors and kinesthetic receptors throughout the body and from gravity, space and time.
- The **proprioceptors** and **kinesthetic** receptors in the bones, joints, ligaments, muscles and fascia, tell us where each part is in relation to the other parts, where each part is in space, and their quality of rest and activity.
- The **interoceptors** in the organs, glands, blood vessels and nerves tell us where the organs, glands, vessels and nerves are and their state of rest and activity.
- **Each cell** experiences its own life process—it breathes, ingests, digests, excretes, moves and receives feedback from itself and from all the other cells of the body.

The Inner Ear

The inner ear registers where we are in relationship to the earth via the magnetic attraction of the pull of gravity. In the inner ear there are little stones called otoliths and little hairs called cilia. The stones fall toward gravity and stimulate the cilia. This stimulation of the cilia by the otoliths tells us where our head is in relationship to the earth. Vision, the contact of our skin on the supporting surface, and gravity receptors throughout the body which register our mass, or our **weight,** also provide us with information about our interaction with the earth.

The inner ear also plays an important role in establishing basic postural tone throughout the body. Postural tone is the readiness of the muscles to respond. I feel that our basic postural tone is an indication of how we are relating to the earth via the pull of gravity. It is reflected in the quality of our movement. Low tone indicates that we are having difficulty meeting the force of the earth's pull; high tone indicates that we are over-reacting to the pull of gravity; an even, balanced tone indicates that we have a comfortable relationship or balance with the earth's force.

Helping us to establish our relationship to **space** is another function of the vestibular mechanism in the inner ear. It receives information, via the brain, from the other movement receptors (proprioceptors, interoceptors, and kinesthetic receptors) throughout the body telling us where we are in space and how we are moving through it.

Changes in **time** are also registered in the inner ear. The semi-circular canals register changes in velocity (acceleration and deceleration) as the head moves through space. Temporal changes are also registered by kinesthetic receptors throughout the body.

In utero, the baby perceives the movement of its mother as inseparable from itself. Both in and out of the uterus, we are registering the movement of the earth and the universe, but until we born from them or separated from them, we cannot perceive their movement separate from our own.

Preconceived Expectations and Pre-Motor Focusing[5]

Our perception of movement, i.e., our interpretation of movement, is dependent upon all of our previous experiences of movement, as it is for every other sense. We develop preconceived expectations based upon how we have perceived similar information in our past experiences. These expectations then precede new sensory input. Thus, we can add the first the additional phases to our sensory-motor loop:

Preconceived expectations – Sensory input – Perceptual interpretation – Motor-planning – Motor response – Sensory feedback – Perceptual interpretation

The second phase that I feel is essential in expanding our potential for choice is based upon our ability to direct or focus our sense organs. This is a motor act. It is the motor component of perception. It is demonstrated by a dog directing its ears toward incoming sound, by the way the hairs of our skin move to pick up sensation, and by the way we focus our eyes in order to see. It is the motor ability to choose which aspects of incoming stimuli we will absorb or attend to.

Another example would be if you're riding in a car with someone. If you are the driver, you have more of a need to see, so your pre-motor focus is more involved, than if you are the passenger. You're looking at the same information, but the driver is having more motivation, concentration, and sense of responsibility than the passenger.

In ourselves we can see this pre-motor focusing as motivation, desire, attention, and discriminating awareness. We can see the absence or repression of it in boredom, resistance, and difficulties in learning.

So, the sensory-motor loop then becomes:

Preconceived expectations – Pre-motor focusing – Sensory input – Perceptual interpretation – Motor-planning – Motor response – Sensory feedback – Perceptual interpretation

Why not call this pre-focusing phase, pre-sensory or sensory planning? Because it is a *motor* act. It is the *active* decision of what stimulation you will take in. However, this "active decision" is usually unconscious, based upon previous experience. For instance, there was a point in my life when I was so fatigued that I realized that I had lost all desire except to sleep and to survive in order to nurture my children into adulthood. I realized that in order to do this, I had no choice but to focus on what I needed, which was to sleep and sleep and sleep. Eventually as I continued to focus on rest, I recuperated and rejoiced as other desires began to emerge and exert their presence. I knew I was surviving.

An example of *conscious* pre-motor focusing is to first gaze around the room randomly. Do it. Now, pay special attention to the color red. Now yellow. Now blue. Green. Purple. Orange. And so forth. How did your perception of the room change as you consciously pre-motor focused?

The pre-motor phase differs from motor planning and motor response in that it directs the organization of the sensory input as far as *how you focus*. The later motor planning phase is how you will organize your response to what you have observed, and the motor response is what you actually do about it.

The Dialogue Between Movement and Touch

I would like to look at another fundamental relationship underlying the development of perception—the dialogue between movement and touch.

In utero, as the fetus moves, it receives immediate tactile feedback from itself and from its environment—its body parts rub against each other, against the wall of the uterus, and against the amniotic fluid. As the fetus moves, it pushes against its mother's organs, which in turn push back against the fetus. When its mother moves, there are changes in the fluid and organ pressures against the fetus's skin.

It is interesting to note that the Vestibular Nerves, which perceive and help organize movement throughout the body, are the first of the cranial nerves to myelinate. The second group of cranial nerves to myelinate are those involving the processing of sensory and motor control in and around the mouth, which is necessary for breathing, sucking, and swallowing—the first survival functions after birth.

It is equally interesting that of the spinal nerves, the motor nerves myelinate before the sensory nerves. When I first read that the motor nerves myelinated first, it didn't make sense to me because it seemed to contradict all the sensory training I had done in my movement and dance training with Andre Bernard, Barbara Clark, and Erick Hawkins. They had taught me to reorganize my motor response by altering my sensory perception. However, I finally recognized that one needs to move before one can have feedback about that movement.

When I work with babies and young children who have neuro-logical dysfunctions and are delayed in their development, I am impressed that along with facilitating their "sense of movement," one of the major keys to repatterning their nervous systems lies in stimulating their tactile receptivity.

If they do not utilize a body part in normal movement and I stimulate that area with a light touch or brushing with a soft brush, they begin to initiate movement with that body part. For example, if the baby cannot turn its head to follow a toy with its eyes or to roll over, and I stimulate its mouth (inside and outside) with the toy, it will usually soon turn its head and follow the toy and roll onto its side.

Another example is a baby who cannot reach for a toy, cannot open its hand and grasp the toy. By brushing the baby's hand with a brush and/or the toy (I have a little bright red rag doll with lots of yarn hair that is wonderful for this) the child will usually soon be able to reach and grasp the toy and play with it.

A third example is a baby who keeps its toes curled under and cannot bear its weight on an open foot. Brushing the top of the foot and usually up the outside of the foreleg, can provide the child with the tactile information it needs to open its toes and to place its foot on the ground in an open position.

In the above examples, touch plays a major role in the opening of the child to itself. However, it is not only a mechanical stimulation, but one aspect of open communication between two people in playful dialogue within a totally receptive, perceptive environment. In this context, the tactile stimulation organizes the baby's *attention* so that it is able to exercise *intention.*

There are numerous reasons why a baby may have neurological dysfunctions. They can be due to genetic differences, in-uterine problems, birth trauma, trauma after birth, nutritional difficulties, and environmental/social factors. One in-utero scenario may be that there was a problem in the fetus's ability to move, which diminished its experience of tactile stimulation, which then limits its skin's ability to let its body part know that it exists and where it is, which prevents the body part from expressing itself (through movement). It is interesting that whatever the initial cause, facilitating the child's experience and organization of touch and movement is fundamental in unraveling their inefficient nervous pathways and establishing a firm foundation for their optimum development through the other senses. Because perception is a cyclic process, it can be entered anywhere in the cycle. Thus, one has many options for facilitating change.

Words remain always an outside viewpoint when describing experience. I do not mean to underestimate the importance of the other senses of taste, smell, hearing, and vision. They are essential and wonderful! I only wish to awaken people—society—to the key role that movement and touch play in the dynamic development of the experience of perception itself, regardless of the particular sense organ being stimulated.

The Interweaving of the Phases

The experience of movement and touch are basic to our discovering who we are and who is other and how we dance this life together. Sensing is not just passively being stimulated; perceiving is not just passively receiving input; motor is not just responding directly to stimulation. There's both perceptual activity in the motor activity and motor activity in the reception of input, in perception.

Learning is the opening of ourselves to the experience of life. The opening is a motor act; the experience is interaction between sensory and motor happenings. When the experience of movement is integrated into our education, our perception of ourselves and the world changes.

Contact Improvisation is a clear example of this opening up of one's perception and thereby one's options (pre-motor focus), sensitivity (sensory), awareness (perception), ability to respond (motor), and to feel successful in your self and in your communication with your partner (perception).

Contact embodies, as a technique, the interweaving of these phases. You change your focus, you receive new information, you discover new possibilities, you open up to the immediate happening, you . . . dance. You touch and are touched—with the head, back, feet. You're moving; you're environment is moving. One minute you're focusing on weight, then on space, on touch, on pressure, on your movement, your partner's movement, on falling, on being supported. . . .

Notes

1. Pp. 63–65.
2. Pp. 99–100.
3. Pp. 114–118.
4. In 1992 I changed this term to "active focusing." While it is actually pre-sensory, it is a motor act. [B.B.C.]

Judith Aston

*J*udith Aston is the founder of Aston-Patterning, a set of methods that involve teaching individuals how to move more efficiently with verbal instructions and light touch; a hands-on manipulative work focusing on introducing more mobility into the joints of the body; and a hands-on work involving gentle subtle moving of the connective tissues of the body. The method also involves redesigning the bodily environment to promote more flexibility and balance: chairs, desks, car seats, keyboards, etc.

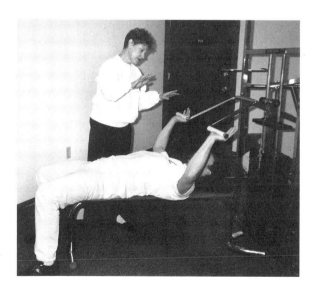

Three Perceptions and One Compulsion

Judith Aston

WHEN I TRY to remember how I became interested in movement education and bodywork, I find it difficult to pinpoint a specific moment. I believe that my interest in this work stems from three perceptions and one strong compulsion that I had even as a little girl.

First, I have always noticed things that are mismatched or out of proportion. I can remember even as a child looking at a picture thinking, "Those arms seem too short for that person," or "Those legs look too long for that body." Second, I seemed to have a skill for imitating people. I could mime movement patterns so that people would know who I was talking about without hearing a name. Third, my awareness of patterns was constant. If I was riding in the back seat of the car and I happened to notice that there were three white houses then one gray house, I would immediately try to guess whether the next three houses would be white followed by two gray ones, or how the pattern would play out. Even now, if someone tells me that 25% of people do something, I'm immediately wondering what the other 75% are doing.

I now think of these three childhood perceptions as part of the abstract thinking process I have been teaching all my life. The sense of proportion is one of the early steps toward seeing how people's bodies might change to make them more comfortable. The ability to take on other people's movement patterns is invaluable in understanding the basic principles of the body in motion. And the fascination with patterns helps me to notice the client's movement patterns and guess what might follow.

This is a newly published essay, a chapter in her forthcoming book.

As for the one strong compulsion, that is my interest in problem-solving. As far back as I can remember, I would always look at things that didn't work very well and think, "There must be a better way." On summer jobs in high school, I can remember noticing ways in which the filing procedure wasn't working and I would offer suggestions to make things more efficient. I believe that my sense of proportion, my ability to mime, my awareness of patterns and my need to problem-solve predisposed me for a career in movement education, bodywork and ergonomics even before I knew these things existed.

My interest in movement brought me to dance training starting at the age of five, and continuing throughout my school years. In grade school I took formal lessons in tap and ballet, and in high school I chose dance for all my physical education classes.

During high school I was a teaching assistant to Martha Walker, an inspiring teacher for the blind students. She was one of my first mentors, and she helped me find my path. She strongly urged me to look at my strengths in teaching and in math. My aptitude tests also pointed the way toward math and abstract thinking. So when I entered college, I decided to go into elementary education and do the "new Math." I continued to take dance classes throughout college and earned a Bachelor of Arts and a teaching credential from UCLA.

I went on to earn a Master's Degree in Fine Arts from UCLA, with a major in dance. My thesis involved three disciplines: psychology, theater and dance. It focused on how movement or stillness created communication; that is, how people communicate with their bodies, through dance, drama or everyday movement and gesture.

During this time I had several mentors who encouraged me to listen to my inner instincts and let the ideas inside me emerge. As a graduate student, I had the pleasure of working with Juana deLaban as my graduate adviser. Her father was Rudolf deLaban, who created the time, effort, motion studies in Europe, as well as the movement notation system called Labanotation. Although she could have taught me this prestigious system, she decided not to. She told me, "I think you're on to something. I think you should pursue your own discoveries for now." Looking back, in some ways I wish I had trained in these other systems, so that I could have continued to work with these wonderful people. However, one crossroads led to the next, so everything felt right the way it happened.

At UCLA I was involved in the early stages of Dance Therapy. Mary Whitehouse was a dance therapist. After my second hour with her, she said, "You don't want to do this work. You want to do whatever it is that's inside of you, and you should do it." I will always remember Mary for encouraging me to develop myself and discover my own life's work. Mary helped me get started as a movement workshop leader at Kairos, a growth center and retreat facility in Southern California.

By 1965 I was teaching dance and theater movement and movement education classes at a community college. During this time, I came to a fascinating discovery that changed my whole approach to teaching. One of my classes was ballroom dance, and this was a requirement for all Physical Education majors. One young man in the class was a track star who won first place in the 440 and 880 races. Though a beautiful runner, in ballroom dance he had two left feet. I tried every conventional method I knew to teach him how to dance, yet we were both unsuccessful.

Frustrated and determined, I finally asked him if I could watch him run. I went out to the track and saw him perform as gracefully as a gazelle. I asked him to run quickly, then slowly. I asked him to run forward, then backward. Then run to one side and then back, and so on. Pretty soon I had him running fast, fast, slow—fast, fast, slow—side to side—until the variations led us to doing the Fox Trot right there on the track!

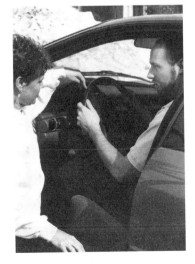

This experience completely shattered every idea I had about how to teach. I realized that if you begin where people already are successful, you can help them transition into the new material, step by step. This method starts with "Yes," the dynamic place where people are already in motion. Rather than stopping their motion with a "No," you can help them move into the new activity from where they are.

"No" is prevalent in most traditional teaching. Often we begin with some form of "No, you're not doing that right. Try this." The problem with this kind of teaching is that the student, this runner, for example, hears the word "No" whether it's stated or not. The interpretation by the rest of his body is "Stop doing what you're doing. Hold on a minute. Now try the new way. Now, yes, go ahead." In essence, the "No" situation causes this person to interrupt his natural fluid movement and become self-conscious. And sure enough, he can't easily do the new activity. When he goes to practice the new movement, he has to stop again at the "No, go on hold" place in the learning and try to recreate the "Yes, go ahead" command. This combination creates jerky, stiff movements. By contrast, if you let him freely get into motion, it is easy to redirect him and build in more tracks for complex movements. Then he can slowly transition, in small incremental steps, to where he wants to be. It's incredible what people can do when they are taught in this way.

I continued developing this technique of building on success as I taught these classes for the next several years. Then in 1966 and 1967 I suffered severe injuries to my spinal muscles and ligaments from two serious car accidents. The physical therapy which was supposed to heal my back injury hadn't really worked. After the second accident, my doctor offered to fuse my spine and suggested I learn how to type because, he said, I would never be able to dance again.

I was not willing to accept either a spinal fusion or a career in typing. And so I found my way to Dr. Ida Rolf. Dr. Rolf introduced me to Rolfing and to the structural changes available through working with the fascia surrounding the muscles. Even though that first session was painful, the effects were very positive. I became hopeful again.

In that first session, Dr. Rolf asked me a lot of questions about my current work, teaching at the college and at the growth centers, and my possible research project with Dr. Valerie Hunt. Dr. Rolf asked me to develop a movement education system for Rolfing to maintain the

Rolf Line and the benefits of the Rolfing sessions. At that time she was using some yoga and a few Mensendyke exercises to supplement the bodywork sessions.

What I developed was a comprehensive system to teach Rolfers and movement teachers how to see each individual body in stillness and in motion, in terms of what structural changes might be most beneficial. Additionally, I taught them how to teach movement, and then how to apply the knowledge and skills to everyday activities. I also taught the Rolfers how to use the teaching principles I had been working with, that is, learning from "yes" and building on success.

I learned the Rolfing method of bodywork in 1968, and modified it to make it less painful for the client and less effortful for the practitioner. From 1972 to 1977, I worked on Dr. Rolf and offered her my newly-discovered bodywork techniques. On a personal level, Dr. Rolf seemed to appreciate the work and the care, and I was pleased to give something back to her. On a business level, I was changing Rolfing as it had been known. Around 1975, Human Behavior Magazine printed that "Judith Aston has developed Soft Rolfing." By 1977, my work was different enough from Rolfing that the changes needed to be addressed. The decision was made that any further changes to Rolfing would depart from Dr. Rolf's vision. It seemed important to keep

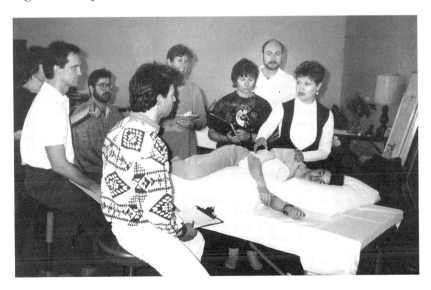

the distinctions clear. And so in 1977 Aston-Patterning® became a separate system from Rolfing.

Aston-Patterning continued to develop and to attract the interest of various people within the fields of bodywork and movement education. I was honored to receive the support and endorsement of people such as Moshe Feldenkrais. My work is complimentary to Feldenkrais' work. We shared the understanding that people usually need to be in a more everyday consciousness to learn to use body/mind changes and improvements in their everyday life.

There are bridges between Aston-Patterning and many other systems as well. In addition to training people to be Aston-Patterning Practitioners, I am also involved in training people to apply certain concepts and techniques to their own disciplines, such as physical therapy, occupational therapy, massage therapy and other health professions such as those associated with the Upledger Institute. I have trained a faculty to teach courses ranging from two-day introductions to five-day workshops to a twenty-week certification training program.

I am pleased with the way that this work can be applied to so many disciplines and activities. I am also aware of how Aston-Patterning is distinct from other systems. The most basic distinction is that Aston-Patterning is a different and unique paradigm (or model) for the way the body can be more optimally aligned, for the way the body can move more effortlessly and efficiently, and for the way the body can interact more comfortably with its environment.

This new paradigm does not agree with the traditional model of the body's alignment perpendicular to the ground, with a plumb line from ear to ankle and symmetry from right to left. Nor does it agree with the linear form of body mechanics that would be more consistent with the perpendicular and symmetrical structure. Nor does it agree with the shape of the objects that have been designed to support the perpendicular and symmetrical structure.

Instead, I find that everybody starts with intrinsic asymmetry, because of the distribution of internal organs in the human structure (one heart, one liver, etc). But more importantly, each individual further develops his or her own unique asymmetries, through adaptation to injuries, work, sports and daily movement habits or patterns.

Rather than working toward making people more perpendicular and symmetrical, this paradigm encourages the negotiation of the body's natural asymmetries through movement, and helps to problem-solve each unique structure according to it's own needs, limitations and abilities. This non-perpendicular, non-symmetrical negotiation is a three-dimensional spiral, and this is the heart of the Aston-Patterning bodywork, movement education and environmental modification.

I made this discovery about asymmetry in 1975 while teaching people how to be symmetrical, as I had learned in posture and dance classes. One day when sitting in a class with 20 people who were all working on their "best" posture, I realized that we all looked the same. Glancing around the room, I thought, "Where did everyone go?" It was then that I realized we maintain our uniqueness when we respect our asymmetries, and we lose spontaneity of movement when we assume a posture that requires tension in the muscles. Often people do not know how to release this extra tension when it is no longer needed. The holding pattern of tension then becomes more permanent, until something can interrupt it and create a sense of ease to replace the tension.

These ideas have become the basis of the Aston-Patterning system. This work helps people find their most natural, comfortable alignment, where the least amount of tension is required. This often requires

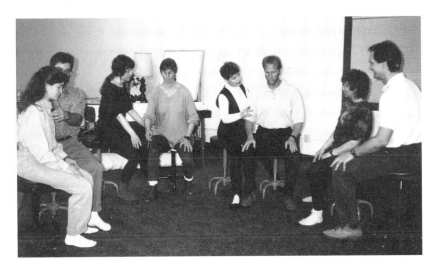

a certain amount of bodywork to release the unnecessary tension that keeps the body in an inefficient pattern. By applying the non-linear idea to the actual way the bodywork is done, I developed a technique of spiraling into the tissue, making the work less compressive and less painful for the client. I apply the three-dimensional approach to the practitioner's body usage as well, to avoid discomfort or injury for the person doing the bodywork.

In addition to receiving the bodywork, the client needs to learn how to use this new alignment in everyday activities. Through movement education, the person is able to maintain the changes that are made in the session by learning ways of moving that do not require the "old" tension-holding patterns. They might also need to learn how to modify their environments, such as shoes, car seats or computer stations, to support the improved alignment and movement pattern.

Each Aston-Patterning session is unique, depending on the person's needs, limitations, abilities and interests. A basic session format usually includes the following:

1. Gathering information
   —hear the client's history and/or interest in seeking help
2. Observation
   —see current alignment, proportion and dimension in standing
   —see current movement patterns in walking or performing an activity such as lifting a child, using the computer or playing tennis
3. Palpation
   —identify areas of hypertone and hypotone
   —make a body map of today's specific pattern of tension and slack
4. Plan
   —hypothesize what areas could change to optimize alignment, improve movement patterns and help meet the client's goals
5. Select the form of work to achieve the desired result
   —choose from bodywork, movement education, fitness or environmental modification

—decide on the sequence and combination of these forms
6. Application
   — put the learning into everyday use by practicing selected activity
   —cue the client to use the changes
   —instruct the client to support these changes in his/her environment by learning the appropriate ergonomic modification

As an example of a series of Aston-Patterning sessions, I'll describe one of my favorite experiences. A 93 year old woman known as M.K. was referred to me by one of my students. M.K. was a vibrant, vital woman who played an active role in her community through such services as volunteering at the Museum of Modern Art. But despite her youthful mindset, the normal effects of aging were catching up with her, and she had taken several falls. Household tasks such as putting away the dishes, vacuuming and making the bed had become more difficult for her. She was faced with giving up needlepoint because of physical discomfort.

I felt that M.K. would fall less if her body were in a more supportive alignment and if she found the unique gait pattern specifically matched to her limitations. In observing M.K., I noticed that she used her body in a way that caused her to lean back as she moved. First, we did some bodywork to release the unnecessary tension-holding patterns that held M.K.'s body in an inefficient alignment. After the bodywork, her tension no longer pulled her into a backward lean. As her alignment became more balanced, she felt more stable on her feet.

Next she needed to learn how to use the new alignment in walking. She found that by using gravity to assist and support her, her new walk was effortless, comfortable and safe. I added a slight modification to her shoes which were worn down into her old pattern. She was amused and delighted that she was learning how to walk at 93.

In subsequent sessions, M.K. learned to stay aligned and supported in all her household chores, using the Aston-Patterning movement techniques that worked best for her specific structure. She was even able to do her needlepoint without discomfort. In the process, she became a very good problem-solver, and was able to do other tasks more comfortably by applying the techniques she learned in her sessions. She summed up the lessons of her sessions by saying, "That makes so much sense. Of course that's why I was losing my balance when I walked and getting so stiff when I sat. Now, dear, why is it that I pay you so much money for COMMON SENSE?"

I agree with M.K. and many of my clients who come to the realization that if we had been taught some of these ideas about our body's optimal movement possibilities when we were children, we wouldn't encounter so many of these problems as adults. Much of what we need to learn is to listen to common sense, our practical wisdom, our "unexamined assumptions as distinguished from specially acquired concepts," as Webster's Dictionary defines common sense. Another part of the problem is that the "specially acquired concepts" being passed along are often outdated. This is most noticeable in the area of ergonomics, the designs of the objects we encounter in our everyday lives.

As I saw people like M.K. change so dramatically, I realized that even with the most comfortable alignment and the most efficient movement pattern, we still have to interact with objects in our environment. I found that no matter how long I worked with people and

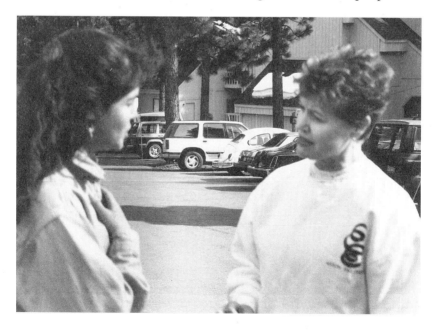

no matter how great the changes seemed, if they climbed right back into the same car seat or the same old shoes, old patterns would be immediately reinforced. I started using duct tape, foam and towels to modify people's car seats, office furniture, kayaks, etc, to improve the relationship between the body and these objects.

I then saw the immense possibility for change, not only in the few things I had modified for people in sessions, but for a whole range of objects that people use in their everyday lives. I realized that most products needed to be re-designed, to allow people to use them in a more natural, comfortable and effortless alignment. This led me to develop The Aston Line of specialized ergonomic products for the car, home, office, gym and anywhere else people want to feel more comfortable.

To date, I have developed over 300 designs. About five years ago I went to a patent attorney to see if I could patent the biomechanical mathematics theory which is at the heart of the Aston paradigm and upon which these designs are based. The attorney told me that "The good news is that you may have discovered a new law of nature. The bad news is that, like the Theory of Relativity, a law of nature cannot be patented. You will have to patent each of your 300 designs."

I took his advice and began patenting my designs. I have produced 15 of them, including seat wedges, furniture and exercise and sports equipment. Many more still await funding to make the products available. I have attempted to get these products out in a number of ways. For example, I met with a leading luggage manufacturer to demonstrate my patented design for an ergonomic handle. My design changes the shape and position of the handle. The purpose is to decrease the amount of body tension and rotation necessary to carry the luggage, thereby improving people's comfort while using the product. The company representatives seemed very interested, but decided that using the design for the new handles would make the luggage with their current handles obsolete. They felt this would not be good business. Perhaps this kind of thinking will change someday.

I continue to be interested in publishing articles and books about Aston-Patterning. Articles have been published in a number of issues of physical therapy and massage magazines, and chapters have been included in books on chronic pain, bodywork, therapy and movement education. I am currently writing a book about trauma and rehabilitation. I thought I understood these challenges from my two car accidents in the sixties and my work with people in these situations. However, my personal experience of trauma and what it takes to transcend it increased astronomically when, in January of 1993, I sustained severe injuries to my right leg in a skiing accident. My knee was broken off across the top of the tibia and my leg was fractured vertically like chopping wood.

In addition to causing debilitating pain and loss of function, these injuries threatened my ability to continue the movement work that has been so central to my life. The book in progress is my exploration of the transformative potential of crisis and healing. I found that regardless of its origin, trauma always leaves a profound imprint upon not only our physical body but on our emotional, mental and spiritual being. The imprint affects how we think, how we use our bodies, how we feel, what we are able to experience and how we relate to the universe itself. A wide range of issues, from self-esteem to spiritual questions, are forged around this imprint.

Depending on what we do with that imprint, it can be a positive or devastating element in our lives. When trauma is experienced consciously, we not only minimize pain and suffering but learn to move deeper into the true meaning of our lives. By contrast, when pushed aside or deeply buried, the imprint of the trauma can greatly limit our lives, perhaps even interrupt our desire to live. I hope that my book will convey the profound inner dynamics of trauma, and how we can literally mine these experiences of their rich transformative potentials.

I believe that my recent journey from darkness back to hope and light both grows out of all my previous experiences, and prepares the way for what lies ahead.

3.
Moving Intelligence

Irmgard Bartenieff

Irmgard Bartenieff (1900–1981), another World War II refugee, brought to New York the body movement work of Rudolf von Laban, which became the origin of dance therapy, widely practiced in medical and psychotherapy communities. It involves exploring the emotional and psychological dimensions of specific movement patterns, a moving-off-the-couch form of psychoanalysis.

Interview with Irmgard Bartenieff

Ilana Rubenfeld

Rubenfeld: How did you start your work and from where did it originate?

Bartenieff: At the beginning I started to study biology.

Rubenfeld: Where was this?

Bartenieff: In, Berlin, Germany. Then I heard about Laban, and I had already done bodywork with Mensendieck. It was the time when all this started, you know.

Rubenfeld: The turn of the century?

Bartenieff: Yes, and Mensendieck was a dominant influence. The Mensendieck organization in the early twenties was very strong. It had actually started before World War I and it was very well organized. but to me that was too static. So I tried a derivative that combined natural living, plus crafts, and living in the country.

Rubenfeld: A more wholistic point of view.

Bartenieff: Yes, and then Laban, of course, was a firebrand. He had just brought out Mary Wigman.

Rubenfeld: What was he like, Irmgard?

Bartenieff: Oh, he was ... (laugh)

Rubenfeld: He was a fiery personality?

Bartenieff: He was a fantastic all around personality. He was origi-

---

Somatics (Autumn, 1977), 9–13.

nally Hungarian and in the Austrian army. He was from a very old military family. His father wanted him to become a military governor and he stood it for two years and then quit and became a bohemian in Paris where he was exposed to painting, architecture, et al. He also began to study biology and some anatomy.

Rubenfeld: When would you say that was?

Bartenieff: Just around 1906.

Rubenfeld: That's fascinating! Just around the turn of the century, together with F.M. Alexander, Sigmund Freud, Elsa Gindler, Jacobi and others.

Bartenieff: Yes, really at the turn of the century. He began to work with dancers in the small cabarets in Paris. He then had an artistic group that was living and working together. That's where Mary Wigman was, in that group. Laban started his whole school around 1920. I went to him in 1925, and that was the time that he really had crystallized his whole space-harmony theory … and the beginnings of what we today call our Effort-Shape work—the quality of movement.

Rubenfeld: Can you say a few words about how Laban developed his work?

Bartenieff: Well, his whole space harmony work resulted from studying the martial arts. In the martial arts he saw that in the situation of survival you have to make adequate use of space and energy. You are forced to. From there, he developed the interrelationship of energy and space to what we call our Effort. It was then called Eukinetics and was developed for the dancer.

Rubenfeld: Who were some people and schools he was exposed to?

Bartenieff: He saw a lot, you know. He was in the Balkans and he saw all kinds of things. In Paris he saw some Chinese and he was immediately comparing their movements. This was the core of work … different styles of movement. He had an enormous sensitivity, and when he began to teach, he first taught small groups of twelve, then he immediately started schools all over Germany. We had at least twenty schools by the mid-twenties. And the interesting thing was that he worked with people personally, and also developed a staff of people that he could use as teachers. A group leader founded the Folkgang school in Essen. He kept those schools together, and every head of a school came together every year. So, the new ideas of Laban were immediately transferred. It was only ten or twelve years really ... I still can't believe it was such a short time. We had very high standards. When he saw a person, he immediately had this kind of "total feeling." He started that person on what they should work on from that feeling.

Rubenfeld: He started them where they were, instead of with a planned agenda. It's interesting that Moshe Feldenkrais also studied the martial arts. When you told me about Laban, I lit up because Feldenkrais told me that he's a black belt in judo. He hurt his knee and that's how he came to develop his work, because the doctors couldn't help him. Moshe at 73 could get an Aikido student in his 30's pinned down so that the man couldn't move. We were amazed watching Moshe's movements in space and time.

Bartenieff: For me the next step was study from 1925 to 1927, and really getting the beginning of the Labanotation; it was then crystallized in the recording of movement and then also called "space-harmonies." The use of space and movement was developed from the core of the defense scale which is a scale of how you successfully protect yourself. The up is protecting the head, the down is protecting the lower quarters, the across is protecting the heart, the out is protecting this flank, the retreating is protecting the belly ... it's all over the body, so the order is important. Last year in Honolulu, I saw a Master group of the martial arts, with a sword, and there was the same kind of concept. They also emphasized the vital points, and how they induct their energy and their space into either avoiding or aiming. You know, it was really fascinating. In the Orient, where they developed these techniques to a great level during the Samurai time they had this idea that you should not just butcher an adversary, but you should really skillfully and quickly deal with him.

Rubenfeld: So you were saying before, that he was able to look at someone and intuit something?

Bartenieff: Yes, you see, gradually through the development of the theory, Laban developed a feel for different qualities of movement, so he could assess people very definitely through their spatial abilities, the energy abilities.

Rubenfeld: So, what I hear you saying is that he begins with concepts of the martial arts, and adds his own way of seeing, which results in his ability to assess the person's energy and movement. This he does by observing a certain sequence of movements.

Bartenieff: Yes, that's how his whole training was built. Exploring your own capacities in the movement. That was what he stressed. Later he taught in England for the English Educational Dance System.

Rubenfeld: When was that, Irmgard?

Bartenieff: That was in 1938. He left Germany and was in Paris a short time. Then he and Lisa Ullman developed dance education in the English school system, or the public school system—what we call here the public school. And, that was an exploratory approach.

Rubenfeld: What was your personal place in the journey?

Bartenieff: After I had a school of my own in Stuttgart and Berlin, I developed my own dance group, and by 1933 we had developed a group in exactly half a year. Then Hitler closed everything down, and I devoted my time mainly to the Labanotation, reviving the notation of the old French dances. I left Germany in 1936 and took the notation with me. I introduced the notation to Hanya Holm who was tremendously sympathetic. I had two children and I had to make a living so I studied physical therapy. I then worked in physical therapy from that point on until almost 1950. But I always gave some classes on the side. I was very interested in the Dance Notation Bureau. I was one of the earliest members when Hutchenson founded the Dance Notation Bureau in 1941.

Rubenfeld: What was the goal of the Bureau?

Bartenieff: To notate the works of dancers for posterity and to create a library of notated dance, which, in fact, they're still doing. They've really greatly increased it! Analysis of the movements necessary to do notation gave me a body of knowledge that I began to use in physical rehabilitation. So, I was a very unconventional physical therapist.

I was for seven years in charge of the polio ward here in Willard Parker Hospital, and that's where I learned the most. The absence of movement taught me what movement is about, so I developed new techniques of rehabilitation. Of course, when I tried to tell the staff what it was based on, they used to say, "She's just an intuitive person." I heard that for many, many years.

Rubenfeld: Instead of the actual hard knowledge and experience.

Bartenieff: Yes, there were really faces behind it. All through the forties and fifties I worked mainly in rehabilitation. I had one marvelous job in Westchester, where I was allowed to change the whole program and work with the coordination of those children who had lost part of their development because they had had to stay a year or two in the hospital. I saw terrible regression in these children, and so I invented dancing in bed and introduced dance rhythm into their program. We organized games for the children that had to stay in bed because of hip diseases. I could coordinate with the staff and that's where I first worked with psychiatrists and with art therapists.

Rubenfeld: So, in the fifties you began to include the psychiatrists in the movement work.

Bartenieff: Yes, I worked on the mental problems as well as the physical.

Rubenfeld: Was Laban and your group familiar with Elsa Gindler in Germany.

Bartenieff: Yes, we all knew about each other. I had only a very fleeting contact. Once, we happened to be in the same place in the summer course. But Laban was very uninfluenced by others. He could see where others were and he didn't condemn them, but he said, "Well, she or he works on just that particular aspect." So there was also the whole rhythmic gymnastics by Broder which go back to Dalcrose. You see, Laban was a contemporary of Dalcrose. They had not really any kind of collaboration. Laban still said that Dalcrose was restricting the body, though of course the Luxembourg people were already freeing their rhythms.

Rubenfeld: I studied with Dora Dubsky who believed in having children move to music.

Bartenieff: Oh yes, she is a good friend of mine.

Rubenfeld: She's a good friend? You know, she helped me develop some of my own ideas twenty years ago back in 1955 and 1956. She started me on my journey teaching music to children. I was then a musician and graduate of Juilliard, and I was very unhappy with the way children sat stiffly in their chairs. She started me on my journey of getting them off and moving. I love her very much. She's just a wonderful human being. She was really the beginning for me in seeing the possibilities of movement. So I really came to my teaching from a different orientation.

Bartenieff: The person in charge of Helleraux is still the professor of music and dance in Vienna at the State Academy. There was also the Gunter School in Munich, a rhythmic school that goes back to Helleraux. That's the school where Carl Orf started.

Rubenfeld: Also there was F.M. Alexander in England. Was there any contact with these other movement?

Bartenieff: My younger son studied in 1950 in London and he had some lessons from Alexander.

Rubenfeld: That's changed a lot. When I visited London I was very interested in the way they teach the Alexander Technique. There was a time when the Technique was very involved with the vertical line. We've gotten into more diagonal and circular movement these days.

Bartenieff: To me, of course, I feel the two principles are the vertical principle and the diagonal principle.

Rubenfeld: I know what you mean. So then, you did physical therapy, and a lot came from watching the children who didn't have complete movement.

Bartenieff: Yes, and I also developed better methods of what they could do to restore functioning. But when you have true paralysis in parts, how are you going to use your whole body to the best effect with some parts missing?

Rubenfeld: Right, what can you use that's already there. How can you develop that to its fullest?

Bartenieff: Yes, and not just in terms of strength. From 1950 on, I went for five summers, every summer, back to the Laban people in England, and I studied the Effort, which was what I didn't tell you. See in 1929, Laban had to conduct a festival for the craftsmen of Vienna. He studied their work songs and their dances, and their rituals, and that gave him an idea of how they related to their own craft through movement.

Rubenfeld: That's beautiful!

Bartenieff: So, when he came to England, he did this work with the educational dance and he worked on the theory as well. Then, in the war he was asked by an industrial manager to do a study of two things: the efficiency of women during war time and what could be done to replace the great lifting tasks of men. How could their effort be altered by different use of space and gravity? He developed this in England and produced his first book, *Effort*.

Rubenfeld: Where does the word come from Irmgard?

Bartenieff: The word comes actually from German where it means *Antrieb*. *Antrieb* is like the motivation of a motor: *trieb* is like "drive" and *An* is "on"—driving on, how your energy drives. That is really the best explanation of effort. We are dealing really with the central motivation in movement, the use of energy—call it space-force-time use.

Rubenfeld: Would the initiation of the movement be an important factor here?

Bartenieff: Yes, the initiation of the energy, not only where it is initiated but how it appears altogether spontaneously in people. People use space-force-time in different combinations that are characteristic of them. And they also relate to outside space in different ways. Of course, his whole idea of the affinity of the two—the space and the effort is involved here. One of his pupils developed the "efficiency" approach not only for the industrial worker and his bodily skill, but he saw this also as an expressive factor. One must not forget that Laban was not just exploring movement per se, but the expressive factors that were closely related to these energy and spatial factors.

Rubenfeld: This, then, united the relationship to expression and allowed expression to come out.

Bartenieff: He defined expression in these energy and spatial terms: that is the core. To him expression is not a separate entity.

Rubenfeld: That's right. It is, again, a wholistic way of seeing.

Bartenieff: Yes.

Rubenfeld: What were some of the ideas about internal space?

Bartenieff: Well, he speaks of internal space, and what he actually means by that is an emphasis on the inner space changes that come through breath. I increasingly emphasize that myself.

Rubenfeld: So, when you brought your work here and got into physical therapy, how did you see the physical therapy in relationship to the Effort-Shape?

Bartenieff: Well, I used it. For instance, I had to teach a child with almost completely paralyzed legs to pull himself up on the next chair in order to get into his wheelchair, and this was a very easy-going, somewhat lazy child. So, I said you have to change your effort. Instead of going always with sustained movement and free flow, you have to be sudden and quick—really sudden and strong.

Rubenfeld: To make that movement to the wheelchair ...

Bartenieff: To really condense that moment so that she could really get up. You see, I changed the rhythmical structure of the phrases in sequence.

Rubenfeld: Like music, the same phrases.

Bartenieff: Yes ... if you change the emphasis in the phrase, you get a different kind of result.

Rubenfeld: And that, of course, would affect also the internal.

Bartenieff: Yes, of course: it would change the breath. Together with a doctor and, later, with the Institute for the Criminally Disabled, I worked with back problems. And so, out of that grew what I now call Fundamentals, which I teach as a separate course. Here the anatomical knowledge that I have from my physical therapy years, and from the spatial and effort knowledge come together.

Rubenfeld: Did you have any connection with Swiegard?

Bartenieff: She did marvelous work and really helped a great many dancers to overcome this hypertenseness.

Rubenfeld: What happened when you left the Children's Hospital? Where did your journey take you then?

Bartenieff: Then I went to work for a doctor in his private practice.

Rubenfeld: You saw people one to one?

Bartenieff: Yes, and then around 1959 or 1960, I started to teach in music school. First, really, movement again for various people, and then somebody brought me to Albert Einstein, to the Jacoby Hospital that had just started to develop more modern approaches to working with mental patients. And that's how I started to work with mental patients. Then they moved away from Jacoby Hospital because they got a grant to start a day hospital on Westchester Square. That's where I developed and did Dance Therapy. You see, this was a department that was still connected with Albert Einstein Medical College, Department of Social Psychiatry. The whole concern was with the short term patient—getting the patient mobilized in many ways and influencing him in many ways. So there, I worked again with an art therapist. I didn't work with the music therapists. I don't know why. It really didn't materialize. It was a small group, and I knew the whole staff because we had to attend every part of the program. There were always weekly meetings where the patients were discussed and where they always wanted a report on the art therapy, which consisted of a group mural, and we were the group that worked with movement. So all together, this really taught us a great deal. The dance alone, maybe, would have been too lethargic, but sometimes it was the opposite. It really reflected always the mood of the ward, the relation of the sexes and so on. It was sometimes very male oriented, sometimes very dominant female. The psychiatrists would see this as a barometer of the structure of the group.

In spite of my physical therapy training and in spite of my emphasis on functional aspects, I always felt that when it came to the mentally ill, there was nothing like the power of dance, like the power of music speaking to the feelings. But, you can work this way only when you have a very deep commitment to dance and also understand the nature of dance, which I got from Laban—how you calm down, or how you excite. That I feel should still be the core.

In psychological treatment, I feel we have not even begun to understand the full range of what one can do with movement. I am very grateful that I had the opportunity of having contact with these psychiatrists. Fortunately, our boss, Dr. Sperling, used to warn us, "Don't accept the jargon of the psychotherapist. You have not yet explored how far this reaches." This has been a golden rule all through, and it still is! In fact, it's becoming very much stronger with every year. So, I feel it should be with dance therapy. There is a great deal of character training in this also, in that a paralyzed person can learn to use crutches and learn to do with very little and learn to perform his daily activities. You see, that's one of the aims of re-education. But there is this additional matter of the influence of movement on the moods when you are depressed, etc. . . .

Rubenfeld: For a joke, I sometimes tell people in the audience to put their arms toward the ceiling and say, "I'm depressed."

Bartenieff: Yes, yes. (she laughs)

Rubenfeld: It's a fun way of demonstrating how movement affects feeling, and how feelings affect movement.

Bartenieff: You see, there's also the spatial thing in that.

Rubenfeld: I remember even in my time (and it must be much longer for you), when people would ask me what I'm doing and I'd say, "I'm combining body-mind work with psychotherapy," and they would be surprised. Today, we're living in a time when everybody wants it fast; they want to learn how to do it fast. It's the "in" thing.

Bartenieff: Here at the Dance Notation Bureau, we have a very demanding program. People come for an intensive year to us.

Rubenfeld: A few of my clients have been in your program.

Bartenieff: It was interesting for me to have one person in particular studying with you and finishing the program. She was coming to me for therapy while she was doing the training. She and I used her experiences at the Bureau to integrate her feelings. The process was revealing and fascinating.

Bartenieff: Some people are what we call body-oriented, and they have trouble with the expressive part of their personality.

Rubenfeld: That's right. They come from a physical orientation.

Bartenieff: Yes, and sometimes it's really difficult to dislodge them from there. It's your relation to yourself and to the outside world that's important and how that is rhythmized. So this is a very intensive time.

Rubenfeld: Yes, I understand, I know my structural changes have greatly affected my life and attitude towards people.

Bartenieff: Yes.

Rubenfeld: When I began to take the Alexander lessons I went for three years totally for my personal benefit. I said, "As long as it takes to change, I'm willing." I didn't ask how fast it would be. I know that from these changes, there was much opening up of my heart, my whole psyche, my whole being. I changed very much.

Bartenieff: It's not just firm muscles that are being changed.

Rubenfeld: Yes, there are some people whose approach is only in terms of body change. Others dealing only with verbal exchanges say that if you talk your body will change. It is in neither one nor the other, it is both.

Bartenieff: Well, I'm very interested in all the other approaches. I'm always delighted that people can start here or there and somehow come to the core. I feel the whole present time is really a rediscovering of some very old principles.

Rubenfeld: Old, basic, obvious principles and truths.

Bartenieff: Yes.

Rubenfeld: We get to the truths from different paths, but we're always coming back to the same truths.

Bartenieff: I always said, for instance, that our work is quite vigorous. We can grade it for different disabilities and so on, as I do personality. But, for instance, if somebody can profit from another way I send them there. I send some of my polio patients that are paralyzed to Alexander people to maintain a balance—also, people that have heart conditions for whom it is very important to open up with no strain on the heart.

Rubenfeld: Did you ever meet Fritz Perls?

Bartenieff: No, I only heard about him.

Rubenfeld: I'm glad I met him at the last years of his life. He mellowed out very much. But he really shocked me into looking at the obvious and going back into just seeing and paying attention to listening and seeing, and not interpreting.

Bartenieff: I feel very strongly about that. And, of course, Laban, also, had such a fantastic temperament. He could roar at you and was the most gentle person. And, of course, he admired women, and many women played a role in his life in various ways.

Rubenfeld: That's interesting. How did he admire women.

Bartenieff: He was capable of having very deep friendships with women. We had a very real friendship which was marvelous. He also had this whole Hungarian vitality.

Rubenfeld: It sounds like he integrated the female part of himself—he wasn't ashamed of it.

Bartenieff: He just lived! Really marvelous! It was interesting that he should have started these schools in Germany with all these problem-ridden people. But, he always used to say, "I feel my work is still best understood in Germany because of the intuitive and sensitive." That was also part of it. What he did in Germany—he also created something that is still a marvel to me. He created the proletarian movement choir. It was full of political background, with a speaking choir possible, and very modern music—unthinkable! Could you see the labor unions dancing? Of course, that was immediately killed when Hitler came, but it was far spread. Hundreds of people would come together at these functions and they would dance.

Rubenfeld: What energy!

Bartenieff: It lasted maybe twelve years. I still can't believe it was only twelve years. but, he had this terrific drive. He himself did several choreographic works. His last job was as ballet master with the State Opera in Germany. It was before he left for England. So he was a terrific comprehensivist. And also the core of everything he did was that everything changes.

Rubenfeld: The *I Ching—The Book of Changes*—the only thing that is constant is change.

Bartenieff: He got you into all of these things that are based on variation and motivation—that's why it is a true movement theory. He speaks about a person going from a state of greater stability to a state of greater mobility—but it is a flux thing.

Rubenfeld: That's fascinating, because in the Feldenkrais exercises—the quality that attracts me to them—is that they are never the same. The brain isn't given a chance to get into the habit of doing a movement in the same way. He never tells you how to do the movement.

Bartenieff: Yes. I was at a conference in Denmark. I met him there. He also has the idea that when you repeat a movement the next time you go further.

Rubenfeld: Each time further.

Bartenieff: Instead of forcing it.

Rubenfeld: One more question—when did the Effort Shape Program start?

Bartenieff: It started—oh, 1959 I gave the first courses, and then I gave the first training programs around 1964–65. It was a very small group; Martha Davis belonged to that class. Since then it has slowly grown; in the last three or four years it has been constantly increasing.

Rubenfeld: And, beside the one-year intensive program are there any other programs?

Bartenieff: Yes, we have in the winter what we call non-certifying courses. The Introduction to Effort, or Fundamentals, Introductory Courses and Special Workshops.

Rubenfeld: That's good to know, so that people who may not have an entire year can do other things at your school. Are there some kind of workshops for professional people who are already working with the body?

Bartenieff: Yes, I give a class for dance therapists in July—a week course. Last year we had a two-week course for practicing dance therapists as we now try to serve different area. See, I tried to do a week course for physical therapists, also. Then I actually had people who were involved with teaching basic movement.

Rubenfeld: I think you would get a very good group of serious people if you were to open it to those who were involved with Feldenkrais, Alexander, Rolf, etc.

Bartenieff: Yes, those that have been practicing for several years! I feel that this is important. First of all, because it comes quicker to them, but also, I feel that it is important because of the richer exchange between us all.

Rubenfeld: That is certainly something worthwhile giving thought to. Irmgard, it has been a pleasure for me to share this time and space with you.

Mary Whitehouse

*M*ary Whitehouse (1911–1979) created the West Coast tradition of *dance therapy, a radically simpler form of body movement, sometimes called "Moving in Depth," or "Authentic Movement." It involves teaching people to move from felt internal impulses rather than imposed forms, and to pay attention to and nurture the feelings that emerge when one moves in that way. While the East Coast Bartenieff work became closely associated with psychoanalysis, Whitehouse's work came to be used by Jungians.*

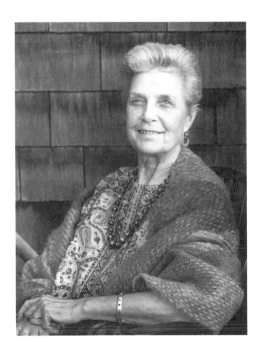

The Tao of the Body

Mary Whitehouse

Movement is the great law of life. Everything moves. The heavens move, the earth turns, the great tides mount the beaches of the world. The clouds march slowly across the sky, driven by a wind that stirs the trees into a dance of branches. Water, rising in mountain springs, runs down the slopes to join the current of the river. Fire, begun in the brush, leaps roaring over the ground. And the earth, so slow, so always there, grumbles and groans and shifts in the sleep of centuries.

So too all living creatures. Birds and fish and insects, animals, snakes, and snails have their being in movement, exist by virtue of it, show forth their nature through it. In the words of the old song, "Fish gotta swim, birds gotta fly"—

And man? Whoever he is, wherever he is, he too lives in movement. His body is a world of movement in itself. Breathing and circulation, digestion and reproduction are all unconscious movement processes, the wonderful motor pattern of his life. Within this pattern he lies down, he sits, he stands, and standing walks and runs. He sleeps, eats, copulates, fights, weeps, laughs and talks. Most of all in our twentieth century civilization, he talks. Words have become his primary means of communication and realization—words that he says, words that he listens to, words in books, words that he thinks with. And slowly, slowly, without his knowing it almost, the words and the talking which are only one kind of movement linked to one kind of understanding, take the place of another quite different awareness of himself and others.

Unpublished lecture given for The Analytical Psychology Club of Los Angeles (1958). 1–17

Two things about physical movement are striking. One is that movement is non-verbal and yet it communicates, that is, says something. Our impressions of people are gathered fully as much from physical attitudes and gestures as from words and clothes. Nervousness often shows itself in little extra movements of hands, feet and face; tension, in raised shoulders as well as voice; depression in downward drooping lines of the whole body; fear in limited and carefully controlled movement, and so on indefinitely. They are all communicated to us by others and by us to others, whether we know it and describe it in words or not. Often other people are more aware of our condition than we are able to be ourselves. Which brings me to the second thing. The body does not, I would almost say cannot, lie. The human being as he actually exists at any moment cannot be hidden, by words, by clothes, least of all by wishes. No matter what he is doing or saying, he has his own way of doing and saying it, and it the *way* that reveals what he is like. The physical condition is in some way also the psychological one. We do not know in what way the psyche is the body and the body is the psyche but we do know that one does not exist without the other. And I would go so far as to suggest that just as the body changes in the course of working with the psyche, so the psyche changes in the course of working with the body. We would do well to remember that the two are not separate entities but mysteriously a totality.

It is difficult to know where to begin. What I want to do is to describe, and later on to let you see, some of the ways in which movement can become direct, subjective experience, and to suggest certain kinds of self-knowledge which are available through it. I am confronted by the necessity of talking about something which is essentially inaccessible to words, but I will try. I have an approach, not a method, much less a theory. In fact, I often feel that the serious and deep things which take place in this way of working with the body happen much more out of what I do not know than out of what I do. Perhaps the fact that they happen is what is important. I well remember my initiation into this truth. I had only recently begun individual appointments. A woman stood alone in the center of the studio. It was her third or fourth appointment. We had been working very simply with stretching, bending, standing and walking. Her movement in general existed in a cloud over her head—the face and eyes nearly always turned up to the ceiling, the arms and hands repeatedly extended overhead, the weight lifted up on the toes, everything going up, nothing going down, everything going out, nothing held. I suggested she clench her fists and bring them up from her sides in front of her. The first time, the hands closed, but there was very little tension in the muscles of the arms, they still floated. The second time she waited longer and pulled harder. Very slowly the arms bent at the elbows, closing upward in front of her body. As the fists approached her face, her expression became one of intense sorrow and strain, and at the point of almost touching her own mouth and cheeks, the whole body turned and pitched downward onto the floor in a violent fall, and she burst into long sobs. A barrier had been pierced, a dam broken, her body had pitched her into feeling.

The core of the movement experience is the sensation of moving and being moved. There are many implications in putting it like this. Ideally, both are present in the same instant, and it may be literally an instant. It is a moment of total awareness, the coming together of what I am doing and what is happening to me. It cannot be anticipated, explained, specifically worked for, nor repeated exactly.

In order that it may happen, one must have a *bodily* awareness of movement. It is astonishing how many people are almost completely unaware of themselves physically. Our personal ways of sitting, standing, moving, eating, smoking, talking, are so habitual as to seem natural and hardly worth noting. The wonderful joy in movement, which children have, has been lost. Movement has become a means to an end, usually a rational and purposeful end, and takes place automatically in response to hundreds and hundreds of mental images of going someplace and doing something. To be sure, first parents, and then friends, have always commented freely on our faulty posture, and lack of grace. "Pull in your stomach—" "Stand up straight." "Don't slouch—" and sometimes when we catch an unexpected glimpse of ourselves in a mirror there is the vague beginning of a realization of something not satisfactory, not alive, but is gone again even as it comes. After all, this is what we look like, and no amount of trying will change it. This latter, incidentally, is accurate since trying seldom changes anything basic—only becoming something different changes what was. It never occurs to us that we have unwittingly lost the body by not experiencing its truth, and that to the extend that it does not and cannot move easily, freely and totally, it is dead; for movement is the life of the body. This life includes the life of the mind, but is not limited to it.

There is a technical term for feeling one's own body move—it is called the kinaesthetic sense and it is just as valuable as the five which inform us of the physical world about us. The kinaesthetic sense is the sensation which accompanies or informs us of bodily movement. Athletes have it, and dancers, also actors, though they often forget to work with it—all the people whom we describe as having natural timing and coordination in motion. It is likely that some people are born with a greater degree of it than others, just as there are greater and lesser visual and auditory gifts, but we all have it. I have an idea that it is connected with the extraordinary capacity of the blind man to move in a world which he can cannot see but can *feel moving*, and that it accounts for the equally extraordinary adaptation some people are able to make in response to serious or permanent crippling. The recent case of a high school girl, paralyzed from the neck down, who has learned to write with a pencil held between her teeth, is an example.

But if the kinaesthetic sense is never developed, or seldom used, it becomes unconscious and one is in the situation I have already described, a situation that I can only call living in the head, which fact the body faithfully reflects, since it must move, by acquiring a whole series of distortions, short circuits, strains and mannerisms accumulated from years and years of being assimilated to mental images of choice, necessity, value and inappropriateness. At this point movement is *in spite of* instead of *with the help* of the mental life.

There is a further interesting reflection in connection with this. In our time there is a widespread repression of all physical emotion, that is, all bodily expression of joy, grief, anger, affection, fear, and an equally widespread fascination with the body's appearance and function. Advertisements of cures for nerves, constipation, colds, headaches, that run-down feeling; recommendations for slimming, trimming, building, developing; diets, gadgets, vitamins, how to sleep, how to wake up, how not to perspire, how to avoid bad breath—the list is endless *and* body centered. All polarized by sex plastered interminably on billboards, in magazines, movies, newspapers, in the form of the female body exposed and as unlikely in proportion as possible. We are embarrassed and irritated when confronted by any form of physical intensity in our personal lives. Joy in the voice and face is all right, grief in the voice and face is understandable, anger in the voice and face will pass, but an exuberant enveloping arm thrown around our shoulders, the sight of a body rocking back and forth with grief, the sudden eruption of a stamped foot or a book slammed violently down on a table, all upset us. Could it be that body *is* the unconscious, and that in repressing and, more important, disregarding the spontaneous life of the sympathetic nervous system, we are enthroning the rational, the orderly, the manageable, and cutting ourselves off from all experience of the unconscious, and therefor of the instincts? Which then take their revenge in the form of an exaggerated, compulsive fascination with the body and all its works? The less the body is experienced, the more it becomes an appearance; the less reality it has the more it must be undressed or dressed up; the less it is one's own known body, the further away it moves from anything to do with one's *self*.

Working with movement is an initiation into the world of the body as it actually is, what it can do easily, with difficulty, or not at all. But it is also, or can be, a serious discovery of what we are like—for we are like our movement. People discover what parts of their bodies are not available, do not move, are not felt. The woman of whom I have already spoken sent me a description, much later, of her first experience. I quote it:

> Together we went out to the studio. [My teacher] said she wanted to see my walk to see how I was built and how I moved. I walked and as I see myself now, it was as if my body didn't belong to me— the very thought of being alone with someone watching me brought a little light to the surface. Putting my feet together was a new

experience and I never forget the feeling of wholeness my hands expressed when I put them together, thrusting them out into space. Perhaps I didn't know it, but my hands contained all that my body did not.

She worked in private appointments weekly until she felt ready to try a class. Shortly after she began she gives this account of another discovery:

> I see an image coming out of the earth. It is a masculine image with arms outstretched to the blue space all about him. His legs dangle in the earth. He must come out of the earth and walk in the blue space that only his upper body knows. he needs legs in relation to his upper body so he can dance in space and love it.

It is interesting that it is a masculine image which needs to dance in the space. Space is a structural element in movement, a principle of definition and order. Walking is a means of moving about in space. It is entirely suitable that the masculine principle be set free to use space as structure. She goes on:

> I realized the only dance I could live now is in this space. I began to dance to the music of primitive peoples. I discovered that my legs were not like the upper part of my body—what a terrible feeling—I'm only half a person, but to know I'm only half a person was not a small thing to me. I had visions of my legs moving like my arms to—so I sat down on the floor and decided I was going to work with my legs. It may take a while I thought but the vision of moving in space as a whole thing seemed worth working for. My gosh my legs felt like two pieces of sticks sticking out of my body. I had found a way for my hands to talk and tell me things, perhaps I could get my legs to do the same. I began to move the legs, letting them do whatever they wanted to do, being sure it was only the legs doing it. It was amazing to see how little they could do—they were so helpless that I was desperately sorry for them. They needed to be cared for like a child. To do this I needed my hands. Now another thought came to me. I had to find my hands first so I could take hold of my legs and help them out of the earth.

Something inside me jumped for joy when I discovered I have something to work with instead of something working with me.

And from another woman:

I feel most of the time a head and shoulders supported by legs that begin just south of my rib cage. This feeling of nothing in the middle has persisted through five different physical culture courses of one kind or another ...

She went on to speak of her husband as a natural born dancer, and I quote again:

... rhythm, flow, light, beautiful, sensitive. Me all these inside, but not connected up with the body. Infuriating to us both as I do feel it as keenly as he does ... he knows it and I do but it just can't get out. I know now why. It's because I haven't a body. It's that something in the middle that's lacking.... Bad balance and awkwardness I used to blame on feet. Now realize it's imbalance inside, and am convinced recently it's something missing in the middle.

The kinaesthetic sense can be awakened and developed in using any and all kinds of movement, but I believe it becomes conscious only when the inner, that is, the subjective connection is found, the sensation of what it feels like to the individual, whether it is swinging, stretching, bending, turning, twisting, or whatever. People can learn movement in a variety of ways; they are not necessarily enabled to feel it when they do so—it is the concrete, specific awareness of one's own act of moving which is so satisfying. The physical culture courses, of which our friend spoke, work with the body as object, not as subject; and while a general release takes place, there is not corresponding experience of the personal identity, its quality and its movement. This seems to mean that something more is needed than simply body mechanics, that the feelings hidden in the body, the source of all its movement, must be involved. People in general are not very interested in abdominal muscles, the diaphragm, the shoulder girdle and the pelvis, but they care deeply about the world in which they must find a way to live and about themselves who must do the living.

You will remember that much earlier I spoke of the ideal moment as the coming together of myself moving and myself being moved. There seems to be two extremes of people. I could describe them psychologically as those who are overwhelmed by the unconscious and those who are cut off from it. Physically, it seems to take the form, in the first instance, of general, overall movement vague in outline, a kind of swimming of the arms and hands particularly, a groping, floating quality, curiously disembodied and unreal. In watching it you have the feeling that it is happening by itself, that no one or almost no one is there doing it. (This is strange, too, because later as the physical awareness grows, one is quite unable to say what has changed. Much of the movement is similar but it becomes indefinably real, three dimensional and somehow in the body.) These people are most at ease when allowed to improvise freely. They do not like form or pattern or any different timing than the one they habitually use, and can only do a specific exercise at first if not required to be exact. In the early stages they seem to experience difficulty in connecting with any given part of the body—you have the impression that a message sent to the foot to move, for example, has to travel a long distance and that the foot responds like an alien thing, slowly, and with surprise at being asked.

At the other end of the scale are the people who cannot imagine a movement which they do not consciously initiate, on purpose, so to speak. They lay great emphasis on understanding exactly what they are doing, and are happiest in exercises, patterns, and forms. Sitting or lying quietly with their attention turned inward on their breathing affects them as boring and when they try to do it, their bodies jerk, their hands place and replace themselves, their shoulders twitch and they give the impression of being thoroughly miserable, restless, and ill at ease. Freedom to move as they please terrifies them because they "do not know what they are supposed to do" and if they do move they are apt to feel self-consciousness more than the movement itself.

When both kinds of people are in a group situation, it presents something of a challenge to the leader. The work has to include a given form for those who are unable to find a form of their own at the same time that they need to be encouraged to find the *feeling* potential of any movement. This is usually done by description of what the movement is like, of the sensation that belongs to it, and since no one image works for everyone, several must be tried. On the other hand, for the people who can only find the form through their feeling, descriptions of recognizable objects or actions provide a form into which the feeling can flow so that it takes an actual shape. Sometimes when both needs are met, the room is suddenly full of real people doing real movement, fully focused and alive.

For the people to whom movement just happens, through whom it pours without any consciousness of the ego's part in it, the liberating experience would be the discovery that "I am moving." Not long ago a young woman arrived in a state of utter confusion, lostness, and depression. She asked if she could talk, and I suggested that if it came to her to say something while she moved, so that it was part of her movement, part of the ritual for moving for herself, and not a conversation with me, it would then be movement, too. But it proved to be unnecessary. She went over and sat down on the rug. We used no music or other accompaniment. There followed what I can only describe as a quite miraculous birth of an actual body. There was a half smile on her face, which appeared very near the beginning and lasted all the way through. She stretched, twisted, touched her own feet and legs, stood up from a sitting position easily and without uncertainty, and went on stretching and bending through all her limbs and torso, finally taking, for her, firm steps on the whole foot into the space around her. When it was over, she opened her eyes and looking at me with the most complete and joyous amazement said, "Do you know what happened? As I sat down, I thought—if I had a body—and then I did."

For the people who are convinced that they do it all, the liberating experience is that "something moves me—I did not do it." The members of a class were improvising one night, individually, but all at the same time. Suddenly one girl who had been working very close to the floor, bounded to her feet and spun around with great rapidity. She was heavy and the movement was totally out of keeping with any I had ever seen her do—if I had asked her turn in that way, she could not have done it. Afterward she told me it was one of the most shocking things that had ever happened to her, she was completely unprepared, she did not know how it happened nor have any image of its happening—"It did itself."

A word about what this way of working with the body requires. There is necessary an attitude of inner openness, a kind of capacity for listening to one's self that I would call honesty. It is made possible only by concentration and patience. In allowing the body to move in its way, not in a way that would look nice, or that one thinks it should, in waiting patiently for the inner impulse, in letting the reactions come up exactly as they occur on any given evening (bear in mind that reactions *are* the movement)—new capacities appear, new modes of behavior are possible, and the awareness gained in the specialized situation goes over into a new sense of one's self driving the car, or stooping with the vacuum cleaner, or shaking hands with a friend. I know one woman who had never found it possible to talk back to her husband, As she discovered what it felt like to carry her body from the ground up, lifted in the middle, the legs firmly beneath her—instead of caved it, the shoulders and the head dropped forward to protect a retreating chest—she found she could no longer avoid speaking up for herself, even when it meant disagreement. She is not, incidentally, in analysis, so the connection is direct, without benefit of dreams.

It would take another paper to go into the question of dance, what it is and how these experiences are related to it, and still another to describe the use of movement as an adjunct to psychotherapy where it becomes a method of active imagination in which there is the possibility of dancing a dream situation and finding out, directly and inescapably (since it happens in the real, that is, the physical world, which is more primary than words and even than painting) a truth about that situation, or a change in it, or a further possibility that one had not known.

I am often asked whether what I am doing is therapy, and sometimes whether this is psychology or bodytraining or dance or what, and why I don't choose one and stick to it. To which I can only answer that any means to self-knowledge is therapy. If that is begging the question. I would be willing to say that I am engaged in professional therapy only insofar as my life, including my training, fits me to mediate experience which is therapeutic to the individual and not otherwise available to him. But it is not my experience and I do not do it. It is done in and by the body, strange as it sounds. As for the question of choice, the whole attempt is concerned with the connections between body and psyche, or between physical movement which is outer, and psychic events which are inner. I have ceased, very recently I must admit, plaguing myself with labels and explanations. I was enormously aided in this by two sentences from the Foreword to the *I Ching*. There, C. G. Jung says:

> Probably in no other field [psychotherapy] do we have to reckon with some many unknown quantities and nowhere do we become more accustomed to adopting methods that work, even though for a long time we may not know why they work. The irrational fullness of life has taught me never to discard anything, even when it goes against all our theories or other admits of no immediate explanation —

There are many other questions which cannot be touched in this space. What is the difference, if any, in a man's experience of his body and a woman's? How much interpretation by the leader or observer is desirable or necessary? Can any correlation be made between the basic concepts of Jungian psychology (persona, ego, shadow, anima, animus, the self, the personal and collective layers of the unconscious) and human movement? When an analysand is also working in movement, what exchange of information and material would be helpful, and would this require at least an introductory experience of his own movement on the part of the analyst? These things and many others wait to be investigated. One cannot even guess at the answers, but that there are answers I feel sure, and that they can help to increase our understanding of what man, in his totality, really is, seems equally certain.

And the Tao of the body? As an ancient sage said,

"Gravity is the root of lightness;
and stillness is the ruler of movement."

Gerda Alexander

Gerda Alexander, born in 1908 in Wuppertal, Germany, is the founder of one of the main modern schools of somatic work, Eutony. Eutony consists of a system of training designed to teach improved perceptual and motor control of posture and movement in everyday life and in the treatment of patients with neuromuscular disorders.

Eutony is part of the course of study in the music, theater, and physical education departments of nearly every major university in Western Europe. In Denmark, where Ms. Alexander makes her home, Eutony teachers are to be found in such diverse contexts as the Royal Conservatory of Music, textile factories, primary schools, institutions for the retarded, the Royal Danish Theatre, expectant mother programs, and physiotherapy schools.

Interview with Gerda Alexander

David Bersin

Bersin: You have been involved with human movement training and therapy since the early 1900s. Could you talk about your first experience and teachers?

Alexander: I was educated in the ideas of Jacques Dalcroze, known in English as Eurhythmic Education. He wanted a new education and development for mankind based on music and movement. His idea was that one should hear music and immediately express it in movement—not by improvising as is very often seen in dance schools, but in an exact following of rhythm dynamics, melody, phrasing and form, working with all the elements of music. He was a pupil of Bruckner and Delibes. While working as a conductor, composer and teacher at the Geneva Conservatory, he noticed that the students did not even feel the basic beat of what they played. They had to help themselves to keep time with their feet. This gave him the idea of helping students by letting them walk in different beats of the music and letting them move with the whole body. The director of the Conservatory thought it absolutely crazy to put music and movement together, of course, but the students felt they were improving their musicality. The students made enormous progress, and not exclusively in musicality. Dalcroze had touched a central point: experiencing music with their whole body in this way, the pupils were touched as a whole. For the students, doing music with intellect and emotions was not enough. The students became more open, better balanced, more creative and happy.

My first contact with Dalcroze's work was some photographs from

---

Somatics (Autumn/Winter 1983–84). 4–10

the first festival in Hellerau in 1911. Although I was only three years old, they impressed me very much. Before their marriage, my parent's were so taken by Dalcroze's new ideas they decided that their child should become a Dalcroze student. As soon as I could walk, I started to dance. My father, who was a good musician, played the piano every day. Even before I was born, I heard music, primarily Mozart, every day. Until the age of fourteen, I never fell asleep without hearing music by Mozart, Beethoven, etc. Later on, when I started to learn Dalcroze movements. I used to dance every evening to my father's playing. Since I danced all the time anyway, my parents avoided telling me about Dalcroze. However, when I started school, I heard about his courses. It took me a year to get my parents' permission to join these classes. Every morning, while my father was still asleep, I went to him asking, "Pa, may I go?" One morning, after a year, he got so angry he said, "Do as you like, but let me sleep!" So I enrolled myself in the Dalcroze school of Otto Blensdorf, where I stayed from 1915 to 1929.

Dalcroze's results became known in the musical world in 1904 when he presented a group of young musicians, trained in this way at an International Congress for new ways in art and school education in Hamburg. His presentation was a great success as well as a revolution. He was invited to demonstrate his work in the main towns in Germany and came in contact with the brothers Doorn. They tried to interest Dalcroze in participating in their project—creating an Art Craft Center in Hellerau, near Dresden. Dalcroze was to take over the artistic development of this new group, and at the same time open a center for musicians, actors, dancers and conductors for this new education of movement through music. The famous architect, Tessenow, built the theater for the yearly festivals of Dalcroze's performances. Very soon, students and artists from all over Europe and America came to Hellerau: conductors, Diaghilev (the head of the Russian Ballet), and great singers and musicians and painters. If you read the list of pupils from those years, you will find the names of all the important people of that time.

This growing work was interrupted by the first World War in 1914, The students returned to their own countries and tried to develop

Dalcroze's ideas of eurhythmic education all over the world. Dalcroze returned to Geneva and opened the Institute Dalcroze, and this institute still exists.

During the years after the first World War, I lived in Wuppertal, West Germany, a center for the development of modern free dance. My friends and I went to a performance or to a new dance premiere every day. I came in contact with all the different schools of modern dance at the great dance congresses, in which our school also participated. I also noticed, however, the limitations of these groups. In the hotel lobbies you could see the persons of the different schools—Wigman, Laban, Lobeland, Mensendieck, Kallmeyer, etc.—and every one of the had the same movement characteristics, typical of their group. Although their idea was to free the personality, they were nonetheless imitating their teachers' expression without expressing their own individuality, just as the ballet style was imitated in older time. Therefore, at a very early stage, I thought that there must something wrong in the pedagogy of these schools.

Bersin: Did Dalcroze use what he was doing with emotionally disturbed people or people with learning problems—with persons other than artists?

Alexander: At a very early stage, Dalcroze became interested in using eurhythmics for disturbed and handicapped children and for grownup patients. He was always interested in the physiological explanation of the musical influence, but at that time neurophysiology and psychology were not yet developed. In Jena, I became Charlotte Blensdorf's assistant and came in touch with many other modern ideas of free school education. I also worked with her at Stadtroda, the first German State Center for developing and educating mentally handicapped and anti-social children and adults, as well as criminals. I worked there for a year. There were about six hundred patients. Teachers, psychologists and helpers held daily meetings at which the effects of eurhythmics were clearly shown. I stayed in Germany, in Wuppertal, Jena and Bonn until 1929. Dalcroze's system was taught in all the large universities and music schools in Germany. Then, I moved to Denmark, having taken my final examinations in Berlin.

Bersin: What motivated you to move to Denmark?

Alexander: It happened by mistake. I was ill and had to give up dancing. My doctor told me that I probably would not survive, and if I did, I would be in a wheelchair for the rest of my life. They advised me to marry a rich man and live in a warm climate. I had this advice about a warm climate in mind when I was working as an assistant to Otto and Charlotte Blensdorf in the courses the school gave at the World Congress for "New Education Fellowship," under its president, Rabindranath Tagore, in Elsinore, Denmark. I thought that through this congress I might find work in a warm climate. At Elsinore, I was invited to give a course in Seeland, which I mistook to be New Zealand. I quickly said yes, not knowing the course was to be given in a part of Denmark called Seeland. It was a summer school for the teacher's training group for kindergarten teachers, and I continued with them in Copenhagen. At the same time I opened eurhythmic classes in Malmo, Sweden, and taught at the Swedish Gymnastics Institute in Lund. In Copenhagen, I also came in contact with singers and musicians at the conservatory and taught the Stanislavsky group which became the Private School for Actors. In 1932, I had been in contact with Germany's most outstanding scenographer, Leopold Jessner, the director of the Staatliches Schaupielhause in Berlin. He wanted all his actors to be trained by me. The contract was to begin in April, 1933, but in January, Hitler took over the regime in Germany. Most of the prominent artists, including Jessner, left the country. I realized that with such a catastrophic development in Germany, it was more important to work towards a new education, to develop the pedagogic work I had begun in 1926 in Jena, and to continue in Copenhagen than to follow my interests in the theater. In Copenhagen, I had taught around 800 children and teachers a week, and this gave me the possibility to influence the system of school education, which was not possible in the Nazi state; so, I decided to stay and work in Denmark.

Bersin: Was it around this period of time that you began to develop your own unique work which you have named "Eutony" or "Eutonia"?

Alexander: Yes, though I had it my mind for a long time—since my student's days. As I said, I had seen all that existed at that time in terms of movement development. Again and again I saw certain types of movement which only were imitative of the teacher or school. It seemed to me to be stereotyped movement, and not living movement which freed the personality. So, eutonic movements are never based on imitation. You stay away from all models, you are given the opportunity to find your own expression by working in a way that gives each person the possibility to experience expression his body's own capacity; its limits and long-forgotten or never experienced expression in his own rhythm. Thus, the student learns how to work with himself. I tried to find out how I could develop every person's own expression without programming him/her. At the same time, there was my personal need to learn how to survive. I needed to learn how to live a normal life with very little energy. I had to somehow learn to develop effort without strain, and in doing so discovered the need for relaxation—economy of action through using principles of bone structure and the postural reflexes. Through their own experiences, anybody can learn to know and use those principles in daily life.

Bersin: And "Eutony" means what?

Alexander: It actually comes from the Greek "*eu*" meaning "good" or "harmonious," and the Latin "*tonus*" meaning "tension." Eutony, then, means well-balanced tension.

Bersin: This brings us to the idea that seems very important to you, the idea of tonus, the distribution of tonus in the muscles.

Alexander: Yes. Tonus as a scientific reality was first explained in 1946 by two Swedish neurologists, Granit and Koda. But as long as man has existed, the tonus has been the system by which you feel and react. Tonus, the capacity of the muscle fibers to change their elasticity, happens in any kind of action. We use high tonus for effort, and medium tonus or low tonus for rest and sleep. In Eutony, we learn to use the best tonus for the action in question. It's interesting to note that when you just *think* of making a movement, just have the *intention* to do it, you change the tonus and circulation of your body, even before the movement is physically done. Tonus changes occur not only with different kinds of effort, but with every emotional change as well, ranging from deep depression with a low tonus, to happiness with a high tonus. This function is called psycho-tonus. Flexibility in tonus change is also the basis for all artistic creation and experience. The orchestra conductor who does not adapt his tonus to the demands of the actual music is not capable of giving a message to his musicians and to his audience. In these instances, listeners hanging on the edge of their chairs miss the experience of freeing unnecessary inner tensions and opening up for the life art can give. What you do not experience in your whole body will remain merely intellectual information without life or spiritual reality. Every social communication remains superficial if you cannot suffer or be happy with others. This adaptation is the basis for Eutony therapy, and also the basis for a real and living contact with your surroundings.

Bersin: So tonus is the way we regulate how we interact with the world?

Alexander: Yes, at all levels—social, artistic, cultural, therapeutic, and in every physical action. The work with tonus regulation and flexibility is so central, so crucial in Eutony. It touches the whole person.

Bersin: Could you clarify how you see the idealized person, and their ability to regulate their tonus?

Alexander: Nature has given us the capacity of tonus adaptation from the first stage of prenatal life where the child lives in total tonus adaptation with its mother—a stage which continues during the first years after birth. The child can also adapt to its mother's tonus state at a distance. Provided that there is no tonus fixation through bad posture or bad movement patterns, through emotional fixation, or through too low or high tonus in the organism, all this adaptation works generally at an unconscious level. To recover the living adaptation of our whole person, we must become aware of the fixations by putting our attention on all the different levels of tonus adaptation. By doing this, the whole range of experience widens and deepens, and creativity opens up. This is the goal of the Eutony work. You see, deep relaxation is only one part of the whole scale. In deep relaxation you are out of contact with the outer world and end by being disconnected with your body as well. That's fine, but for daily life you need to have access to any situation on every level and in all circumstances.

Bersin: I've heard you describe a relationship between hypotonus and certain kinds of characterological traits, and hypertonus and certain kinds of characterological traits.

Alexander: Yes, if your tonus is too low, you can be so low that the inner organs hardly function at all, and you may have a hormonal depression. A fixation of too high a tonus will make you restless, sleepless and irritable, and this, naturally, will overwork the heart. With depressive patients, we have obtained very good results through working on the bony structure. By administering vibrations which enable patients to feel the transport of anti-gravity forces in their organism, they often change their emotional state in a few minutes. This is one of the fascinating results with tonus change. I could not have imagined such results, but found them by chance. This gave me the interest to work with Eutony in therapy. At the beginning of my teaching, I worked solely with people who were music or movement oriented. Often they told me they felt changed in their way of living. They were less irritated, happier, and their families noticed the change, too. I did not discuss their psychological problems with them, but could see that working to liberate the tonus fixations influence the whole person—bodily, emotionally and spiritually. The students' dreams changed, too, even in persons who had gone through verbal analysis. To me, this proved that even the unconscious is touched by Eutony.

Bersin: So then you began to use the work more and more in therapy?

Alexander: Yes, I had many psychologists and psychiatrists among my pupils, so I got the patients with whom they did not succeed. I got all the cases I had never dreamed I would work with which gave me a broad range of possibilities for the application of Eutony principles. For five years I worked at the University of Copenhagen, and occasionally in the neurological clinic. The professor who invited me to work there got much resistance from the other doctors and physical therapists because we got very good results in a very short time. You see, I had to find out what was really wrong with these cases, why they did not function. The reasons were often unexpected—not to be understood from the diagnosis given by the hospital—yet, by working with the basic regulation of tonus and circulation, the symptoms soon disappeared. In Eutony, every lesson is based on the reality of the student's difficulties and never repeated in the same way. Our goal is to make the person capable of adapting to the reality of the moment.

Bersin: Let's talk more concretely about the pedagogy of Eutony. There are different aspects to your work, and perhaps the most general aspect is bringing the person into greater awareness and contact with himself. From what I've read, this seems to be the groundwork of Eutony.

Alexander: Yes, that is the basis of Eutony. We call this state "presence," consisting of awareness of mind, sensation of the outer form of the body, in contact with the surroundings, awareness of breathing, circulation, tissues, inner space with organs and bones.

Bersin: Were there any other significant influences on you during this early period of Eutony?

Alexander: I was very much influenced by the school of Clara Schlaffhorst and Hedwig Andersen, the Rothenburg school. They were two singers who had lost their voices. Through their own research, they looked at the basic function of the voice in connection with the whole organism, and also in connection with breathing and movement. Though I achieved more strength, I could not agree with some of their basic rules. For example, one rule stated that one should always move in rhythm with the breathing. I felt that it was impossible to apply that rule in daily life, and especially in art. In an opera, if the singer waits with his aria until his breathing impulse is coming, the orchestra will have gone ahead. Still, their way of stimulating breathing and circulation through a light, swinging movement had inspired me to find the importance of the anti-gravity forces and the postural reflexes for free flexible posture, and every for great efforts. At my school, we now talk about "transport" of force triggered by our own weight on the feet—going through the bone structure and the tissues from the legs up to the small pelvis ring, to the upper part of the sacrum, through all vertebrae bodies and the ribs up to the atlas. We look at ideal posture as being given by reflexes from the feet up to the head through the bone structure, needing neither contraction from the great outer muscles of the back, nor an isolated regulation of the position of the head. It took me years of observation to come to this conclusion. It's interesting that the scientific explanation for this basic principle in Eutony came only ten years ago: the discovery of the mechanoreceptor system with four different receptors reacting on different levels of pressure in every joint capsule of the articulation and in the skin.

Bersin: It seems to me that many schools take awareness as a discipline in itself, where for you, it's always awareness in relationship to the environment and awareness in relationship to other human beings.

Alexander: Yes, but on the basis of the awareness of your own person, your own form, your own inner space with the invisible radiation zone of your own bone structure. In your contact with your surroundings, you stay as much as possible in yourself and then you widen your awareness towards other objects through other materials or other persons. You see, with all this, what I want is to make it possible for everybody to experience the reality of the spiritual part of themselves here and now, included in our body, in connection with the spiritual part of the universe. That is a reality we can get more and more aware of—consciousness about our body in all details as a manifestation of spiritual creation. Spirit is always present, it does not exist only when you meditate or pray.

The next step after becoming more in touch with the surroundings is noticing the distance from side to side to find the outer form of your body, and to become aware of the inner space without waiting for a special experience. If you put enough attention to the inner space, you can suddenly have the experience of the reality of the skeleton, of your inner organs, of the flow and the wholeness of circulation, or suddenly you feel your heart and lungs present by themselves. This experience comes most unexpectedly, perhaps after years of clear awareness of your inner space. This phenomenon of presentation of skeleton and inner organs is part of the maturation of the person. It's a development you cannot force. Everybody has to take his own time for maturation, and if you feel the resistance of the person, you know that he or she is not ready, not sure enough of his/her own reality and inner security. At some point, they have security in themselves, a security which is greatly connected with the experience of their bone structure, of their skeleton. Once they have this basic experience, they can let go the resistance. I am very much against the aggressive way to attack a person practiced by many of the Reichian and post-Reichian schools. They believe they can force maturation. In fact, the results are not long-lasting. I never met Wilhelm Reich personally, but I learned from the patients who came to me after he had left Denmark never to break down a person's resistance. You yourself may feel great as a powerful person, but with this attitude you only weaken the other person still more. You do not help him to stand on his own feet, to liberate himself to find his own security. This is a rule for all Eutony pedagogy and therapy. Inner maturation has its own laws and is never reached by overwhelming the person with outer pressure.

Bersin: I agree with you that a person's sense of security is connected with their experience of the skeleton, and recently I've become interested in the psychological importance of the skin. The skin is the membrane or boundary by which we differentiate ourselves from the outer world, and may be the medium with which we begin to develop a body self-image.

Alexander: Yes, this awareness of the skin is so important. A sense of self begins with this differentiation between the surroundings and the outer skin, and gives a basic body security. In our work with dancers, physical therapists, and all kinds of people working with the body, we see how poorly their body image has developed. Even among people whose profession it is to work with the body—medical doctors, physiotherapists, etc.—I have never seen anybody who had a complete body image. Really, it doesn't exist.

Bersin: Would you describe the dancer's self-image as very flat, unidimensional?

Alexander: Yes, very often ballet dancers, who are used to training before a mirror, will make a body image with clay by putting the clay against the floor flatly and forming the human being as a relief. You can be almost certain that a person who forms such a body has danced ballet in his childhood, or is a professional dancer. I created this body image test using modeling clay by chance. In a group of professional students, I noticed that their drawings of certain control positions, even when they drew stick figures, always showed the body form typical of the person who drew it. So one day I asked the whole group to model with clay some control positions without explaining my reason. There I obtained confirmation: Everybody made his own body. In my book, *The Discovery of the Total Person,* you can see some exquisite examples of my collection of drawings and modelings. These facts have something to do with a missing link in our culture—we do not have enough real experience with our bodies. I think in other cultures it would be different. The only group in Europe I saw with complete body images were my Greek pupils. Perhaps this was because they jumped into the sea several times a day.

Bersin: That gives a more three-dimensional experience?

Alexander: Yes, they feel the skin as a totality of the volume. There was really not one of those pupils who was missing the outer skin.

Bersin: You differentiate a lot in your book between touch and contact. Could you describe that?

Alexander: There's a world in between: if you touch, and you hold your attention only on the limit of your outer skin, or if you contact the other through his skin into the deeper part of his organism, you obtain two different results. The latter can attack and stimulate other organisms and give the other person missing vitality; the first, where one only touches the outer skin of the other person, we call "neutrality." With neutrality, you give the other organism the possibility to liberate his contractions in his inner space and open up his own radiation zone. These are two very different ways of helping another person. When you help the other person by your own will, you invade him and usually make him even more tense. It is very important to begin all treatment with this in mind: what does the other body need? If you give too much, you press the other back to his own limit and you reinforce his state of hypertension. If you widen up into your organism for the outer space of the other, you help to relieve him profoundly. In cases where the person has less vitality, you can stimulate through contact, and at the same time observe the needs of the other. It is a constant dialogue between two organisms. This form of treatment needs long training to be capable of controlling the actions of the other organism and of yourself. It calls for respect for the other person, not to make him dependent on your help.

Bersin: I know you use contact a lot in your group and have people interacting in movement.

Alexander: We begin by studying contact with the floor, with bamboo sticks, instruments, clay, with everything we touch in our daily life. To touch and make contact with another person is only allowed when you are balanced in yourself. Usually, with daily training, being balanced in yourself comes at the end of the second or third year, although it often takes longer. Afterwards, you can make contact with more than one body, a real contact with every member of a whole group. This group contact should be in Eutonic movement, where they create a form and expression together.

Bersin: Being able to regulate tonus and to maintain one's balance is a prerequisite.

Alexander: That is absolutely necessary. If balance within oneself is not established first, it causes many disturbances, and the pupils fall back into imitating movement patterns instead of opening up to free creation. But when that *is* established, it is a gift, a wonderful moment, to become able to move and to improvise movement forms together as a whole, where everybody is in contact with everybody. We work toward this state from the beginning. In their weekly studies, the students have the opportunity to make their personal research of a given task at the different levels of movement development—alone, with two, later with a group—creating together movement forms which can be repeated. At this level we touch all hidden psychological difficulties of each person; for every part of the organism, every hidden resistance of the person is touched.

Bersin: So I gather that you don't, in the course of the studies, deliberately bring people into a regression—it's something that comes from within themselves?

Alexander: Yes, the moment they are ready for it. If they are not ready, we do not force them. The reaction from the other members of the group helps the person better understand his/her own fixation.

Bersin: It must take some time for an individual to develop this type of awareness.

Alexander: Yes, but the awareness is stabilized, and does not fall back. To become a help to others, you must have solved your own problems. Sometimes this process is finished in four years, sometimes not, so the students stay in contact with the school for a longer time. The school can only give them a basis for their own work on themselves, and here lies the difference between Eutony and other body work. It's not only mastering a movement technique, but coming into the depth of your self and growing towards a total person. It's a maturation process.

Bersin: There's third aspect of your work, which is working with people who have limitations in their movement. We would call this a hands-on approach, even though I understand that you're just barely making contact. What kind of people do you work with?

Alexander: I personally have not treated very many strokes, but my pupils have. I have worked with people paralyzed from polio—old cases, twenty to thirty years after the acute phase, where no movement is possible. I think it would be much easier to begin work soon after the infection is over, but we have people who have not been able to move for thirty years, and in a short time, they succeed. The same is true with paraplegics and quadriplegics.

Bersin: Do these people join your groups, or just have individual treatments?

Alexander: Both. The results are much faster if we can combine group work with treatments. Especially for the paraplegics, it is a wrong idea to treat only the paralyzed parts. They need all the basic work with touch and inner space. First of all, they have to normalize the circulation. If you try to make too much effort in weak muscles, you disturb the circulation. Instead, try to use the wholeness of whatever movement is still possible. I prefer to let the patients participate in normal groups, and they make unexpectedly quick process. The body then gets the chance to find the motor units that are still capable of functioning. We train them to *intend* movement they really can't do. The intention changes tonus and circulation. A person can clearly prove the difference in the weight of the body if they will turn the paralyzed person, and then turn him when he intends to make the movement himself. You will see from day to day the amelioration of the disability and new movement patterns. In paraplegics, the sensation is mostly missing. In private lessons, we do more helping with our hands, using different possibilities of pressure and light touch of skin to awaken circulation, thereby beginning superficial and deep-lying sensation. We do this also through vibration. We delicately vibrate the skin, bones, tendons, and muscles. For paralyzed patients, we use special contact with the skin to stimulate the mechanoreceptors to help restore a complete body image. My first paraplegic patient was a director from the Copenhagen Broadcasting House. He was burned deeply on his thigh. He couldn't feel anything if you pressed against his skin. These wounds had been several months old and couldn't heal. I first used contact with his skin surface without touching him, using only the communication though the radiation zone, and the would healed in three or four weeks. He got one private lesson weekly, and worked daily by himself on his whole circulation and skin contact. It is absolutely necessary to stimulate the patient to work daily several times to get him to feel responsible for the healing process.

Bersin: Has your wealth of experience led you to certain notions about how the brain functions? Obviously, you were restoring functions with people about whom a doctor would say, "This person is going to spend the rest of their life without being able to walk."

Alexander: You know, I would always say: "Try to adapt to the situation. Try out what is still possible, what is still functioning in the organism." Everyone reacts differently, and we always have to try what is possible. The body is in itself organized to recover, so if you help the circulation to normalize, and recover the sensitivity by stimulating the skin, then the body begins to recover in its own way. The brain needs stimulation from the body.

Bersin: And when you are working with people individually, if people remember a situation or feelings from their early life, do you take the time to let them speak?

Alexander: Yes, if they talk spontaneously, but we only interface if they ask us directly. Otherwise, we hear often what a person speaks, thinking aloud, without being conscious of it. Usually, we try not to interpret it. Sometimes you can support them in what they are saying, sometimes you only remain open to them without criticism, only listening honestly, so the person feels he/she is accepted. I think it is more important to help a person to find the origin of his/her difficulties, it makes the student more independent.

Bersin: What is your experience with people who've worked in Eutony for some time and then gone into some psychotherapeutic work? Do you feel that perhaps the Eutony opens them to a certain place where they can benefit more from psychotherapy?

Alexander: Yes. That is surely dependent on their own difficulties, though. Some problems need verbalization—but we have had people who go through analysis, and yet they felt they touched much deeper layers in their unconscious the moment they worked with their bodies—layers they didn't reach with verbal analysis. If trauma comes early, even prenatal, then Eutony is more helpful. All prenatal trauma experiences come from preverbal influences, but conflicts which arise after the preverbal period need verbalizing. All influences in the preverbal time are received though the body, through the sensibilities of the mother's tonus, which is imitated by the child. If you work on these problems, the verbalizing does not enter deeply enough, doesn't touch the sources. We have again and again seen people going through the long analysis and therapies—Freudian, Jungian, and others—and when they begin with Eutony, completely new dreams and rememberings come up from the unconscious from the preverbal period. To have a trained psychotherapist who is also a professional Eutonist, that would be the idea. I've talked to the French analyst, Madame Dolto. We met at a world psychodrama congress in Paris in 1964. She agrees with my idea that if the preverbal experiences are satisfying and don't cause a trauma, the person generally has enough resistance to overcome difficulties later in life. That is also the explanation for our results with neurotic persons, working without any verbalizing. With Eutony, the symptoms disappear and the person is standing on his own feet and is then capable of solving his own problems.

Bersin: Have psychotherapists always been interested in your work?

Alexander: Yes, since the beginning of the school in Copenhagen. I had pupils who were psychiatrists. The first was the neurologist, Thorkild Vangaard. Dr. Vangaard, who was educated here in America as a psychoanalyst, became the head of the Freudian group in Denmark. I personally had very little sympathy for this form of analysis, but after reading Freud's *Lectures*, I had the idea that it might be possible to use the psychic energies manifested in hysteria for healing. Later, when I read the work of Jung, I felt the connection between his work and Eutony. Jung got interested in Eutony through the parents of one of his students, and followed her development for many years. He invited me several times to see him in Zurich. I didn't go, because I thought I had to know and understand more about his work. In any case, he seems to have understood my work, so I always feel very connected to his approach.

Bersin: In some ways, in reading your book, I identified more and more with what we would call free education—free schools like Summerhill.

Alexander: Well, I was invited to give Eurhythmic and Eutony lessons in 1934 to the pupils of Summerhill through my friend Elna Lucas, a specialist in children's analysis. Neill had his first school in Hellerau before 1914—at the same time Dalcroze worked there. As we talked the first day about lessons, A. S. Neill told me, "My boys here, they never will listen to classical music; all they want is jazz." As I couldn't teach with jazz music, I devised a little test. I saw a piano in the big room as we were waiting for tea, so I began to play a little. After a time, the door opened and a boy came and sat down on the floor and listened. After a while, a second came, and so on until I had at least 20 boys and girls sitting around listening to my music when Neill came in for tea. He was absolutely astonished to see them all quietly listening to classical music. As I ended, one asked, "Was that Bach? That's so beautiful." The next day, they all came to the rhythmic lesson and they liked it—even without jazz.

Bersin: Did you ever work with Elsa Gindler?

Alexander: No. I was only once allowed to see a lesson. This was in Berlin. I was sixteen, and came too late to her lesson. I was terribly shy, but at last I decided to open the door and glide to a seat nearby. In the middle lesson, Elsa Gindler said to all the pupils: "If you are shy, you should always think, 'the other is just as a great a donkey as I am.'" After the lesson, we spoke some words together, but not a word about my coming too late. Gindler's advice about a donkey helped me very often in my life. In 1957, I wrote to her and told her how many times in my life I've been thankful to her for this good advice and that I would like to talk to her in Gstaad about an invitation to give a workshop in Copenhagen. So I went to Gstaad on a free day from my yearly summer courses in France. I was also to talk with Heinrich Jacobi to whom I had sent a young gifted music pedagogue who got a stipend for half a year study. I told him the best advice I had to give him was to work with Jacobi. I had to take a train at 4:00 in the morning to arrive at Gstaad at 10:00, the time Jacobi had given me. I could tell a long story about this meeting. Jacobi, who was also a pupil of Dalcroze, let me wait one hour and a half and was very cross with me that I had sent this pupil as he only wanted to work with persons who wanted to change their lives completely. Well, everybody has a right to choose their pupils, and we finished as friendly and still good colleagues. Then I saw Elsa Gindler, who told me that she had got my letter, but she didn't want to work with persons who taught gymnastics. So . . . Gstaad is a beautiful place, and I enjoyed my lunch in a beautiful garden in the open air.

Bersin: Did you ever meet Mary Wigman?

Alexander: Yes. You could feel her charisma the moment you entered the theater. She was originally a Dalcroze student also, though influenced by the ideas of Rudolph Laban. Laban was married to one of the first Dalcroze teachers and she is still teaching today in Zurich. Laban went to England after the war where his work for free movement got included in school education. I think Irmgard Bartenieff worked with him at that time. Laban has been the great creator of dance without music. I agree with his idea that if you move only to music, it is difficult to develop your own expression. For this reason, we use music in our Eutony studies only after we have developed our own dynamics and our own intentions. This is at a late stage in our studies. After Mary Wigman met Laban, she used music very rarely. Her great creations for herself and her group of dancers had only percussion accompaniment. She came back to music only at the end of her career, and her creation to Bach's music was one of the greatest impressions of my life. It was beautiful. In the beginning, I saw her at the International Dance Congresses. but during the last period of her life, I met her several times in Athens in the home of my friend Zouzou Nicoloudi, the dancer and choreographer who had made the festivals for classical Greek drama, with her music and choreography in Herodes Atticus in Delphi and Epidaurus. She is a pupil of the Dalcroze school in Athens, and later she studied with Rosalia Chladeck (another Dalcroze teacher and dancer). Nicoloudi was a great friend of Wigman's who came to see Nicoloudi every year. There she saw the film made of my school. She understood the meaning of Eutony at once, and was moved to tears. She said: "If I had seen your work before, I would have changed many things in my life."

Eutony: The Holistic Discovery
of the Total Person (Excerpts)

Gerda Alexander

The Principles of Eutony

Even if it were possible, it is not my intention to describe all aspects
of Eutony in this book. Such an attempt would fail because Eutony is
in no way a special system to be practiced separately from everyday
life. Eutony keeps one in constant contact with all aspects and realities. It concerns the healthy person just as much as the sick one, the
sportsman just as much as the dancer, the intellectual as much as the
physical worker. I have given particular emphasis to those aspects of
my work which I consider to be essential and which at the same time
are fundamentally different from and contrary to other systems of
individual and body development.

Let us recall briefly some of the principles of Eutony in order to
clarify this assertion. First, it should be remembered that release from
tension, one aspect of the control of tonus, constitutes in fact only a
partial aspect of Eutony. Eutony depends on conscious tactile perceptions and the development of both superficial and deep sensitiv-
ities. Eutony avoids any teaching by suggestion. Eutony also avoids
active breathing exercises, but works through indirect action on the
autonomic nervous system. Eutony's teachings are based on the uncov-
ering of the personal biorhythms of each student by the setting of
tasks for which he must find his own solutions without following a
set of patterns. Personal awareness in contact with the environment,
a vital aspect of Eutony, is developed from the beginning. Physical
touch and contact between two persons requires prior regulation and

Great Neck, NY: Felix Morrow, 1985.7–33

control of the tonus in order not to harm the partner by transferring one's personal way of behaving or any psychological or psychosomatic disturbances. Thus the practice of Eutony helps one to be open and receptive to others without diminishing one's individuality. This is in contrast to other methods which use mental suggestion, regulated control of the breathing process, the setting of patterns to follow, and fixed rhythms of action or directed forms of meditation. In this book, I have, in fact, tried deliberately to present only the principles and not the practice of Eutony.

I have separated the principles from the practice because a presentation of a series of exercises, such as one usually finds in instruction books, teaching breath control, would very probably result in errors or misinterpretation when no teacher is available for expert supervision. Experience shows that the same exercises, apparently carried out in the same manner by a number of people, result for the most part in different kinds of experience. All students naturally react in a different way depending on their personal history and culture, prejudices and unconscious inhibitions.

Action is the result of conscious or unconscious stimulus. It cannot be reduced to a series of independent movements, as if the body were merely being directed by outside factors. Traditional gymnastics do in fact make possible a more-or-less perfect execution of a set of movements. But such exercises have only a limited significance: nothing essential happens within the person. These types of training have nothing in common with Eutony, because Eutony depends, on the contrary, on restoring and increasing the capacity for conscious individual awareness.

Sensations and observation are different types of perception—it is necessary for them to interact one with the other. In order to achieve a deep relationship with oneself, with another person, and with the environment, it is necessary to experience one's total person consciously in stillness, in movement, and in contact with the physical environment. My long experience in many countries has taught me that a predominantly abstract training does indeed increase intellectual responsiveness, but at the same time it encourages the trend toward self-centered imagination; the result may be purely intellectual without any reference to physical reality. Such abstract and imaginative concepts are an expression of the inability to remain present within an actual situation and to achieve conscious sensations. The tendency to emphasize intellectual considerations rather than felt experiences frequently places people outside the reality.

The teacher can distinguish easily between a student who is really working in the eutonic manner and is totally present and one who is merely pretending. The constant correlation between the total person and the environment is, from our point of view, the indispensable prerequisite for a conscious awareness of reality which is basic to achieving a healthy state. To learn to feel oneself consciously in relation to the environment, and to be able to cope with the stress and strain of everyday life, are benefits obtainable by Eutony.

One should best start along this path with the help of a teacher. If a teacher is not available, then the prerequisite for independent work is the ability to discover by oneself, through one's own authentic bodily experiences, the true sense of conscious sensation which forms the basis of Eutony.

I have emphasized the astonishing significance of the skin as an organ, as a living envelope, with countless nerve-links throughout the whole organism. Contact through the skin, which gives us information about the outer world, makes us aware simultaneously of the essentials about ourselves. What we touch also touches us. This interaction, which influences blood and lymph circulation, breathing and metabolic processes as well as the muscle tonus, is the source of the reassuring sensations of oneness and well-being which the work on "touch" and "contact" taught in Eutony makes possible.

The work of "contact" which we propose produces immediate effects. It develops a sensitivity which reveals a part of ourselves and in so doing helps us to discover our physical, mental and spiritual oneness.

To this end, the basic exercises represent a very favorable starting point for discoveries. One must not, however, try indiscriminately to feel everything which our body touches. When we learn the distinctive qualities of the touch of clothing on the body, or sense surrounding objects in a global perception of the body in its environment, this situation already presents many opportunities for personal discoveries. Whoever is successful in realizing that presence to himself is a reality, soon perceives that "touching" reveals a wealth of working perspectives without endangering the psychosomatic equilibrium.

All these personal discoveries are now supported scientifically by discoveries such as that of the fusimotor nerve system by Granit and Koda (1946) and the work of Barry Wyke, M.D. England (1977), which have provided explanations and scientific proof. History teaches us that many discoveries often receive scientific corroboration long after the empirically discovered facts have become known. Today's knowledge of different disciplines and modern research makes possible new forms of scientific cooperation and the formulation of fundamentally new concepts.

In writing this book I have constantly tried to express my ideas as simply as possible, and to place the accent on a way of working, and an attitude, which everyone can incorporate into everyday life. To express oneself simply does not mean to simplify. The primary is often of the greatest importance, as in making every sense organ feel as vividly as it did in the first contacts a child has with the world.

Gradually the physiological sciences are discovering interactions which explain the extraordinary effectiveness of Eutony, pedagogy and therapy. Certain discoveries with respect to the structure and function of the nervous system have provided Eutony with scientific support of which it has made extensive use. Twenty-five years ago, it was not clear how we could succeed in restoring to some paralyzed patients, whose motor nerve paths were destroyed (considered indispensable for locomotion) their ability to walk through making them conscious of their reflex mechanisms. There remained nothing more for us to say than to paraphrase irreverently the words of the great Galileo: "And yet it moves." Eutony helps the individual to discover the possibilities contained within his biological reality and to adapt himself in a continuous constant, dynamic and creative process to the wholeness of life.

The effects of a responsiveness reduced by tensions and restraints are well known today. When a situation requires a response which exceeds our capabilities, a kind of panic takes over and we behave like a kicked dog which does not know whether to bite or run away. In the last analysis, certain forms of opposition are only an admission of importance and are not a sign of greater freedom. Henri Wallon[1] showed brilliantly that the emotions and muscular tonus influence each other. That explains the importance of the ability to react to life and other people in full possession of a total adaptability of the muscles tonus and not to overreact or not react; it must also be said that not only hypotonic and hypertonic persons are restricted in their emotional life. Anyone who is fixed in an intermediate muscle tonus is equally limited. We have sometimes described responsiveness, which is made possible by the maximum adaptability of the tonus, by the expression "to be in order." This does not mean being subjugated to an external order but, on the contrary, having control over a maximum of possible responses, both in social as well as in personal areas. In this way a latitude of freedom is attained without which neither potential for expression or creativity are possible. We also know that the limits set by a rigid structure are among the main causes of our difficulties in communicating with our fellow men. Since Eutony depends on permanent contact with the environment, it enables the individual not only to discover himself but it also contributes at the same time to break down the barriers of his natural isolation.

After the first working steps, the essential components of Eutony—the training, the rehabilitation, and even the therapy embedded in the interpersonal and general dynamics between the individual and his environment—may not be immediately obvious to an outside observer or a beginner. However, careful observation of group processes shows the vital importance of these first steps. To give only one example: is it not of fundamental importance for a student to discover, after his first session of Eutony, that his sense of perception and his experience of the world and himself are frequently quite different from those of his neighbor and can even be in conflict? This reaction is neither right nor wrong and contains no element of judgment, but is a step toward personal independence and to the recognition of basic differences between people.

It is of equal importance to a person working in a group to discover by means of a simple object, such as a bamboo rod, that it is also possible to relate to ever-new situations by a continuous mutual adjustment in group action without guidance.

What the students experience during their session of movements and what they express verbally at the end of their work often reveals unexpected depths. Even their words seem to take on an expressive and communicative force. What they previously expressed in the form of mimicry and preconceived attitudes is thus conveyed clearly across all linguistic boundaries.

This relationship between body expression and speech, a sign of a subtle encounter between the manifestations of consciousness and unconsciousness, happens all too seldom in daily life; such encounters are all the more important as a preparation for achieving a unity of the total person. Eutony originated in Western Europe and opened up to people—particularly the sick—the possibility of experiencing the present consciously and meaningfully. It allows people to detect unnatural methods and limitations. This is essential if people want to preserve that force which enables them to work toward spiritual development and future progress. Eutony is relevant to the problems and needs of our time.

As to the spiritual movement to which Eutony belongs, it is a part of the great flow of ideas and research which has distinguished the twentieth century. Another book, however, would be required to demonstrate this relationship precisely. Were I to try to describe the ideas which guided me, I would draw attention to the relationship between Eutony and the creativity which developed in Europe and the United States of America after the First World War toward a new pedagogy and whose representatives joined together in the New Education Fellowship. I came into contact with leading exponents of these new educational ideas through studying at the Dalcroze Rhythmics School of Otto Blensdorf, one of the first followers of Emile Jaques-Dalcroze, and his daughter Charlotte Blensdorf-Mac-Jannet. I was especially inspired by my working experiences at the first Science of Education Institute at the University of Jena, under the direction of Peter Petersen, and also by my experiences in the first free schools and kindergartens in Denmark.

Although I pursued the ideas and research of the times with inward sympathy, I always kept myself free from dependence on any fixed theory or established school. This striving after spiritual and professional independence is in fact a part of my personal history. I had an inner urge to find new paths and forms of expression. My state of health on entering professional life—heart troubles resulting from rheumatic fever—supplied me with the necessary motivation. My natural way of being kept me from being completely involved in the spiritual movements of that time. It was only in this way that I succeeded, over the course of years, in creating and developing a new conception of work.

I hesitated to write this book, whether from an apprehension that what should be a discovery made anew each day could become rigidly structured, or because of the difficulties of expressing in words the nature of inner experiences, which are our basic tools in Eutony pedagogy, and the danger that this living, unique and changing process would get deformed into a mechanical technique.

For it is characteristic of the practice of Eutony, that everyone experiences it differently, as a path by which life reveals itself. The unity for which it strives is brought into being through the interplay of countless internal and external forces which allow each of us to achieve a dynamic equilibrium in continuously new ways. It is an illusion to believe that one can, for example, train individual capacities in isolation by movement education and then afterward unite the individual parts into a whole without losing the body-soul unity which is the object of movement. This insight came to me early, when I discovered the barriers great artists had erected for themselves as a result of strictly stereotyped training.

Can one help man find again the source of his spontaneity, can one awake in him the desire to create in the various artistic areas, in drawing, in painting, in music, and in movement? Valuable aid in discovering oneself and acquiring self-knowledge is available to us through free movement improvisations which lead to the creation of one's own style of movement within the framework of established forms and so release spontaneity. In cooperation with a partner and a group, we experience social behavior. We learn to accept the other person in his uniqueness of feeling and to adjust to him without loss of our individuality. It would be valuable if many adolescents could make use of such opportunities, to the investigation of which I have devoted a lifetime of work. In this area, a constant reference to reality is of paramount importance as the main source of personal spontaneity and its objectification.

The way in which you realize yourself is unique. If you do not undertake the quest of finding your own way, you run the risk of losing yourself. One of the essential elements in the shaping of our destiny is developing the capacity of managing ordinary life situations. It is the fundamental outlook of Eutony that relates it to the great spiritual movements of the twentieth century, leading to a new culture.

The attempt to experience being in one's wholeness, starting from a living contact and from experiencing the environment, stands in relationship to the fundamental thinking of the new pedagogy as the path to self-awareness through complete trust or confidence toward men and all the phenomena of life. Yet another thing becomes clear from this parallel between Eutony and the new pedagogy: the respect for the individual. The similarity between Eutony and the new pedagogy consists in their shared rejection of any standardization and any ritualized pattern of gestures or mechanization of movements or of any coercive aims.

This presupposes that the main role in eutonic training devolves upon the students. They must make their own discoveries and work toward their own development. Training and reintegration into everyday life are therefore, above all, the concern of the students and not of the teacher, whose role consists mainly in orientating their work

Eutony is by no means a method in the traditional sense of the work, but offers man a new approach toward life. The specific ways which Eutony offers and which today form a coherent plan, are a new holistic way for an integral education and further development.

What Is Eutony?

The word Eutony, from the Greek prefix *eu* meaning good, well, harmonious, and the Latin *tonus*, meaning tension, was adopted for my work for the first time in 1957. Tonus is the level of tension of all striated and smooth muscle fibers in the body. Such fibers are controlled by the peripheral nervous system and other physiological regulators such as the limbic system and the reticular formation, all of which can be affected by a person's psychological condition.

Eutony is a Western way of experiencing the unity of the total person. This feeling of unity and integrity liberates the creative forces and develops the capacity of contact with others without losing individuality. This totality manifests itself though the body's autonomic and motor nervous system. The autonomic nervous system creates a balance between the sympathetic and parasympathetic nervous systems, establishes stimulus and regeneration in the organs, and influences physical functions such as circulation, the basic metabolism and breathing. The motor nervous system controls voluntary movements throughout the spinothalamic and dorsal column. Through these two functional systems, both the conscious and unconscious parts of the body are made manifest. Our posture and movements, the way we breathe and speak, are all expressions of our physical, emotional and mental states and are in turn influenced by them. A change in our awareness can influence these life manifestations and functions, and a malfunction in any of them can affect our physical conditions, emotions and our awareness—that is to say, our whole behavior.

The different functional systems in the living organism cannot be separated from each other. They interlock and influence each other without being aware of it. Just as in music where the elements of melody, harmony, rhythm, dynamics and form can be perceived separately, leading to a deepened appreciation of music, so can our distinguishing between the individual parts of the body lead to a deepened awareness of the whole person.

In Eutony, the general involuntary tonus regulation and the autonomic balance can be consciously influenced. In the beginning we develop awareness and sensation of the body surface, then of the inner space, including bone structure, internal organs, breathing and circulation.

Dysfunctioning can be eliminated and an optimal tension balance can be obtained leading to the Eutony of the total self. Such training requires a particularly acute ability to observe. Awareness itself can become the object of observation, while tracing at the same time the effects of this observation on the whole organism and registering any change in tonus, circulation and breathing, whether the body is still or moving, and the manner in which these functions are affected by emotions and thoughts. We call this state of awareness "presence." It calls for a deliberately neutral attitude so that the observations are not affected by expectation of any particular results. Being "neutral" is a chief prerequisite for the successful practice of Eutony. Encephalographic readings have shown that "presence" occurs in a fully conscious state and thus differs considerably from the levels of awareness obtained with the Autogenic Training of Professor Schulz and through yoga.

The degree of sensibility that the students possess at the beginning of their training can be ascertained by the models and sketches they make of the human body. It is alarming to see how stunted this sensibility has become today although its role is so important in our overall body development and in experiencing our own individuality. Thus, more often than not, these modeling and drawing tests show that students rarely have an image of their body corresponding to its actual form. This is so even in the case of gymnasts and dancers, physiotherapists and doctors: people who have a professional concern with the human body. This is indicative of the general alienation from the body, the lack of real contact, and the isolation to be found in our society.

The first step is to develop sensibility over the whole skin surface and so normalize the student's image of his body. Only then can we induce that total person awareness which includes muscles, organs, joints and bone structure, as well as Eutony. "Control positions" are used as a test for the optimal muscle length at rest. Like the modeling, they can be carried out by the students themselves. They show whether there is any shortening of the normal muscle length through chronic muscular tension. The students may find it difficult or impossible to maintain the "control positions." Muscle shortening impairs the optimal suppleness of the joints and the natural, unconscious upright position of the body becomes hard to achieve. To remedy this, in addition to a regularization of the general tonus, students need eutonic techniques to stimulate metabolic processes and to facilitate lymphatic and blood circulation.

Tonus

By tonus we mean the state of tension of the striated and smooth muscles of the living organism. Tonus is heightened by any movement lowered during sleep. anyone who has lifted a sleeping child from its cot knows that it appears to be heavier than when it is awake. Its actual body weight is the same in both cases, but its body elasticity changes with any alteration in tonicity. It takes more energy to move a relaxed and therefore flaccid body than one that is braced and rightly tensed.

Tonus can also be affected by emotional changes such as fear and joy (psychotonus), by all states of excitation, by overfatigue of the body or the mind. Everyone experiences changes of this kind. A stairway which we find easy enough to climb when there is something pleasant awaiting us at the top will seem to go on forever if we are depressed and our body feels heavy.

Tonus may be influenced by other people's behavior and attitudes. A gentle, relaxed personality can have a beneficial effect on a whole group whereas a nervous one will set others on edge. Young children and animals are particularly sensitive to such influences; their ability to communicate lies essentially in their capacity for picking up and imitating the tonus of others.

All adults too, whether watching a football match, entranced by a play or film, or listening to stimulating or soothing music, react with tonus imitation. Wallon refers to this in his work, particularly in "De l'acte à la pensée."[2] The results obtained through music therapy and the catharsis produced by Greek drama, are, in large measure, due to this phenomenon.

All fluctuations in the range of human feelings, from ecstasy to apathy, are followed by changes in the tonus which, after extremes of tension have died down, reverts to an intermediate position. This may be too high or too low—hypertonia or hypotonia—depending largely on individual constitution and temperament. Remaining at an intermediate level with no ability to move up or down under emotional influences constitutes a pathological condition.

In its concern with tonus adaptability, Eutony is aware of the importance of keeping the tonal balance. This is done through:

Tonus regulation, which changes the fixed positions of certain groups of muscles and gives the back their tonus-flexibility.

Tonus equalization, when fixations in muscle fibers are removed. Such action on the tonus is taken by directing attention to specific parts of the body; to its volume, inner space, to the skin, the tissues, the organs, the outer form of the bones and periostea.

A normal, flexible tonus enables a person to adapt to all life situations and to have a whole range of feelings and not to be fixed in one state.

A voluntary and immediate change in tonus can be achieved in practice. It is experienced subjectively as a feeling of heaviness or of lightness. Objectively, it is verified by controlling the myotatic reflex, that is by voluntary suppression or, on the contrary, by the reinforcement of the patellar reflex, and a low tonus can eliminate it. The proof of the capacity of tonus regulation is to lower the tonus of the thigh in such a way that even a strong electric current cannot contract these muscles.[3]

While manipulating a subject who is immobile but can alter his tonus at will, the teacher can note easily the variations in tonus from the weight differences in his body. This enables us to understand better why Eutony is not only a method of relaxation, though it enables the pupil to gain control over his tonus at all levels down to deep relaxation and sleep, but also gives him the ability to find the correct tonus in all circumstances.

When all fixations of muscle tone are eliminated, voluntary change of tonus is achieved as follows:

Hypertonus Lightness: By the awareness of three dimensional bone form.
Awareness of bone structure
Inner body space.
Normal Tonus: Through touch of skin.
Hypotonus Heaviness:By contact with the ground.
Mass of the body.
Mass of muscles and bones.

In Eutony training, the teacher constantly watches the pupil's breathing, its rhythm, and the duration or near-absence of the respiratory pause. Any rapid change in tension can cause an emotional upset or lead to an anxiety situation.

Action on breathing is not carried out through direct breathing exercises, but indirectly by releasing those tensions which prevent the fullness of a normal, free, unobstructed respiration. This is obstructed by tensions which may be found in the pelvic musculature, perineum, diaphragm, intercostal muscles, shoulders, neck, hands, feet, the digestive and intestinal apparatus. If those tensions can be eliminated, breathing becomes normal by itself. If, however, voluntary breathing exercises were performed, these obstructions are apparently overcome but they reappear as soon as the exercises are discontinued. Confirmation of this observation is to be found frequently among pupils who have done breathing exercises, such as physiotherapists, actors and athletes. In general, it takes longer with such pupils to normalize tensions since their muscular and organic fixations resist more.

In spite of the great importance we attach to breathing, we avoid mentioning it—especially in the beginning. In a group, when the word *breathing* is mentioned, the breathing of everyone changes. It becomes voluntary, loses its individual nuances and is then less adapted to the real and constantly changing needs of the person. For the teacher, too, it loses its value as a source of information about the psychosomatic state of the pupil.

We are aware that it is extremely difficult to observe our own breathing without exercising any influence on it, even if body consciousness has become relatively well developed. since the act of breathing is unconscious most of the time (except when speaking or singing) the normalization of this involuntary breathing is very important. It is through breathing that the unity of the total personality is observed and influenced easily. Once an equilibrium of tonus has been attained, no special exercises are necessary to adapt breathing to the needs of the moment, whatever they may be.

There are other methods through which this kind of breathing can be attained. The Schlaffhorst-Andersen School in the Federal Republic of Germany, to which I am indebted for a number of original ideas, and the practical and scientific work of Professor Horst Coblenzer and Professor Franz Muhar, Vienna, are in this respect closely related to Eutony. Eminent teachers have obtained good results through totally different approaches. But without competent guidance, mistakes are made which can lead quickly to the kind of mechanical exercises too often seen in sports, physiotherapy and other disciplines

Many of the respiratory techniques taught today are from cultures other than our own. Their exercises, developed over thousands of years, are based on psychosomatic effects suited to a certain time and a particular culture, and they were taught by masters working with their disciples under special conditions. Our situation is very different. We have to find methods that correspond to our culture, that can liberate the breathing process. People should be capable of understanding the physiological and mental influences of breathing with the help of the latest scientific findings.

Circulation

It is well known empirically that the temperature in the different parts of the organism rises when attention is given to that area. From the beginning of Eutony work this fact has been used to improve the circulation in various parts of the body, in the outer and deeper skin, the outer and deeper layers of muscles, the inner organs and the bone structure. The modern electronic skin thermometers show that this change of temperature begins at the moment that attention is focused. Research made at the University of Louvain-la-Neuve in Belgium with three groups of physiotherapist students shows clearly that the group which had followed 90 Eutony lessons during a year had developed a greater capacity to raise the temperature than the two control groups without knowledge and practice of Eutony.[4]

Touch and Contact

In Eutony, a distinction is made between "touching" and "contact." In touching, we experience the boundaries of our organism and our external body form. Touching also gives us essential information about the surrounding world, its shapes, temperature, consistency and the numerous sensations coming from outside.

In touching we do not reach beyond the surface. In eutonic "contact" we move consciously beyond the visible boundaries of the body.

Through this "contact" we can include also the surrounding space in our awareness. Thus, without touching, we are able to make real contact with other human beings, animals, plants and objects, passing through external boundaries.

This conscious "contact" has greater influence than "touch" with regard to changes in the tonus and the circulation. Eutonic "contact" of the feet with the ground or of the hands with tools or materials, during modeling for example, produces a harmonization not only of the tonus but also of emotional tensions.

A conscious influence on the equilibrium between the orthosympathetic and parasympathetic nervous systems, its effect on the circulation and hormonal equilibrium, is attained by the technique of "contact." This technique permits stimulation or inhibition of the autonomic functions and reestablishment of the equilibrium of the autonomic system.

"Contact" is also used in life situations. Good craftsmen contact objects through their tools; good musicians become one with their instruments. The Swiss psychiatrist J. de Ajuriaguerra calls this expanded consciousness "the delegated function," and this consciousness can be developed and strengthened with training.[5]

With eutonic movement, which incorporates total body awareness, we widen our "presence" through space by means of "contact." We include also the other person's space or that of the group, plus the three-dimensional space underneath the feet.

Aside from its effects on breathing and circulation, this multidirectional contact with the ground has a clearly perceptible and specific influence on movement. The use of ground contact has particularly impressive results with movements and actions demanding great efforts. These can be performed with the minimum expenditure of energy by a very precise use of direction and angles of the lines of forces.

The unconscious ability to make contact is innate. It is first manifested in the mother-child relationship. The faculty of becoming one with another person, like the baby with its mother, can be learned and experienced through the eutonic "contact." But this is only the first level of work in Eutony.

The conscious contact with a partner whose personality one respects, and the space around him in which one does not lose oneself in spite of a total opening toward him, is another stage which can be attained through the development of this capacity.

The next step, which involves the ability to contact two other persons simultaneously, without losing the awareness of oneself, is more difficult. Another simple example of the difficulties of contact is, when people do not like to be invited together, because they cannot deal with different people simultaneously. This kind of difficulty may become a serious problem for couples when they have their first baby; the mother is not able to have contact with them both. Either the father feels left out, or the baby lacks a real contact.

Lack of contact is clearly to be seen during movement in space. Once the ability to make contact is acquired, the widening of it to include two, three, four or five persons does not raise any problems, if each has been able to reach the same degree of maturity and understanding.

If we have two persons or a group walking together in "contact," even if they are separate in space, and the dynamic and the rhythm are changed, the contact can be kept, and in fact it opens the way to a dynamic expansion of each individual member of a group toward a genuine togetherness. So to be three persons, and simply two plus one, capable of simultaneous opening each toward each other, is a sign of developing maturity.

Such togetherness should not be confused with that which can be obtained through a musical accompaniment or drumbeat. In that case, it is the domination of the music or rhythm which creates a pseudo-liberation and group feeling, while the real contact between individuals is weakened. Movement groups of this latter kind are far easier to set up. They are used in ballet, theater, Dalcroze, eurhythmics, and other performing arts. Used in therapy, they are valuable as a first step toward group experiences. But even if there is a certain feeling of unity in these groups, the dynamic exchange between each member of the group with others is missing.

A certain impression of togetherness also appears in social gatherings where the consciousness of the group members is lowered by socially acceptable drugs. But the aim of eutonic movement and "contact" is to increase and expand individual dynamics into a conscious contact interchange between each member of the group.

Conscious contact with another person has also a therapeutic application. Once you have acquired the capacity of balancing your own tonus, you are in a condition to observe and to influence others, feeling their disorders and blocks in your own body by making eutonic contact with them.

Eutony Education

Eutonic movement and eutonic forms need a conscious presence—in both pupil and teacher—similar to that in meditation. A Eutony teacher and a therapist must learn much more than the intellectual and technical aspects of this art: he must learn to experience Eutony in his own body. For the pupil, this means at least four years of study as a rule in order to develop the sensibility essential in Eutony. The development of this faculty is primordial, and the pupil must be able to exercise it in all circumstances, not only in sheltered isolation, but in any external conditions found among the distracting influences of urban life.

One of the most important tasks in Eutony teaching is to develop in the pupil the capacity to observe objectively and nonjudgmentally the reactions of his own body. He must be able to distinguish between imagined and real sensation and not be deluded by fantasies which are as harmful for the body as for the mind.

The experience that all thought, however abstract, has a real effect on the entire organism is basic to Eutony work. Geometric forms such as straight lines, waves, zigzags, circles or triangles, which are all forms habitually conceived of as having no effect on the body, actually do produce palpable and measurable changes in the muscular tonus and circulation. Our understanding of this phenomenon is confirmed in our daily observations in the school.

Similarly, it is known that negative feelings such as distress, hatred and jealousy are accompanied by body changes. Distress is often accompanied by hypertension in the lower pelvic muscles, the muscles of the stomach and the diaphragm. For most pupils, the objective observation of body sensation is a very important first experience, especially if it is intensified by teaching giving rise to changes which can be measured: pulse, temperature, tonus. It is necessary only to direct the attention to a foot and its various parts: toes, metatarsus, instep, sole, joints, to produce, even among the noninitiated, perceptible and measurable changes in the circulation and muscular tonus. In making slight movement with one foot only, pupils notice a distinct difference in sensation from that of the other foot.

With the same exercise, sensation can vary considerably according to the state of the individual. The hypotonic person will feel his foot lighter and more alive, whereas the hypertonic will feel some heaviness; another will feel a slight tingling heat and a fourth will feel cold. In any group, only a few pupils will report the same sensation. Eutony avoids suggestion as much as possible. Methods based on suggestion rely on a weakening of the consciousness and therefore prevent an accurate observation of processes manifested by the organism at any given moment. For this reason, during the period of learning, Eutony is incompatible with other body-work techniques.

A similar exercise may also lead to different or contradictory reactions in the same person at different times. The reaction must therefore be noted in relation to the existing situation which depends on the psychological state and the various conditions of the environment, such as atmospheric pressure, or radioactivity. These experiences condition the whole pedagogical and therapeutic method of work. They show teachers and pupils that there is no permanently valid solution. One cannot forever rely on formulas which once gave good results; it is important to reexamine them constantly in accordance with the reality of the movement.

The teacher must develop the capacity to observe the pupil's behavior, posture, movements, tonus, breathing rate and quality of voice, circulation—i.e. all the nonverbal manifestations which indicate his physical and psychic state. The teacher must also feel in himself the pupil's tonus condition.

All these observations and the teacher's subjective impressions can be confirmed objectively by the tests referred to in the preceding chapter. Among these, the "control positions" make it possible to observe the condition of the joints and of the muscular elasticity, whereas the "passive movements" show the subject's capacity to master the motor innervation and myotatic reflexes.

The group training and individual lessons are drawn up on the basis of this information.

In the process of speaking, the teacher experiences each set task in his own body. Each time, therefore, his indications are based on his actual feeling and personal experience and are not just mechanical repetition. He rarely demonstrates what is required since it is not a question of initiating, but of allowing the pupil to make his own experience. The pupil must feel in himself the laws of tonus change and good posture reflex or the consequences of a consciously directed effort. In proposing a new task, the teacher allows the pupil to discover these laws and to reexamine them in ever new situations so that in each one the pupil becomes conscious of his psychosomatic unity.

The teacher should give indications in clear terms with no suggestive overtones, enabling each pupil to experience his own reality. Reference may be made to a change in temperature but not to heat or cold. The pupil is asked to feel his body with no suggestion of the quality of the feeling.

In any case, the departure point of the practical work must differ according to whether it is a matter of professional training in Eutony, of people having difficulty in exercising their professions (musicians with technical or rhythmical problems, actors suffering from stage fright, dancers or athletes with overworked muscles and joints), people who are ill and have tried many other treatments before coming to Eutony, and those who are trying to develop and grow harmoniously as integrated, creative persons.

Group Work

There are great advantages to be found in group work. A group is enhanced by the diversity of the personalities which compose it. For this reason it should consist preferably of not less than eight participants, provided that the teacher has enough experience to perceive and understand each member's personality. Group teaching can be supplemented if necessary by individual lessons and treatments. But although the profound and manifold possibilities of individual therapy can rapidly produce results through Eutony, the beginner is rarely capable of consciously integrating the transformations of his body image and body gestalt, which is a primary condition for acquiring long-lasting results from the treatment. Instead of becoming independent, the pupil runs the risk of becoming dependent on the teacher. It is only at a later stage, when the pupil has developed the ability to observe his own reactions that treatment, carried out by the teacher, will greatly improve the pupil's body image. Over the past fifteen years, however, group lessons have achieved results for sick pupils who formerly needed individual treatment.

In a group, the pupil has less feeling of being watched. He has time to develop his own working method which will prepare him for working alone later. The teacher observes the pupil's reactions and adapts the work proposed until the pupils themselves become conscious of their reactions and that of the other members of the group. The varying individual ways of reaching the same goal are an enrichment to everybody in the group. This result cannot be obtained to the same extent through individual treatment. Group work is most important in the training of a eutonist. The whole range of possibilities of mutual observation within the group, close contact with the other group members, whose development is assisted by the trainee's own development, deepens the understanding of differing personalities and prepares for an essential quality in future teachers, i.e. the capacity to observe the person as a whole through body expression and behavior. The observation of movement in a group provides unsuspected richness and opens up possibilities which the individual cannot find alone. This improvement comes from the need to adjust one's own tonus, tempo and rhythm to that of the group without losing one's identity. We shall go further into this concept when we study movement.

Notes

1. Henri Wallon, *De l'act à la pensée* (Paris; Flammarion, 1978)

2. Henri Wallon, *De l'acte à la pensée* (Paris; Flammarion, 1978).

3. Research done in C.N.R.S., Paris (Centre National de Recherches Scientifiques), 1979, Prof. J.G. Henrotte.

4. Research conducted by Pierre Debelle, licenciate, for a thesis of Mme. Paulette Friedman, Supervisor: Dr. Georges Marechal, Professor of the Medical Faculty. Measurements were taken with Digitec Datalogger manufactured by DIGITEC, 918 Woodley Road, Dayton, Ohio 45403.

5. J. de Ajuriaguerra: *"Méconnaissance et hallucinations corporelles"* (Corporeal Misperceptions and Hallucinations), (Paris; Masson & Cie., 1942).

Emilie Conrad Da'Oud

*T*he founder of the school "Continuum," Emilie teaches a primal form of movement awareness, involving exploring the reverberations in awareness of the smallest movements, breaths, and sounds. She has used the work to enable seriously disabled people to create previously unimagined kinds of movement.

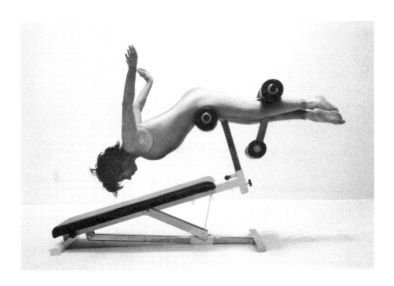

Life on Land

Emilie Conrad Da'Oud

> *If Martians were looking at us through some interstellar resonating device,*
> *I am sure they would marvel at how our planet has arranged us.*
>
> *"Look, look," they would say, "Their bodies are mostly water, and yet*
> *they move about the earth in this apparently solid way."*
>
> *"Just look at how each organ is maintaining its link with all of its*
> *undulating strands."*
>
> *"They are like fish out of water, but they carry it with them."*
> *"How amazing these humans are!"*

I have worn a path searching for a spiritual link that was not offered
in the world around me.

My spiritual struggle and my theories of movement are like the
Caduceus—eternally intertwined, facing each other, falling into each
other, then distancing for another embrace later on.

The question I asked myself when pushed to the walls of my own
psyche, was in what unknown ways are we in rapport with our atmosphere? And if we were to experience this unknown "rapport," would
it matter?

The question rose and fell. It made me tired just to have it linger
in my neural catacombs.

The question haunted me for years. From the tenements of New
York, to the huts of Haiti, to the Spanish stucco of Los Angeles, the
question grew more urgent.

In what ways do we commune with our biosphere? And how
would we know?

This is a new piece, a chapter of a book in progress, published here for the
first time.

A voice comes to us, a pressure on a shoulder, a message in a dream, a person in an airport—innocent moments glistening like eggs in a sea of fertility. An idle remark, a shadow from the eyes—an orchestration of creativity takes place in the magical moments of the unseen, between the lines.

Discovery takes place within a context of circumstances in which mysterious forces guide us, prod us, and invigorate our darkest moments.

The unknown is the invitation   come enter   come closer
Yes

1939 Brooklyn

Grandmother spent most of the day at the kitchen sink, peeling, washing, slicing what must have been food, but the plate before us was sadly populated with bleeding tomatoes, fainting cucumbers, and whispy potatoes slightly tinged from resting in an old pan. The meat was held over an open fire in a wire grate, so that it would dry out completely and become like leather. One could say the meat was tanned rather than cooked. Staring down at this sad plate, meat stiffened with rigor mortis, bloodless, it scratched my throat as it struggled to be swallowed. One could track its journey from mouth to colon easily, the meat marking its path with little agonies.

The matzo that was at all meals was a perpetual flight from Egypt— never to be forgotten. Relived daily, the dry wafer lay on my tongue waiting for some moisture to soften it, praying for saliva as if for rain, to drench the poor stiff thing with heavenly dew so that it could drop gracefully.

Life at Grandma's house was destitute of any warmth or love or care—no laughing, no touching. Only sad little immigrant meals, Diasporic meals, wandering in space, no homeland for these plates, suspended over the earth, waiting for the messiah.

The lesson I received was that life was a harsh brick wall onto which one hurled oneself till one was dead.

On one side of our tiny apartment was a window staring blankly at a Brooklyn landscape of utter desolation. The grey asphalt of the street, the chain link fence of the playground, the dark tar, the grunge grey of the El trains that rattled by—trains ran every ten minutes—they would shake our windows and interrupt every phone call. All our activities were timed by the schedule of the West End El. Certain faces as they whizzed by became familiar to me. For a second we would make contact and then gone.

Grey, bulky figures burped out of the El train like chunks of undigested food. Scooped up every morning—spilled out every evening. They tumbled from the train and made their way toward their grey tenement cells, sitting before grey plates with grey leaky food, and the sky, oh yes, the sky—grey sky barely seen above the tenements, barely seen from the view of the street; the border lines of the grey asphalt met the relentless sky.

It was always night, even the sunniest July day seemed like night. A blanket worn snugly over my heart, the grey covered any hope at all.

My child eyes took this in. My child eyes saw everything.

Our part of Brooklyn was called Gravesend. Well named. The Greenwood Cemetery was close by. Dead Dutch immigrants nestled in their final peace with great trees comforting them and guarded by ornate headstones with flying angels. The cemetery was my refuge. It went on for miles, and I would wander there for hours, sometimes sitting by the lake hearing the sighs of leaves, being very quiet. I don't recall any visitors. The graves were so old—all the Dutch were gone from "Broeck Land" by then—leaving the dust of their bones to Italians and Jews with their salami smells, pizzerias and bars and grills.

Among all the muted grey, a pink hope blasted out from the fog. Port Alba Pizzeria neoned through the streets. The "greys" clutched their glasses, singing old Italian songs, as their eyes got redder, lips softened, and wet drops oozed from their tongues. I, small, watched men and women huddled around the dark wooden bar, a coffin turned upside down—I smelled disinfectant mixed with beer, saw sawdust rippling the floor; a blue and pink juke box swinging its lights, a trapped hep cat wailing Harry James and Sammy Kaye. Slow dancing in the night. Hard-ons pressing tight skirts. Words whispering huskily, "I'm gonna be a cop." "I'm gonna get married, get a fridge, have a coupla kids."

Dark skinned kids from Italy's boot, dark skinned kids with kinky Sicilian hair, born to drive trucks to New Jersey, born to stir endless sauces for spaghetti, born to live with smoky blue mirrored fake fireplaces, naked bulbs swinging over sinks, blood-brown mohair living rooms, windows fogged with stifling steam heat—tropical forest inside, freezing cold outside.

The bright pink of the Port Alba Pizzeria shone like a spark of heaven coming to meet this puzzled earth.

I think back to this time as a kind of initiation. The kind that can only take place in childhood. Wrapped in innocence, with no defenses, the universe can converse with you, shed its tears, whisper its lament, and only the child can hear.

My mother tells of how, bringing me home newborn from the hospital, I choked and turned blue. On the verge of death, a friend of hers put her hand down my throat and pulled out a huge wad of mucus. Later on, I choked on the darkness of my childhood—off to hospitals with exotic somatic responses that were diagnosed as disease.

Looking back, I see these illnesses as sorrows of the soul.

The struggle for breath became the hallmark of my early life. Imprisoned by breath, I stuttered and gasped. My stuttering clogged my chest, causing words to stand on top of each other like the rush hour scenes I knew so well.

Words colliding in my throat, clinging to each other in lumpy embraces. My throat became a BMT door in which words would tumble out like giant centipedes all tangled inside each other—great lumps of words rushing to get out before the doors closed. Rushing to make it to the exit. Pushing and shoving each other with odd matings. Words struggled to exist on the slim threads of breath that I poorly provided.

Better to keep my mouth shut.

I knew even at a tender age that my breathing problem was a form of incarceration. I felt imprisoned by childhood. I was doomed to serve my term as a "small person" amid the purgatory of the screaming adults around me. Trapped, I stuttered and gasped.

Daily my ribs contracted and my throat become a tiny hole; the more I struggled the less breath there was. This led to chronic sighing. Like an elm tree withering in the dust, I sighed and sighed, my words punctuated with gasps which finally escaped from my pinched throat with puffs of sadness. Sometimes the sighing would be over right away, sometimes it would just go on and on.

I measured my sanity by the amount of sighs that percussed the air. I had bad days and I had less bad days. Humid days were the worst. The oppressive steam of New York heat in the summer was a bronchial challenge. I learned to get up at five AM before the cooked streets and tarry rivers came to life with their gurgling vapors. I learned to rise early, snatching clean breaths before my daily gasping would begin, before my lungs got clogged with tenement dust.

I knew that my perpetual hyperventilation and my feeling of incarceration were the same. My breath was as trapped as I was.

I knew I was catatonic way down where coffins lay at the bottom of the ocean, where El trains ran through tombstones.

I knew where faces jarred in glass cages stared at me through my own glass cage.

I knew the waste of my grandmother's life as her gnarled hands shaped the pyramids of Egypt as she prayed over the Friday night candles.

I knew I was banished, wandering in the desert.

I recall the child sitting at the window, and I can feel the child's despair, knowing that the world was much more than this.

This could not be why dinosaurs roamed and stars burst.

This could not be why oceans sprayed and forests clustered.

The movement of water on land is represented by the symbol of the snake.

We learn to live on land,

But it is in our aquatic home that all life emerges.

An octopus stirs, a snake moves and hatches its eggs on land. Far away from the primordial ooze it struggles out of its muddy home and stretches itself   past rocks and crevices—its belly shapes the dirt with elegant markings—markings of ocean on land. The swirl is remembered in my fingertips as I write this page.

I had an intuitive sense of how I wanted movement to feel. I never saw it in a human but I recognized it in the octopus.

Watching those undulating fluorescent ripples, I recognized the *quality* of what I was looking for. The iridescent fluttering of life stretched and undulated, rippled and curved. As the complexity of this shiny wet dance caught me, I felt that movement, and I knew.

I stood in a pool of recognition, and I knew.

Below the sea, before light, swim prehistoric forms, ancestors—ancestors gleaming with iridescent quivers—creatures living so far down—so far, far, I stand, they swim, but we are the same.

I entered the darkened pool, up to my knees at first, then hips, fingertips, chest, shoulders, neck, ears, until all there was only silent water.

quivering

iridescent memories beneath the water, resting.

I wade into the water.
Wade, but not like Virginia Woolf, to die.
I drown, but not to die.
I drown, to answer the call.
But not to die.
How do I know about breathing?
How does the snake know to move its belly?

A struggling prisoner, I bang the bars with my spoon.
Is anybody there?

When I was fifteen I was rushed off to have my appendix ripped from my belly. Igor, the mad doctor, did such a ghastly job, I needed to be sewn up again three times. My belly looked like I had been run over by a tractor, and a gaping hole looked at me in my bathroom mirror.

Not only did I struggle with layers of scar tissue, but I had massive adhesions as well.

For twenty years I was greeted with the same screaming pain in my appendectomy scar. It would constantly gnaw at my right side—insatiable for my attention. The pain was so severe that I could not touch my own abdomen. I felt the thick gristle of scar tissue strangling my organs and swallowing my intestines. Pain led to numbing, and I would deaden myself from shoulders to knees—to keep it at a low throttle. But it was always there. No matter how well I muted myself I could feel its constant gnarling. All of my pain converged in my scar, a convention of memories thronged on my right side. I had deadened my emotions enough to create a generalized state of agony that was a souvenir of my childhood, with all the long dark hallways and no light at the end.

From my shoulders to my knees was a zone of protection.

My stomach muscles, cut in surgery, lay immobilized within the ice cube of myself. Winter spread its snowy stillness until I was completely frozen: my eyeballs, my toes, my heart, nothing left but icy vigilance. I gave the "impression" of being alive. I managed to maintain a certain acceptable coordination, to compensate so well that no one could tell I was an ice cube.

Fully petrified, I hung like a stalactite from the ceiling of a cave in a perpetual state of dropping—no movement could be completed.

1967. Los Angeles.
My gasping and sighing kept increasing all through the years, until my chest felt like a frozen fortress.

I had to teach myself to breathe.

I rode my breath, sliding and falling over snowy peaks and crevices; a Saint Bernard was bringing warm whiskey to the frozen traveler.

My life was being saved.

I breathed, and small rivers of warmth brought blood to the surface. At first the pain would rise up to meet the breath and scream even harder—shouting down the breath—petrified tears circling a fire. The pain rose to clutch the breath, to kill it—no movement here. "Stop at once," I say.

"No! "

The battle rose, sometimes to monstrous proportions.

A war between ice and heat—life and death.

It felt like two vultures were fighting over an almost dead carcass. A voice inside said, "Do not give this any value. Keep going, keep going."

I lay there as pain tried to swallow breath.

I lay there as life crashed.

Then, ice cracked—a trickle of feeling.

The Saint Bernard struggled toward the stranger, pushing through the snow.

Rivulets of sensation were recorded by my nerve fibers, and brought me to "feel" the heated life inside me.

It was difficult for me to feel pleasure. I could only tolerate it for microseconds before the pain would rise to demolish it. Microseconds, as I stayed the course, grew into minutes. An achievement was to have a "good" feeling for more than ten seconds.

Over a period of time the waltz of the vultures subsided, and little by little the ice age ended, and as rosy blood coursed through my heated cave I was able to accept more breath.

I traveled on my breath through centuries of despair. Not only *mine,* but ancestral despair, a mantle passed from generation to generation, a mantle of suffering, passed like a bowl of peas. Not only *my* scar, but all of it lay there inside me—so many generations, shaping the course of my life.

My overwhelming sadness was bound, not only by my own misery, but to centuries of ghettos and isolation. The foot of the Jew, never permitted to touch this earth—somehow always lifted, always wandering. Desert after desert, always wandering. Those women stared from my eyes, those hands formed pyramids of fingers before Menorahs. "Boruch Atou Adonai" echoed in my throat—voices, hundreds of voices.

Black clad ghosts fled as heat from the sun warmed the rocks of the cave; lungs opened, and air breathed against rock.

As I taught myself to breathe, I concentrated on exhales—expiring, the dissolving of form.

I would sink my body with every exhale, taking the burden off my lungs—my body would take on the whole expression of breathing—sinking in as completely as I could with exhaling, and receiving the breath as best I could with inhaling.

Inspiration—the taking on of form.

It made sense to let my whole body take on the movement of breathing.

Everything inhaled.

Everything exhaled.

The first music is breath. Music is movement. The basis of all music is inhaling and exhaling.

The octopus and snake shaped my movements. They were my teachers.

Lying on my back, bringing a wave motion to my belly—getting my diaphragm to move, trying to become more fluid, was completely different when I incorporated breath.

I explored breath as a musician would experiment with music.

The movement became the outcome of the breath.

If my breath was dynamic and heated, a wave motion would reflect that: it would be larger and quicker—if my breath were more subtle, the wave was more internal, softer, finer.

I could tell, as I slowly began to sense more distinctly, that if I changed the textures of my breath, I could bring about deeper sensation. It was as if the shifting of breath magnified occurrences that usually lay beneath the threshold of my awareness. The stimulation of dramatically shifting my breath brought me closer to feeling internal movements—sensations that were organismic—not about anything else.

The more I recognized sensation, the deeper inside myself I could be. Sensation was about itself—a textured palette of many qualities, not imbued with any content.

The feelings were like an umbilical cord connecting me to the world of the sperm and the egg, the world of love itself.

But the inside of me maintained a stony silence, until one day, a miracle, something moved from inside!

Something moved that wasn't filled with pain.

I didn't even know that a person *could* move from the inside.

I continued with my breath, my attention watchful—not knowing what to look for, I was simply alert.

Gradually, slowly, incrementally, more movement occurred internally. Further and further I could go, feeling myself as a wave joining a multiplicity of waves—multidirectional—some, perhaps tiny, barely a ripple, some stronger, more determined.

As I softened, I was filled with whispers of sensations which were subtle and permeating.

I had to teach myself to not run away from myself and what I was feeling.

Over a period of time my experience of sensation went through a drastic change. My sensation vocabulary had been rudimentary: sexual, menstrual, pain. Sensation was something I had tried to avoid. Now I made myself stay.

Attentive breathing, day after day, I could feel the snow turn to water.

One day I felt wave motions moving inside my spine, my face, my fingers.

There was no inside, no outside, no up or down, no "body" only wave motions, many kinds—short waves—long waves—dancing waves.

I wept with deliverance. I was home.

I dwelled in the marvel of this world.
Breath—a thread hovering between life and death.
I am joined with all creatures in breath.
Breath pneuma spirit
Shiva, the god of dance, stirs
Nostrils quiver

Inhale, the Creator meets exhale, the Destroyer
The dancer turns one face then the other until life and death embrace
A snakeskin hangs from a cross, molting, shedding
The great dance begins.

Breath is the movement of wind on water—it becomes a beckoning of our origins. As amphibians that developed legs to pursue life on land we return to our watery beginnings to resurrect.

As breath moves more freely, a softening occurs, what once was a barrier now becomes a threshold and life can go on. As breath brings waves of movement into soft tissue and to the bones of my sternum, I feel love entering me, I feel as delivered as a new babe lying hummed in the wrappings of a cosmic love. The waves enter my pelvis, deep into the subterranean chambers where prehistoric anemones twirl. I permit myself to welcome the undulating caresses of love. It spreads into my legs, my arms, my face. Tenement dust is kissed from my eyelids, as I begin the "cosmic drowning," the relinquishing to love.

Like secret agents from a distant star, we are born out of water, shaped by its liquid love, protected, adored, we bring our oceanic heaven to earth.

Water shapes our bones, our organs, our brains, and finally nestles inside our cells waiting—waiting for the call of earth.

Waiting for the first burst of air.

Water waits.

Dolphins and whales swim calmly as the aquatic human awaits destiny.

The moment comes, throbs increase as the space ship struggles to land, slipping, sliding, screaming. The pulsing amniotic softens the arrival.

Cut from the placenta—the ship has landed!

Breath enters the tiny human cargo a cry the song begins

The juke box twirls

Harry James lifts his trumpet

The whales sing out

Happy Birthday

This wet being will soon learn to live on land.

Its fluid memory will be erased, the membrane between lives barely felt. A dorsal fin shudders as our oceanic past is remembered in our internal movements. These ancients who arrived before light—they swim quietly, waiting.

Our organs undulate with rhythms of the first algae. Our tissue sways like kelp, furling and unfurling—eternal sway—dark ocean sway—deep in the middle of the dark, where photosynthesis never occurs.

The kelp of our tissues remembers the ancient ones.

On land now, remembering the dark, dark water where light never is, the silent ones move.

Blood memories like oceans of dark

Blood moving the Red Sea parting

the Red Sea coursing round the Cape of Good Hope

the Red Sea of blood moving through vessels and tunnels

The membrane between lives is barely felt, except in dreams, perhaps.

If we lived on Mars or Jupiter, the atmosphere of those planets would shape us very differently.

We breathe the way we do because we are on this planet, and not on any other. Our lungs develop in such a way because of this earth and not another—we crawl, we stand, we move with confidence. Our bodies are stabilized by invisible fields that keep us from floating off. Born into another atmosphere with the same DNA, we would breathe differently, our organs would orchestrate differently, and our neuro-muscular development would interface with the requirements of that planet.

In short, our bodies behave the way they do because we are here. On Earth, all existence begins in water. Whether we speak of the amniotic and the world of sperm and egg, or we speak of the primordial soup—in either case, on this planet, water and life are one.

It is our guide and our prayer, this atmospheric substance that is the movement of love.

As we lie in our watery cradle the pulsations and signals of life creating life start their sculpture. Buds appear, the liquid pulsations bring forth a shape, the cues and chemical signals pulse and dance as this shape continues to grow. This liquid being has entered a new atmosphere, and as it hesitates, still wet with its memory, terrestrial urgings begin. The atmosphere of the earth calls forth its own chemical responses, and this extraordinary water enters the amphibian stage. The movement of water to earth.

We lie in our grass hut, or brick house, we lie on leaves, on cotton, on wool, or straw, and we become.

We are lifted, we are touched, liquid eyes meet earth eyes, we make contact. We have arrived.

The water, undulating with memories, begins grasping, and the tiniest pulsations of muscles begin. We have arrived.

As we take on the callings of our new environment, our grasps become firmer, our fluid movements become more stable, and we become more adapted to flexing, grasping, shoving, reaching, falling away.

An alphabet of movements spill forth. Gushings of muscles learning the laws of earth.

This amphibious stage continues, and only the intrinsic movements maintain their oceanic memory. The organs undulate as they have always done, unaware of the hardening of muscle and the demands of new reflexes—organs pulsate in rhythms more ancient than we; our connective tissue dances like sea anemone.

Unaware of any change in existence, the interior life remains true to its watery origin. The amphibious human continues to stabilize itself in its new environment, testing out new strengths and capacities as it wiggles its way into its new world. Each movement brings about an identity of body. Liquid pulsations become random thrashings, little reflexes awkwardly begin humming, a bud becomes a leg. As each limb adjusts itself to its new atmosphere—a body image begins to emerge.

A sense of "body" comes with experience. The identifications that accumulate around "body" come from use over a period of time.

All of our identities around "bodies," what they are, what they do, come from use and experience, and outside of that framework we go no further.

The "shock of arrival" creates a kind of amnesia—a blank. Like mountains scored with sea etchings, so we are etched—strangers in a strange land.

Perhaps, like reptiles that peered out from the primordial mud and squirmed on land to find a new frontier for hatching their eggs, we are like them, following signals of which we have no idea.

For me the message of God can be felt in the movement of water. The fluids in our cells are the liquid presence of our spiritual birthright. The ocean—our blood—the water inside the planet—amniotic and spinal fluid—are all the same.

All fluid activities are in resonance. They mutualize and inform each other. The fluid inside this biosphere called earth and the fluids of our bodies are in constant rapport. Inexorably mutualizing in ways that we have barely discovered.

The recapitulation of our biosphere by the embryo is the greatest spiritual message of all. Take the sage off the mountain and put him back in utero, have him feel his skin fall away and the undulating memories of his umbilical tie to his planet.

These undulations, cosmic perturbations, are carried by the movement of water in which electrical impulses impregnate the soft waves with an immanence of what can be possible.

An ocean of probability for planet, for human, play out this theatre of fecundity as messages merge and reverberate, perhaps even having a separate purpose from the hardened shell of the biped stalking the savannas, questing for fire.

Perhaps human beings are engaged in a process that is "other" than our muscular meanderings on earth. Is it possible that we are participating in something vaster than our limited brains can realize? Perhaps the mitochondria are running us? Perhaps it, or they, are participating in a cosmic drama that goes far beyond our hairy bodies and smart drugs.

Amnesia sets in as earth greets us.

The shock of arrival wipes out all traces of our watery birth. We now take in the shapes around us, trees, rocks, grass. Textures call us to be touched, walked on, eaten, smelled. We are called by the gurgling of brooks and the roaring of mountains, we are called, and we never look back.

Eyes stare straight ahead with wonder and delight.

Fragrances fill the nostrils and the aromatic earth seduces us toward her. Forever clasped, we stand tall, our frog legs firmed up now, ready to walk, to kneel, to climb, to run, to kick, ready for earth and all its delicious temptations.

Like a cosmic joke our tendrils become fingers and we forget.

Ah yes. I see it now. The hardening of our bodies deadens us to our home.

We are no longer wet.

It took me a long time of deciphering to realize that the amniotic, the oceanic, *is* the movement of love.

Not emotional love but an encompassing *atmosphere* of love

A love that has its own destiny—perhaps using humans as its messengers, this love is trying to land on earth.

Water is the substance for all life forms on this earth.

Love is the substance in which all life form is expressed.

Oceanic memories continue among all humans who have landed. The pulsing waves of ancestral amphibians is recorded in every undulation of an organ, in every sweep of tissue, in every course of blood.

What we call "body" is not "matter" but movement. The body is a profound orchestration of many qualities and textures of movement, interpenetrating tones of fertile play, waiting to be incubated. What I see as body is the urging of creative flux, waves of fertility. The cosmic play that we enter this atmosphere with still goes on at an intrinsic level—we are mostly not aware of the world we carry.

It is *there* in this cosmic soup disguised as organs and cartilage and tissue that the universe is moving in its creative flux like a giant egg waiting to be fertilized. The amniotic matrix moves with the same undulations that started this cosmic swirl that we call earth in the first place.

Our intrinsic world *is* our cosmic connection, it is our legacy of love and wonder—it is where God plays at midnight, it is the big bang, the splitting of atoms, and the message of Jesus.

4.
Piecing Together

Elizabeth A. Behnke

*B*ehnke is a phenomenologist who has created the Study Project in the Phenomenology of the Body. She edits a bi-annual publication that represents some of the best attempts at making theoretical sense of these various practices by engaging a dialogue between practitioners of embodiment practices and phenomenologists. This particular article, published some years ago, has had an enormous impact on the self-understanding of these various schools of practice.

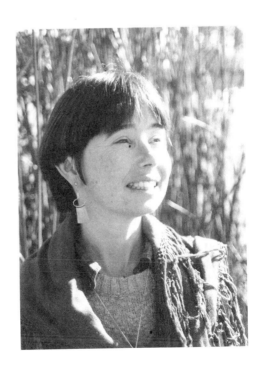

Matching

Elizabeth A. Behnke

T HE PURPOSE OF this essay[1] is to single out a feature of somatic education that is already in use in a number of bodywork and body
awareness disciplines and is potentially of value to other approaches
as well. Don Johnson has distinguished between principles and techniques in the field of somatics: *Principles* are fundamental "sources of
discovery" that "enable the inspired person continually to invent creative strategies for working with others," whereas *techniques* are specific methods arising from such principles.[2]

The feature I would like to discuss may be considered a principle,
and I will indicate some of he ways it has been applied in existing
approaches as I go along. However, in order to center the discussion
in a more concrete way, I will focus on a specific somatic technique
based on the principle in question. I shall begin by describing this
technique in its simplest form before moving on to some variations
on the technique and a few comparisons with other ways in which
the same fundamental principle has been applied. Toward the end of
the essay, I shall take a more philosophical look at the technique and
what it implies. Thus, this essay is both practical and theoretical.

A word of caution is in order, however. What this essay as a whole
is about is something to be lived or felt or done in your own body.
Even the philosophical reflections presuppose direct, first-person,
somatic acquaintance with what I am discussing. My job is, therefore,
to put a somatic technique into words as well as I can, so that you can
learn the technique (and grasp the principle) by reading my descriptions. And your job, as I see it, is to test my descriptions by actually

---

Somatics Spring/Summer 1988. 24–32.

"cashing in" the words for the experience itself. Only then will this essay be more than "just so much hot air."[3]

I have termed the feature I am concerned with *matching* because of the way the word is used in a *Somatics* interview with Judith Aston. After talking about her training as a Rolfer and her initial development of Structural Patterning, Aston describes an experience she had when working with a little boy who was paralyzed. None of the bodywork techniques she had ever learned seemed to have any effect. But when she took his hand and gently tried to feel into and *match up* with the stress pattern she felt there, his hand let go and moved a little bit in the way it could not move before. Then, as she goes on to say:

The very next day I was to give a lesson to a teacher who had one hip high and the other low. Usually I would have done a whole session sitting, lengthening the short side and then have her walk lifting out of the short side so she would appear to be more symmetrical.

I said, "Susan, your right side is shorter than your left, and that creates asymmetrical movement. That's the given condition. So let's see if we can find a way for you to incorporate this asymmetry of the hips into a movement that feels good. So walk on your short side, the right, and let yourself feel that it's shorter, also accepting the height of the left. Consciously *match* your asymmetrical condition. Since the right side is short, *don't resist it,* just feel it." At first she walked down the hall looking very lopsided, then gradually she began to look less asymmetrical. She said, "Judith, it's lengthening! This certainly is different from my other lessons—but it works!"[4]

Note that matching takes on two different forms in the two examples mentioned. In the first case, the bodyworker is matching the shape of stress in the little boy's body; in the second case, the client herself is consciously matching her own asymmetrical shape. The matching principle can indeed be used when working with another person, as in the story about the little boy. And as Aston points out, many times we do need the help of another person to release holding patterns we cannot let go of by ourselves.[5]

In this essay, however, I shall emphasize the kind of matching found in the second example, where the woman herself matches her own experience in a particular way. It is the kind of application of the matching principle that I shall term the *matching technique*. This technique is not something that I do to another person or another person does to me, but something I do for myself. Although it can be used in conjunction with specialized bodywork practices, the matching technique described below is first and foremost something I do on my own: it is a way of taking responsibility for my own somatic experience.

In its most schematic form, the matching technique may be said to consist of three parts: (1) awareness of something in one's own body; (2) an inner act of matching or aligning oneself with this; and (3) allowing something to change. In actual practice these can flow together, but I will comment on each separately for the moment.

(1) Matching presupposes that there is something there to match, some feature of my own bodily experience—such as a shape, a feeling. or a movement—of which I am aware. This seems obvious, but deserves mention because there is the widespread impoverishment of the experience of one's own body in our culture. As numerous writers have indicated, the ability of many people in Western society to experience their own bodily feelings is profoundly impaired.[6] Matching can help to recover and improve the capacity for somatic perception (by which I mean somesthetic/kinesthetic/proprioceptive experience in general,[7] and I will return to this question later in the essay. For now, however, I will assume that I can indeed feel some of my own body from within, simply by turning my awareness to the shape of my limbs in space, the quality of tonus in this part of that part of my body, the sense of my movement being free or restricted, and so on and so forth.

Let us say, then, that I decide to practice matching. Perhaps I begin by setting aside whatever I am doing and allowing the feeling of my own body to come more fully to awareness.[8] I do not *try* to relax or to correct my posture in any way, but simply let myself be conscious of whatever is there to feel, just as it is, welcoming it with a calm, "oh, how interesting" attitude rather than a critical, fault-finding attitude. Typically, something or other will stand out—a feeling of tightness somewhere in my body, for example, or an awareness of a particular shape, such as the feeling of one shoulder being higher than the other or the feeling of my upper torso being slightly turned to the left. Sometimes, the tightness will loosen up, the shoulder will drop down, or the torso will untwist of its own accord—once I have noticed what is going on. At other times, I can easily change whatever it is that I have discovered—realizing, for example, that I have scrunched myself up while doing a particular task and am now uncoiling with relief. But there are also times when the shape or the feeling of tightness is *just there*. It is, quite literally, the shape I am in; it *is* the way I feel, whether I like it or not.

(2) At this point, there are various things I can do. I can try a variety of relaxation techniques, or I can stretch, or massage the tight area, and so on.[9] But in matching, I do not try to change the shape or the tightness: I match it. This does not mean, for instance, that I consciously try to tighten this area of my body still further, as with some relaxation exercises. Instead, I *enter* the shape or the tightness, feeling from within as clearly as I am able, and I begin to *appropriate* it as something I myself am doing—tightening myself precisely here, or holding myself in exactly this shape.[10]

What is crucial is that even if in fact I cannot voluntarily change the shape of the feeling at this moment, I can pretend that I am maintaining it on purpose, just as it is. Perhaps I imagine that I am an artist's model, and must deliberately maintain this configuration (this shape and this quality of tonus) for a few moments while the artist sketches or photographs me. This does not mean that I imagine what I would look like from the outside; instead, I get in touch with the *feeling* of holding the pose and I consciously *inhabit* this feeling, putting myself into the position, as it were, of the active doer of whatever it is that produces this felt shape and this quality of felt tonus in my body. I match it—but I do not try to control it. I simply *join with it,* not as a static fact, but as something ongoing, something that is continuing to be just this way. And I do so not from the vantage point if a spectator, but from that of a participant.

(3) What happens when I do this? Sometimes, nothing happens. But often, what happens is that I feel myself spontaneously shift myself in a slightly different way, with a new shape and a new body feeling. The change often seems to be directly related to whatever it was I was matching: a tightness eases, a stuck place begins to come unstuck, etc.

At other times, however, a shift will take place somewhere else in my body than in the area I was matching. Yet whatever happens, it generally seems to be move in the direction of greater openness and ease. If I want, I can go on to match this new shape or feeling, and see if this leads to a further organization.[11] But for matching to work, I must be genuinely focused each time on simply matching what is there; trying for a specific outcome only gets in the way. Thus I have to allow myself time just to feel whatever presents itself and to match it just as it is, or getting caught up in comparisons between the way things are and the way I think they should be.

One can, of course, use the "golden moments"[12] of bodily awareness to try out new ways of organizing one's body, first sensing what is there and then consciously changing into a new configuration. But the matching technique I am describing is a process in which one allows oneself to change spontaneously, rather than attempting to direct the processing in a particular way. Sometimes the shift will be a familiar one; I may even get what I expect. If, however, I am able to set aside both my specific expectations about will happen next and my desire to control what is going to happen, the spontaneous shifts can be a surprise, as well as a delight.

Now that I have described the basic stages of the process, I will indicate some variations on the matching technique. In the example above, I matched a salience—something specific (a tightness or a shape) that stood out against the background of bodily experience in general. But I can also include more of this background itself, in several ways. I can begin with something salient—for instance, a certain feeling somewhere around my ankle—and then instead of matching only the gesture I am making at this joint, I can begin to match the inner "felt shape" of my whole leg, perhaps even following this up into how I am in my torso, at the other side of my pelvis, and so one. Or, instead of starting with something that is already salient, I can match the *pre*-feeling (i.e., the general ambience in a certain area or in the whole of me before anything specific stands out, the background normality) in contrast to which a specific place might feel tight or stuck. In fact, when I first began working with matching, I nearly always found myself matching a tension that was calling out for attention, as it were; now what often happens is that I "come to" after a period of being unaware of my body and sense my normal postural pattern for what it is: a bodily *signature* that has taken on a characteristic and habitual form—but it need not stay that way forever, for I am free to match it and to allow myself to change.

When I begin to explore the whole of this habitual body signature, however, I find that there are gaps in my proprioceptive awareness—numb spots, or places I can almost but not quite feel my way into or move independently. One approach to matching such areas is to sense as clearly as possible where the borders of these missing pieces are, and then to match these boundaries, these "edges." Another possibility is to match the missing area itself, inwardly aligning myself with it, imagining that I am numbing myself precisely here.

There is yet another approach, one that uses what has been termed bodily reflexivity.[13] When we touch our own bodies, the sense that we are *living* in the touching hand can predominate; I can touch myself in much the same way as I might palpate another person's body, feeling the structure, the tonus, the degree of resistance to movement, and so on. Conversely, I can give myself over to the feeling of being touched, receiving the touch from myself in the same way as I might receive a massage from another person. Sometimes, both roles intermingle: I massage my foot, and I am both the active touching hand and the receptive, touched foot. But another variation is possible.

Let us say that part of my foot seems stiff to the touch. I look at it, and seem to see years of tight shoes still invisibly in place, even though I am barefoot at the moment. But when I try to feel the shape of my foot from within, what I actually feel is vague and truncated. The inner felt shape is hardly there enough to match: it lacks vivid presence and clarifying detail. At this point, I touch my foot lightly somewhere in this "no man's land." It does not matter if I touch it with my hand, my other foot, or even with an object I am holding,[14] because what I do is to put my awareness on the side of the touched foot. Perhaps I can then say, "Ah, I am being touched precisely *here*," or perhaps all I can really tell at first is that I am feeling the touch nearer the toes than the heel. But I match the feeling of being touched just so.

Then, however, I shift gears: I reinterpret the very same sensation as though I am the *toucher,* touching something else with this part of my foot, rather than the *touchee.* If, for example, I have begun by touching my foot with my hand, I leave my hand where it is, but reinterpret the situation so that now it is my hand that I am touching with my foot—or, and this is the point, I can begin to feel how my foot feels, from within, in the act of touching my hand. In this way, the sensation in my foot becomes, however minimally, a sensed gesture that I myself have appropriated—an active gesture of touching, with just this part of me and just this degree of pressure. And matching this gesture becomes a way to break the cycle of sensorimotor amnesia that clouded my awareness of this part of myself in the first place.[15]

So far, I have described matching a shape or a feeling, turning it into a gesture of continuing to hold myself in precisely this way, with just this feeling. In the examples I have presented, I have assumed that my body is more or less at rest. However, I can also match while moving, as in the case of the woman matching the asymmetry of her hips while walking. This kind of matching is especially helpful in practicing motor skills, e.g., in learning to play a musical instrument with more ease and freedom. By consciously matching, say, my habitual way of raising my shoulder as I play the violin, I open the door for new possibilities to emerge of their own accord. But matching may be equally useful for more basic matters, such as the habitual way my foot meets the ground as I walk. Indeed, some shapes and patterns that are difficult to match when I am still can suddenly make a lot of sense when matched as a *frozen moment* in a habitual (and habitually out of awareness) movement pattern.

And the possibilities do not stop here. For example, Carl Ginsburg describes how a person who had sustained a spinal injury but could still feel her own body "learned to begin to control spasms by internally moving herself in the direction the spasm was already taking her; in other words, she turned the spasm into an intention. The intention in this case did not produce movement but did result in a rapid subsiding of the spasm."[16] And Ninoska Gomez describes how we can begin to "transform into" or "merge with" all sorts of somatic data, consciously embodying, say, our heart pumping or our blood circulating in a spirit of "pretending and seeing what happens."[17] In other words, matching is a way of reinterpreting what is happening *to* me or *inside* of me—not only by feeling my way into it, but also by experiencing whatever is going on *as if* it is something I myself am doing.[18] The limits of what we can learn to match in this way—even without the aid of biofeedback equipment—are not yet known. Clearly, though if something is at all present to me kinesthetically, somesthetically, or proprioceptively, I can find a way to match it and see what happens. For as a way of appropriating something as ongoingly my own, matching blurs the distinction between the voluntary and the involuntary; I can use the *as if* to align myself even with processes and functions I would have thought were outside *my* control.

Up to now, I have focused on matching as a solo venture, but the matching principle can be applied in the way one works with another person, as well. What Thomas Hanna has termed *kinetic mirroring* can serve as an example. Here the teacher does not attempt to break down a student's habitual patterns, but actively goes along with them, guiding the student's body into the very same resistance pattern which is normally assumed unconsciously. In this way, the student not only begins to become aware of the habitual pattern, but also "somehow [becomes] voluntarily free to control the formerly programmed pattern of muscular contraction."[19]

The same principle is evident in Judith Aston's description of how somatic learning happens in general:

It's not a matter of adding concepts and effort on top of what is already there. In this work we analyze how a body is in structure and function, evoking the person's awareness of it and then expanding the pattern to unveil and reveal a new truth. In this way we provide the option for a new pattern to emerge and grow. First, you have to match what it, then you evoke expansion of movement, then you progressively multiply this into new movement patterns.[20]

Another way of putting this is that matching what is, just as it is, *possibilizes* it.[21] Something that is initially given as simply actual ("this is the way it is") is maintained as being precisely *this way.* But the act of consciously maintaining it (or imagining that one is doing so) helps turn this actual way-it-is into a *possibility*—the particular possibility that happens to be actualized here and now, in this particular case.

And by transforming the given condition into a possibility—into one possibility among others, the one that happens to be actual at the moment—it is as though we have made these other possibilities thinkable, feelable, doable.[22]

Matching, then, turns out to be a kind of "prescribing the symptom"[23] that surrounds the actual—even the habitual—with a "halo" of other possible ways to be. But it is more than this. The matching technique I have described is a way of overcoming an ingrained dualism; it involves a dynamic and participatory appreciation of time; it is predicated on a tendency toward health and wholeness; and it encourages autonomy and responsibility without isolating the individual from the context. Again, these points are interlinked, but I will comment on each of them in turn.

(1) One of the most pervasive features of contemporary experience might be termed the *I-it* structure of bodily experience. This structure can take on many forms, ranging from the "notion that perhaps oneself and one's body are two separate entities"[24] to a tendency to organize one's perception of one's own body as though I, the perceiving self, am *up here* (in my head) while my own body, the thing perceived, is *down there* (with my foot being farther away from me than, say my, shoulders).[25] These and other ways of carrying on the tradition of mind-body dualism find both expression and support in everyday language. Thus one can say, for example, "I have a feeling of tightness in my body," without noticing that this way of speaking drives a wedge between *I* and *my body*. The discourse of disembodiment is particularly obvious when we are ill or injured: "It hurts," I say, or "It's not getting any better" (or, more optimistically, "It's going to take quite a while to heal").[26] But even if I avoid referring to my own body as *it* and say something like "I have a pain in my right foot," my language distances me from my own foot.

Matching, however, is a way of reappropriating *my body* as *me*. At the beginning of the matching process, something (e.g., an inner felt shape) is present *to* me, as an object of my experience. Even if it is woven of a special class of sensations that can refer to no other object in the world, but only present a unique object of experience, *my own lived body*—even if these sensations are distinguished above all by a certain quality of *mine*ness (as the word *proprioception* already indicates)—the shape I perceive can still seem other than, or external to, the perceiving self. But when I *enter* this shape, joining with it, aligning with myself with it, as if *I* were doing it on purpose, the whole structure of the experience shifts: the shape is transformed into a gesture *I* am participating in. Even the tonus of a particular bodily region becomes a subtle gesture of holding on here, tightening up there, bracing myself in just this way. With matching, then, it is as though I begin to melt the boundary that the I-it paradigm imposes between me and my own body, and I can begin to let *me*-ness flow more fully into the whole of me.[27]

(2) Furthermore, with matching, something relatively static—a shape or a tightness that is just *there*—is transformed into something that ongoingly continues to be just this way.[28] Bodily experience is not only appropriated as mine, but it becomes dynamic. We speak of "keeping ourself in shape," and we know what we mean: keeping fit, so that we can move with grace and strength, endurance and ease, flexibility and precision. But in another, more literal sense, we are always *in a shape,* with our limbs at this or that angle, our torso buoyant or droopy, and so on. This shape is not a *fait accompli,* but an ongoing achievement, a self-shaping and a "keeping ourselves" in this or that shape, for even a seemingly frozen feeling or shape is an ongoing temporal phenomenon. And habitual shapes are habitual precisely because they are reiterated. Thus with matching, what I do is get inside the skin of this reiteration, maintaining it as an ongoing, dynamic process. Again, however, I do not *try* to keep myself in this shape; I simply match the continual renewal of it that is already going on, leaving the door open, as it were, for other possibilities to emerge.

And there is a certain way of appreciating the flowing *now* that facilitates this process. One can begin to get in touch with the leading edge and the trailing edge of the now moment, experiencing the way it spills into the future while remaining connected with the just-past.[29] When I do this, it not only helps me to become more aware of the ongoingness of somatic experience, but it also helps me to stay with the living now, rather than fantasizing about, predicting, hoping for, or trying to produce certain future *results.* In matching, not knowing what will happen next is of the utmost importance, for it keeps me from limiting myself in advance to my repertoire of known possibilities—all of which may reinstate a pattern that might otherwise be free to shift spontaneously. But such not-knowing also involves a trust—sense that whatever spontaneous release or reorganization may occur will turn out to be a good thing.[30]

(3) It is here that the matching technique I have presented perhaps differs most from other approaches that use the "golden moments" of bodily awareness as opportunities for correcting faults and replacing old habits with new patterns. In such approaches, I might match with what is in order to lead it consciously in a new direction—or better, to lead *myself* as a whole in a new direction (rather than bringing the I-it paradigm back into play in such a way that an ego, mind, or self tells the body what to do.) But matching is a way to allow the whole itself to lead.

As I have already mentioned, there are limits to what can be achieved through self-help. Peter Koestenbaum points out that self-help in general is usually based on the very premises that have contributed to the problem in the first place;[31] if I try to "stand up straighter," for example, I will rely on my usual sense of what standing is in the very act of trying to stand up straighter. Yet it may be these deeper bodily assumptions about what standing is and how it is accomplished that need revision. Furthermore, some holding patterns may also be so much a part of me that they are simply not present in my awareness at all; I cannot imagine changing them because I do not even know that there is anything there to be changed. At other times, I am all too aware that something is amiss, and so I try to fix it. But I may not notice that I have my own bodily style of *trying*(and if at first I don't succeed, trying not only again, but *harder*).[32] Yet my somatic pattern of trying may be intimately interwoven with the very best pattern I am trying to correct, so that the more I *try* to change, the more I let my old pattern sneak back in. Finally, as F. M. Alexander pointed out years ago, my sense for what feels *right* and what feels *wrong* may not be trustworthy, for what feels right to me is likely to be some version of the same old age pattern I thought I was learning to change.[33] What all of this adds up to is that there are indeed times when self-help does not get to the root of the problem; we may genuinely need the other person to help.

But there is another side to the story, for it can be debilitating to relinquish one's body to "experts," whether they be physicians, bodyworkers, parents, gym teachers, or other "authorities." Don Johnson has set forth in great detail the difference between two sorts of "techniques of the body": the "technology of alienation," which "trains people to be disconnected from their sensual authority," the "technology of authenticity," which is based on what one directly experiences with one's senses.[34] The matching technique I have presented here is unequivocally meant as a technology of authenticity. It is not only a way of taking responsibility for the shape I am in, but also a way of empowering myself—as a whole, not just as a reflecting ego— as the "expert" who will decide what needs to happen next. Thus I am assuming that the spontaneous shifts, which I experience when matching, stem from a tendency toward health, wholeness, and optimal functioning, a tendency that permeates every cell of me.[35]

Moreover, the open-minded attitude of matching—the not-knowing what will happen next or where a shift might occur—not only assumes that I can trust my own somatic wholeness, but helps me actually experience myself as an articulated whole. As I have mentioned, the spontaneous shifts are not necessarily confined to the area I am actively matching; they can reverberate through other parts of me, as well. I may begin to feel what else has to accommodate for this to let go, or I may begin to sense that this shape is the tail end of a larger gesture, and so on. Thus, rather than considering myself to be a collection of separate parts—this muscle here, then that one there, and so on—I begin to feel like a creature of one large muscle, elegantly differentiated into many intricate details, contract here and lengthening there, but always moving as a whole.[36]

(4) This shift from thinking in terms of isolated parts to perceiving articulated wholes suggests yet another dimension to matching. There are many things in life that go better if I match with the situation as a whole, moving with it as a participant instead of separating myself from it in a resolutely I-it kind of way. Simply being with what one is doing in a matching way can open up the process and allow it

to flow freely, whether one is performing in a concert, skiing down a slope, or washing the dishes.[37] Matching an impasse with awareness can allow it to melt, and matching a painful emptiness can allow it to become a "fertile void."[38] Somehow the simple experiential move of consciously aligning with what is already going on anyway and gently illuminating it with awareness not only brings some clarity to the situation, but also eases it—loosening up, as it were, the invisible lines of force that had set the situation up in just this way. Then whatever needs to happen next can emerge naturally, and I find myself moving with the situation as a whole, rather than confronting it and trying to control it. Here matching is not so much a strictly somatic technique as an attitude toward life.

But even in a more literally somatic sense, matching is more than a matter of individual awareness of one's own body. It is not merely a solipsistic procedure, but has intercorporeal reverberations as well.[39] Many writers have pointed out that somatic experience is a matter of *shared* rhythm and tonus.[40] We are who we are in interconnection with one another.[41] It is as though, on some deep level, we are matching one another all the time. For instance, if I enter a room full of tense and anxious people, my own tonus and breathing may be affected— often without my realizing it. But if I am able to tap into my own somatic awareness, matching allows me to reclaim my autonomy. I need not automatically continue mirroring the prevailing tension, but can allow a small shift to happen on my own. And if I find myself calming down and easing up, I may notice this spreading to the others as well, just as I *caught* their tension in the first place—all without any attempt on my part to manipulate them actively. Thus although we are intercorporeally connected with one another, we are neither completely nor irrevocably determined by what is going on with the people around us. We do move in concert with one another, adjusting ourselves to each other in a "mutual tuning-in relationship"[42] that is thoroughly somatic. Yet I am free to move in a new way, too, and one way to do this is by consciously matching how I already am in the intercorporeal situation.[43] Matching, then, fosters autonomy and self-responsibility without ripping us out of the human context: it honors both our individuality and the way we are linked in larger wholes.[44]

Some final comments may serve to place the notion of matching itself in a broader context. Thomas Hanna has characterized the "shared vision" of the discipline of somatics as involving two fundamental factors: recognition of the importance and power of awareness (in particular, of direct awareness of our own somatic processes); and respect for the person as autonomous and self-governing.[45] The matching technique involves precisely these factors, and is thus an undeniable expression of an approach in a somatic style. But as Hanna indicates, the "common vision of the emerging present" found in the somatics field is itself the expression of a "new world, just now appearing, that beckons to be discovered, explored and created."[46]

Among those who have charted this new world in the greatest detail is the European philosopher of culture Jean Gebser (1905–1973). His monumental "history of the structure of consciousness" culminates in the description of a new, integral world and consciousness that is emerging in our times, for which he finds evidence in every discipline and every aspect of life. Among the clues to this new world-perception are the supercession of dualism; the full incorporation of time as a dynamic feature of things, as well as events; and a turn toward wholes and wholeness. The matching technique involves overcoming habitual I-it dualism; awakening our sense of the ongoingness of somatic experience; and relying on the wholeness of the soma while realizing that somas are interconnected in larger wholes. Thus matching fits Gebser's requirements for being a manifestation of this new consciousness; it is a way toward embodying integrality.[47]

In fact, the discipline of somatics as a whole may be fruitfully linked with Gebser's work. The somatics field not only overcomes dualisms, such as mind v. body and theory v. practice, but also integrates first-person and third-person approaches to the soma, rather than conceiving them as opposites. And somatics not only deals with the soma as living process and function (rather than as corpse or machine), but it does so in a way that situates the wholeness of individual somas within more encompassing cultural and cosmological wholes.[48] Somatics itself may thus be seen as a manifestation of the integrality Gebser writes about, and his work provides one way of elucidating the broader context within which the emergence of this new discipline makes sense. On the other hand, somatic education offers a bodily praxis that can foster and sustain the emerging world of wholeness that Gebser speaks of. The matching technique I have described here is but one of many approaches to such a practice of wholeness. Other articles could well be written to show, for example, how the matching principle can enrich existing somatic techniques and generate new ones. But the point is not just to read and write about it—the point is also to *do* it.[49] Only then are all these words fulfilled in the experiential evidence that alone justifies them; only then is what I am talking about present, not abstractly, but in the flesh: in our flesh and in the "flesh of the world" we share.[50]

Notes

1. This essay is a revised and expanded version of one section of a previously published essay: Elizabeth A. Behnke, "'How we shout into the woods is how the echo will sound': Remarks on the Reintegration of Projections," *Gebser Studies* 1 (1987), 59–143. See section 9, "Bodily reintegration of projections: 'matching,'" pp. 111 ff. The present version is part of a larger research project, the Study Project in Phenomenology of the Body, founded in 1987. For more information about this project, please contact the author at P.O. Box O-2, Felton, CA 95018.

2. Don Hanlon Johnson, "Principles versus Techniques: Towards the Unity of the Somatics Field," *Somatics* 6:1 (Autumn/Winter, 1986–87), 4.

3. Edmund Husserl, *Introduction to the Logical Investigations,* ed. Eugen Fink, trans. Philip J. Bossert and Curtis H. Peters (The Hague: Martinus Nijhoff, 1975), p. 57. The necessity of cashing in the words for the appropriate experiential evidence is one of the cornerstones of Husserlian phenomenology, as I see it. Husserl (1859–1938) was not only the founding father of the 20th century discipline of phenomenology, but contributed many important descriptions of somatic experience as lived in the first person. See, e.g., Edmund Husserl, *Ideas Pertaining to a Pure Phenomenology and to a Phenomenological Philosophy,* Second Book: *Studies in the Phenomenology of Constitution,* trans. Richard Rojcewicz and André Schuwer (Dordrecht: Kluwer Academic Publishers, 1989). In addition, he sketched out a discipline he called "somatology," which combined "the direct somatic perception that every empirical investigator can effect only on his [or her] own body" with scientific-physiological investigations into "the material properties of the animate organism." See Edmund Husserl, *Ideas Pertaining to a Pure Phenomenology and to a Phenomenological Philosophy,* Third Book: *Phenomenology and the Foundations of the Sciences,* trans.

Ted E. Klieg and William E. (The Hague: Nijhoff, 1980), section 2b. (Both the Second and the Third Books of *Ideas* were originally written in 1912.)

4. "A Somatics Interview with Judith Aston," *Somatics* 3:1 (Autumn, 1980), 12. Although I subsequently realized that the matching principle had been used by a number of bodyworkers, it was reading this passage that initially set me on the path of trying out matching for myself; the present paper is based on what Aston asks the woman to do in the story cited.

5. Aston emphasizes (ibid., p. 14) that although some bodily "holding patterns" can be changed "at will" through education and awareness, other chronic holding patterns "require another person to help unravel the accumulation of abuse." She characterizes the latter type of holding pattern as "structural" and the former type as "functional." For another approach to the question of self-help and the need for the other in somatic reeducation, see Elizabeth A. Behnke, "Practical Intercorporeity," forthcoming.

6. See, for example, Sidney M. Jourard, "Some Ways of Unembodiment and Reembodiment," *Somatics* 1:1 (Autumn, 1976), 3–7; Thomas Hanna, "What Is Somatics?" [Part One], *Somatics* 5:4 (Spring/Summer, 1986), pp. 7–8, on "sensory-motor amnesia"; James J. Lynch, *The Language of the Heart: The Human Body in Dialogue* (New York: Basic Books, 1985), pp. 223–240, on the "disconnected body"; Gerda Alexander, *Eutony* (Great Neck, N.Y.: Felix Morrow, 1985), pp. 112 ff., on impoverished body image.

7. See, for example, the inventory of possible kinds of somatic sensations in the Shaun Gallagher, "Hyletic experience and the lived body," *Husserl Studies* 3:2 (1986), p. 142, based in part on the discussions in Russell Mason, *Internal Perception and Bodily Functioning* (New York: International Universities Press, 1961).

8. I say "more fully" because often it is an incipient sense of bodily discomfort that has moved me to let go of the task I've been engaged in and take some time for bodily awareness. However, matching need not be motivated by discomfort, but can be done at any time—seated at one's desk, standing in line, practicing a skill, etc.

9. Of course, I can also ignore or repress my bodily feelings, or treat them as symptoms to be brought to the attention of a doctor or bodyworker. Here, however, I am presuming that I am not only aware of my own body, but willing to take personal responsibility for my own bodily feelings rather than consulting an "expert." I will return to this point later in the text.

10. The root of the word "appropriation" is the Latin *proprius*, "one's own"; "appropriation" literally means "making something one's own," which connotes as Edward S. Casey points out, *"making it one with one's ongoing life"*—Casey, *Remembering: A Phenomenological Study* (Bloomington: Indiana

University Press, 1987), p. 192. *Proprius* is, of course, also the root of the word "proprioceptive."

11. The notion of using matching as a sequence of small shifts, matching each new configuration as it arises, is modeled after the use of similar sequences of steps in the Focusing process developed by Eugene T. Gendlin. See, e.g., his *Focusing,* 2nd rev. ed. (New York: Bantam, 1981), pp. 62–63. Cf. also Aston (see n. 4), pp. 12, 14, on the progressive "unraveling" of holding patterns.

12. I have borrowed this lovely phrase from Alexandra and Roger Pierce, *Generous Movement* (Redlands, California: work in progress, 1986 version), Chapter 8, "Transformation," where the concept is discussed at length.

13. See Elizabeth A. Behnke, "World without Opposite/Flesh of the World (A Carnal Introduction)," unpublished (1984), especially pp. 14–19.

14. I can also begin simply by becoming aware of what I am already touching anyway with the part of myself concerned. In addition, the experience of being touched by another can be used in this way as well. Cf. Carl Ginsburg, "The Shake-A-Leg Body Awareness Training Program: Dealing with Spinal Injury and Recovery in a new setting," *Somatics* 5:4 (Spring/Summer, 1986), pp. 40–42, where Ginsburg describes how a client he is touching gradually reintegrates her somatic perception into her body image; cf. pp. 35–36 on transforming amnesia and lacuna into embodiment. The use of a "matching" attitude on the part of a client while being touched by a practitioner is a wonderful way to make the latter's touch facilitative rather than merely manipulative, and allows the client to participate more fully in his or her own somatic reeducation, rather than just "receiving therapy."

15. See Hanna (see n. 6), p. 8.

16. Ginsburg (see n. 14), p. 38; cf. p. 37.

17. Ninoska Gomez, "Embodying the Structures and Functions of the Body," *Somatics* 5:4 (Spring/Summer 1986), p. 52.

18. On the efficacy of the "as if," cf. the well-known benefits of imagined movement. See, e.g., G. Alexander (see n. 6), pp. 38–41, and Lulu E. Sweigard, *Human Movement Potential: Its Ideokinetic Facilitation* (New York: Harper & Row, 1974); cf. the general notion of practicing a movement on one side of the body, then imagining it on the other side (one of the most potent strategies in the Feldenkrais Awareness Through Movement Approach).

19. Thomas Hanna, "Moshe Feldenkrais: The Silent Heritage," *Somatics* 5:1 (Autumn/Winter, 1984–85), p. 26. As Hanna points out (pp. 23, 25, 27), Feldenkrais' use of kinetic mirroring in Functional Integration is an application of a basic principle in Oriental martial arts, such as jujitsu and judo (which Feldenkrais, of course, was thoroughly familiar with).

20. Aston, (see n. 4), p. 12. Cf. the general formula "pace, then lead" used by many psychotherapists, notably those whose work is modeled on that of Milton Erickson. See, e.g., Richard Bandler and John Grinder, *Patterns of the Hypnotic Techniques of Milton H. Erickson, M.D.,* Vol. 1 (Cupertino, California: Meta Publications, 1975), pp. 15 ff., 202; John Grinder and Richard Bandler, *Trance-Formations,* ed. Connirae Andreas (Moab, Utah: Real People Press, 1981), pp. 14–15 (where the term "matching" is used as synonymous with "pacing"), 27–28, 35, 43; Mark Reese, "Moshe Feldenkrais' Verbal Approach to Somatic Education: Parallels to Milton Erickson's Use of Language," *Somatics* 5:3 (Autumn/Winter, 1985–86), pp. 23–24, 25.

21. On "possibilizing," see Richard M. Zaner, "The Leap of Freedom Education and the Possible," *Main Currents* 28:5 (May/June 1972), pp. 177–178; *The Context of Self: A Phenomenological Inquiry Using Medicine as a Clue* (Athens, Ohio: Ohio University Press, 1981), pp. 175 ff.

22. To describe matching in terms of possibilizing is, in a sense, to describe "how it works" in terms of the structure of experience in general. A more precise phenomenological explication of how matching works might focus on (a) the shift from "the lived body given as an object of experience through 'body feeling'" to "bodily subjectivity as kinaesthetic consciousness'—i.e., the shift, in Ludwig Landgrebe's terms, from the "body as constituted" to the "body as constituting"; and (b) the horizonal nature of kinaesthetic consciousness, i.e., its status as a coherent system of possibilities. On the body as constituting, see Ludwig Landgrebe, "The Problem of Passive Constitution," trans. Donn Welton, in Landgrebe, *The Phenomenology of Edmund Husserl,* ed. Donn Welton (Ithaca: Cornell University Press, 1981), especially pp. 56 ff. On kinaesthetic consciousness, see Ulrich Clesges, *Edmund Husserls Theorie der Raumkonstitution* (The Hague: Martinus Nijhoff, 1964), and on kinaesthetic systems see, e.g., Edmund Husserl, *Ding und Raum, Vorlesungen 1907,* ed. Ulrich Claesges (The Hague: Martinus Nijhoff, 1973). Note that a physiological approach to explaining how matching works is also possible; indeed for researchers in somatics, phenomenological explication of the relevant structures of experience would be incomplete unless complemented by an account of the biological processes involved. For instance, it has been suggested by Thomas Hanna (personal communication) that certain techniques using the matching principle can be understood with reference to different parts of the brain involved in voluntary and involuntary actions. However, a neurophysiology of the "matching" type of awareness is beyond the scope of the present essay, which is written solely from the phenomenological side.

23. Cf. Reese (see n. 20), p. 28.

24. Lynch (see n. 6), p. 11; cf., e.g., Deane Juhan, *Job's Body: A Handbook for*

Bodywork (Barrytown, N.Y.: Station Hill Press, 1987), pp. 335–36; Zaner, *Context of Self* (see n. 21), pp. 48–57. for more on the identity/difference of self and body, see Sally Gadow, "Body and Self: A Dialectic," in Victor Kestenbaum, ed., *The Humanity of the Ill: Phenomenological Perspectives* (Knoxville: University of Tennessee Press, 1982), pp. 86–100, and especially Phyllis Sutton Morris, "Some Patterns of Identification and Otherness," *Journal of the British Society for Phenomenology* 13:3 (October, 1982), pp. 216–25.

25. See Erwin W. Strauss, "The Forms of Spatiality," in his *Phenomenological Psychology,* trans., in part, Erling Eng (New York: Basic Books, 1966), p. 26; cf. Herbert Spiegelberg, "On the Motility of the Ego," in Walter von Baeyer and Richard M. Griffith, ed., *Conditio Humana* (Berlin: Springer, 1966), pp. 289–306.

26. On such "disconnected language," see Lynch (see n. 6), pp. 213, 226 ff.

27. Richard Heckler is applying the matching principle in a similar way when he says, "Working with the person living in the body, we say 'Relax yourself around your jaw' instead of 'Relax your jaw'"—Richard Strozzi Heckler, *The Anatomy of Change* (Berkeley, California: North Atlantic Books, 1993), p. 16

28. On the "ongoingness" rather than "one-and-for-all-ness" of embodiment, see Richard M. Zaner, *The Problem of Embodiment* (The Hague: Martinus Nijhoff, 1964), pp. 249 ff.; *Context of Self* (see n. 21), pp. 57 ff. Cf. Juhan (see n. 24), pp. 10, 19.

29. Here I am relying on Edmund Husserl's description of retentional and protentional horizons; see his *On the Phenomenology of the Consciousness of Internal Time* (1893–1917), trans. John Barnett Brough (Dordrecht: Kluwer Academic Publishers, 1991). For a convenient presentation of these concepts in a less technical context, see Thomas Clifton, *Music as Heard* (New Haven: Yale University Press), pp. 59–65.

30. Thus although I may disengage myself from specific expectations about what will happen next, a general expectation that it will be a move toward more optimal somatic functioning is swung into play. On the role of expectation in shaping health, see Thomas Hanna, "What Is Somatics," Part Four, *Somatics* 6:3 (Autumn/Winter, 1987–88), pp. 57–58.

31. Peter Koestenbaum, *The New Image of the Person* (Westport, Connecticut: Greenwood Press, 1978), p. 245. It is nevertheless noteworthy that many of the major approaches to somatic education are founded on what pioneers such as F. M. Alexander, Elsa Gindler, Moshe Feldenkrais, and Gerda Alexander discovered in their own efforts at self-help.

32. See, e.g., Roger Tengwall, "Towards an Etiology of Malposture: A Social Scientist Looks at Postural Behavior," *Somatics* 3:3 (Autumn/Winter, 1981–82), p. 26.

33. See, e.g., F. Mathias Alexander, *Constructive Conscious Control of the Individual* (New York: E.P. Dutton, 1923), where he uses such expressions as "unreliable sensory appreciation" and "debauched kinesthesia." On the entire issue of self-help, cf. also his general critique of "end-gaining" where what is needed instead is attention to the "means whereby."

34. See Don Hanlon Johnson, *Body: Recovering our Sensual Wisdom* (Berkeley: North Atlantic, 1992), pp. 68 ff., 142 ff., 152 ff., 167 ff.; the phrase quoted is from p. 80.

35. See, e.g., Sweigard (see n. 24), pp. 3, 227–228, and cf. the principle of homeostasis, in general.

36. I have borrowed this notion from Deane Juhan. Cf. Juhan (see n. 24), pp. 113–15.

37. Cf., e.g., Eloise Ristad, *A Soprano on Her Head* (Moab, Utah: Real People Press, 1982), Chapter 13; Denise McCluggage, *The Centered Skier,* rev. ed. (New York: Bantam, 1983), pp. 178–79; Mildred Portney Chase, *Just Being at the Piano* (Culver City, California: Peace Press, 1981), pp. 6–8. Cf. also the kinds of aikido notions of "entering" and "blending"; see, e.g., Heckler (see n. 27), pp. 90 ff., and cf. n. 19 above.

38. See, e.g., Fritz Perls, *The Gestalt Approach & Eye Witness to Therapy* (Palo Alto, California: Science and Behavior Books, 1973), pp. 96–100, especially p. 99; cf. Oliver Sacks, *A Leg to Stand On* (New York: Summit Books, 1984), Chapter 3.

39. The term "intercorporeality" is derived from the writings of the French phenomenonologist Maurice Merleau-Ponty (1908–1861). See, e.g., his *Signs,* trans. Richard C. McCleary (Evanston, Illinois: Northwestern University Press, 1964), pp. 19, 168, 173.

40. See, for example, G. Alexander (see n. 6), pp. 21–22, 48, 55, 57, 61–62, 150, 169 on tonus imitation and transmission; Edward T. Hall, *The Dance of Life* (Garden City, N.Y.: Anchor, 1984), pp. 177 ff., and George Leonard, *The Silent Pulse* (New York: E.P. Dutton, 1978), pp. 13 ff.; on the synchronization of people's microrhythms in the "entrainment" phenomenon studied by William Condon; and Jourard (see n. 6), pp. 3–4, on bodily communication of vitality.

41. See Lynch (see n. 6), especially chapter 6 on blood pressure and dialogue and the Chapter 7 on the "social membrane."

42. Alfred Schutz, "Making Music Together: A Study in Social Relationship," in his *Collected Papers,* Vol 2, ed. Arvid Brodersen (The Hague: Martinus Nijhoff, 1964), p. 161.

43. See G. Alexander (see n. 6), pp. 8, 48, 50–51, 53, for application of this principle of working with another.

44. Although I have mentioned only the human context, the interspecies somatic dialogue must be considered as well.

45. See Thomas Hanna, "Backing Into the Common Ground: Reflections of the Editor," *Somatics* 3:1 (Autumn, 1980), inside front cover; see also his four-part series, "What Is Somatics?" *Somatics* 5:4–6:3 (Spring/Summer, 1986–Autumn/Winter, 1987–88), especially Part Four on awareness.

46. Hanna, "Backing Into the Common Ground" (see n. 45).

47. Gebser's major work, originally published in two parts in 1949 and 1953, is *The Ever-Present Origin,* trans. Noel Barstad with Algis Mickunas (Athens, Ohio: Ohio University Press, 1985). For introductions to his work, see Georg Feuerstein, *Structures of Consciousness* (Lower Lake, California: Integral Publishing, 1987); Elizabeth A Behnke, "An Introduction to the Work of Jean Gebser," *Gebser Studies* 1 (1987), pp. 1–29.

48. See, e.g. Johnson, *Body* (see n. 34) on the cultural, and Hanna, "What Is Somatics?" (see n. 45), especially parts Two and Four, on the cosmological.

49. I would be interested in feedback from persons who have tried out the matching technique or taught it to others, as well as from those who have devised different ways to apply the matching principle.

50. The notion of the "flesh of the world" stems from Maurice Merleau-Ponty; see his *The Visible and the Invisible,* ed. Claude Lefort, trans. Alphonso Lingis (Evanston, Illinois: Northwestern University Press, 1968).

Thomas Hanna

*T*homas Hanna (1928–1990) wrote several books and a journal which have been major factors in creating a community of understanding and dialogue among the many schools of embodiment. As both a philosopher as well as a practitioner of the Feldenkrais method, out of which he eventually created his own method, he had the unusual standpoint from which to see not only the practical healing significance of these works but their larger implications for understanding reality. This first of a long series of essays on the these works of embodiment represents a seminal moment in articulating the unity of the seemingly diverse works represented in this volume.

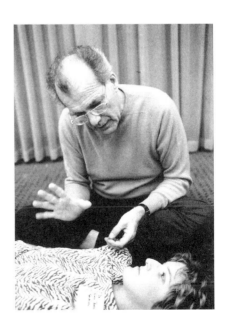

What Is Somatics?

Thomas Hanna

1. The Distinction between Soma and Body

Somatics the field which studies the *soma:* namely the body as perceived from within by first-person perception. When a human being is observed from the outside—i.e., from a third-person viewpoint—the phenomenon of a human *body* is perceived. But, when this same human being is observed from the first-person viewpoint of his own proprioceptive senses, a categorically different phenomenon is perceived: the human soma.

The two distinct viewpoints for observing a human being are built into the very nature of human observation which is equally capable of being internally self-aware as well as externally aware. The soma, being internally perceived, is categorically distinct from a body, not because the subject is different but because the mode of viewpoint is different: it is immediate proprioception—a sensory mode that provides unique data.

It is fundamental to recognize that the same individual is categorically different when viewed from a first-person perception than is the case when he is viewed from a third-person perception. The sensory access is categorically different as are the resultant observations.

The categorical distinction between these two viewpoints establishes the ground rules for all studies of the human species. Failure to recognize the categorical difference between first-person observation and third person observation leads to fundamental misunderstandings in physiology, psychology, and medicine.

Somatics, Part I: Spring/Summer 1986, 4–8; Part II: Autumn/Winter 1986–87, 49–53; Part III: Spring/Summer 1987, 57–61.

Physiology, for example, takes a third-person view of the human being and sees a body. This body is an objective entity, observable, analyzable, and measurable in the same way as any other object. The universal laws of physics and chemistry are brought to bear on this body, because—as an observed body—it richly displays universal physical and chemical principles.

From a first-person viewpoint, however, quite different data are observed. The proprioceptive centers communicate and continually feed back a rich display of somatic information which is immediately self-observed as a process that is both unified and ongoing. Somatic data do not need, first, to be mediated and interpreted through a set of universal laws to become factual. First-person observation of the soma is immediately factual. Third-person observation, in contrast, can become factual only by mediation through a set of principles.

It should be understood that this difference in data is neither a difference in truthful accuracy nor of intrinsic value. The difference is that the two separate modes of recognition are irreducible. Neither mode is less factual or inferior to the other: they are coequal.

Psychology, for example, takes a third-person view of the human being and sees a body of behavior. This bodily behavior is an objective datum that is observable, analyzable, and measurable, as is any other behavioral datum. The universal laws of cause and effect, stimulus and response, and adaptation are brought to bear on the behaving body, because—as an observed body—it richly displays these behavioral principles.

But, from a first-person viewpoint, quite different data are observed. The proprioceptive centers communicate and feed back immediate factual information on the process of the ongoing unified soma—with the momentum of its past, along with the intentions and expectations of its future. These data are already unified; they have no need to be analyzed, interpreted, and later formulated into a unitary factual statement.

Medicine, for example, takes a third-person view of the human beings and sees a patient (i.e., a clinical body) displaying various symptoms that—when observed, analyzed, and interpreted according to universally known clinical principles—can be diagnosed, treated, and prognosed.

But, from a first-person viewpoint, quite different data are observed. The proprioceptive centers communicate and feed back immediate factual information on the continuous and unified past of the soma and its expectations for the future. The somatic appreciation of how this past led to ill health and how the future may restore—or not restore—health is essential to the full clinical picture. Ignorance of the first-person viewpoint is ignorance of the somatic factor that permeates medicine: the placebo effect and the nocebo affect.

Thus, the human being is quite unlike a mineral or a chemical solution in providing, not one, but two irreducible viewpoints for observation. A third-person viewpoint can only observe a human body. A first-person viewpoint can only observe a human soma—one's own. Body and soma are coequal in reality and value, but they are categorically distinct as observed phenomena. Somatics, then is a field of study dealing with somatic phenomena: i.e., the human being as experienced by himself from the inside.

Interlude: How This Distinction Affects the Sciences

Apart from the requirement that it have a methodical discipline, science has validity in both its research and theorizing exactly to the degree that all data are considered. To ignore essential data, either willfully or innocently, automatically calls into question what one claims to be factual, as well as what one speculates to be so.

The fact that two modes of cognition on the same generic subject will lead to two distinct sets of data has no bearing on the validity of the physical sciences, whose subjects are inanimate and lack the proprioceptive awareness that the scientist himself possesses. But this fact does bear directly on those sciences dealing with subjects who are just as consciously observant as are the scientists who are engaged in observing.

The life sciences in general and the sciences of physiology, psychology, and medicine in particular lack valid grounds for what they assert to be established fact and sound theorizing exactly to the degree that they ignore, willfully or innocently, first-person data. To avoid evidence that is "phenomenological" or "subjective" is unscientific. To dismiss such data as irrelevant and/or unimportant is irresponsible.

2. The Soma Is Self-Regulating as well as Self-Sensing

When you, as a scientist, are looking at a subject who, unlike a rock, is looking back at you, it is not easy to pretend that the subject is merely a complicated rock. If one insists on doing so, it is certain that no valid scientific conclusions will be reached, nor will they have genuine applicability to anything at all—unless, perhaps, to a complicated rock.

Thus, the first step in understanding somatics is to recognize—and never cease to remind oneself—that somas are not bodies and the objective scientific verities concerning the latter are not *ipso facto* applicable to the former. To do so would be what logicians refer to as a "category mistake."

The second step into the somatic realm is just as significant: it is the recognition that the factor of self-awareness is only the first of several distinctions of the human soma. The human is not merely a self-aware soma, passively observing itself (as well as observing its scientific observer), but it is doing something else simultaneously: It is acting upon itself; i.e., it is always engaged in the process of self-regulation.

When we play the role of scientist and observe a rock, nothing thereby changes for the rock (except, as Heisenberg reminded us, there are minute changes caused by our body heat, shadow, etc.). But the soma that is being observed is not only aware of itself through self-observation but it is also simultaneously in the process of modifying itself before the observer's eyes.

A fundamental finding of physiological psychology is that humans perceive a sensory impression only of that for which they already have an established motor response. If we cannot react to it, the sensory impression doesn't clearly register; it is shunted away from perception. This happens because in the perceptive process the sensorium never operates alone, but always in tandem with the motorium.

The indissoluble functional and somatic unity of the sensory-motor system is testified to by the obvious structural and bodily unity that is built into the human spinal column. The column is composed of descending motor nerves and ascending sensory nerves which exit, respectively, to the fore and aft of the vertebrae. This fore and aft schema continues all the way up the spine to the top of the brain where, just to the fore of the central sulcus of the cerebral cortex, lie the motor tracts and just to the aft the sensory tracts are aligned. It is a schema that is at the center of our being.

The sensory motor system functions as a "closed-loop feedback system" within the soma. We cannot sense without acting, and we cannot act without sensing. The indissoluble unity is essential to the somatic process of self-regulation; at all times, it allows us to know what we are doing. And also—as we shall presently discuss—it is at the core of our unique way of learning and forgetting.

It is not possible to have a distinct sensory perception of any external objective situation without having a distinct motor response already established. This also happens to be the case with the internal sensing of somatic perception: *to sense what is happening within the soma is to act upon it*, i.e., to regulate it.

When, for example, we focus our awareness internally on some portion of our body—our right knee, for instance—the sensory perception of the knee is, indeed, more distinct. But this distinctive highlighting of a bodily part takes place only by selectively relaxing the cortical motor neurons of all the muscles attached to the right knee while contractively inhibiting all the other motor areas of the body. This is to say that focused sensory awareness occurs through focused motor inhibition as a negative "ground" against which a "figure" stands out. Thus, the sensing is not passively receptive but is actively productive, involving the entire somatic process.

This interlocking reciprocity between sensing and moving is at the heart of the somatic process—a process that constitutes its own unity and continuity by constant self-regulation. The externalized "body" seen by the third-person observer is the living product of this continuous somatic process. If that process ceases, then the human body—quite unlike a rock—ceases to be: It dies and disintegrates.

It is the soma's internal process of self-regulation that guarantees the existence of the external bodily structure. Hence, the dictum that is universally valid in somatics: function maintains structure.

The second step in understanding the distinctiveness of the human soma is, then, that it is both self-sensing and self-moving and that these interlocked functions are at the core of somatic self-organization and adaptation.

The soma has a dual talent: It can sense its own individual functions via first-person perception, and it can sense external structures and objective situations via third-person perception. It has the distinctive talent of possessing two modes of perception.

When a human soma looks at itself in a mirror, it sees a body—a third-person, objective structure. But what is this same body when looked at from an internal, somatic perspective? It is the unified experience of self-sensing and self-moving. From the mode of first-person perception, the soma's "body" is a body of functions.

Descartes was not sufficiently thorough. *To think* is not merely "to be" passive; it is *to move*. "I am self-aware, therefore I act," is a more accurate description of first-person perception. *Cogito, ergo moveo* is a statement accurately reporting the data of first-person experience, which always perceived "mind" and "body" in an indissoluble functional unity.

In passing, it should be noted that, by concluding his famous phrase with "... therefore I am," Descartes was incorrectly depicting himself as a passive observer, whereas he was—like all humans—an active observer: a sensing-moving self. It is insufficient to say, passively, "I *am* myself." Inasmuch as "being" is a self-organizing, self-regulating activity for all living beings, it is sufficiently thorough going to say actively, "I am *being* myself."

Interlude: Human Somas and Other Somas

The phrase, *all living beings,* used in the preceding paragraph implies that more is being referred to than human beings alone. This merits a comment.

All members of the animal kingdom are somas, because all animals are self-organizing beings with sensory-motor functions. Many of the things said in this essay about human somas are applicable to all other living beings—with increasing quantifications as one descends the evolutionary scale.

We must not ignore the fact that plants are somas. One needs only to observe the daily opening and closing of petals or the determined striving of a cloistered plant toward the open sun in order to recognize the sensory-motor functions busily in operation.

What does not—as far as anyone knows—occur in any living creature other than man is the ability to focus awareness volitionally, i.e., without an external stimulus being necessary to cause this focusing. This ability, plus the immense learning capacity of the unique human cortex, is the foundation for the extraordinary sensory-motor capacities of the human species, not the least of which is the ability to recognize and actively replicate symbols through vocal speech and manual writing.

3. Consciousness and Awareness

What has been said already about "consciousness" and the focus of "awareness" shows them to be prime somatic functions. Consciousness is basic to the human soma: it designates the range of voluntary sensory-motor functions acquired through learning. Humans learn these functions from birth onward, the motor skills expanding sensory recognition and greater sensory richness potentiating new motor skills.

Consciousness is "voluntary," because its range of skills are learned and, therefore, available for use as familiar patterns. To learn a skill is to learn to employ it at will. Consciousness should not be misunderstood; it is not a static "faculty of the mind" nor a "fixed" sensory-motor pattern. To the contrary, it is a learned sensory-motor function. And the range of this learning determines 1) how much we can be conscious of, and 2) how many things we can voluntarily to.

Involuntary somatic events—such as autonomic reflexes—are not necessarily subject either to conscious sensory recognition or to conscious control. But these involuntary functions can become included in the repertoire of consciousness by the human learning to recognize and control them. This, for example, the established procedure of biofeedback training, just as it is also the practice of those who teach sensory awareness techniques.

Human consciousness is, therefore, a relative function: It can be extremely large or extremely small. As the soma's achieved state of sensory-motor learnings, consciousness cannot perform beyond its self-imposed limits. The states of consciousness lurking within individual somas is variable and unpredictable: it can range from an animal level to a godlike level and, in either of these cases, cannot be made to perceive or respond beyond its achieved level.

Because it involves accumulation of voluntary sensory-motor skills, the greater the range of consciousness, the greater will be the range of autonomy and self-regulation. Human consciousness is, in fine, the instrument of human freedom. For this reason it is important to remember that it is a *learned* function, which can always be expanded by further learning.

By insisting that consciousness is not a fixed mental faculty, we are making it clear that it is not an empty "lens" that focuses on outside objects—this is obviously a third-person conception. Rather, consciousness is the soma's available repertoire of sensory-motor learnings that springs into action when provoked by external stimuli or when caused to act by internal needs.

"Awareness," on the other hand, does function somewhat like a lens that can be pointed and focused. Awareness is a somatic activity that is exclusionary: it uses motor inhibition to exclude any sensory recognition other than that upon which it is focused—which could be something external in the environment (third-person awareness) or internal within the soma (first-person awareness).

The activity of awareness is, one might say, ninety-nine per cent negative and one per cent positive—a "nothing-but-this" function that is the only way for the soma to isolate perceptive events. It is a most useful way of exercising voluntary control over one's repertoire of sensory-motor skills.

Awareness is the function of isolating "new" sensory-motor phenomena in order to learn to recognize and control them. It is only through the exclusionary function of awareness that the *involuntary* is made *voluntary*, the *unknown* is made *known*, and the *never-done* is made *doable*. Awareness serves as a probe, recruiting new material for the repertoire of voluntary consciousness.

The upshot of this is that *somatic learning begins by focusing awareness on the unknown*. This active focusing identifies traits of the unknown that can be associated with traits already known in one's conscious repertoire. Through this process the unknown becomes known by the voluntary consciousness. In a word, the *unlearned* becomes *learned*.

4. Somatic Learning and Sensory-motor Amnesia

Somatic learning is an activity expanding the range of volitional consciousness. This is not to be confused with conditioning, which is a bodily procedure imposed upon a subject by external manipulations. Conditioning deals with the human as a object in a field of objective forces, and thus it is a form learning reflecting the typical viewpoint of third-person science, notably of psychology.

The Pavlovian and Skinnerian models of learning are manipulative techniques of forcing an adaptive response on the body's involuntary reflex mechanisms. Conditioning is an engineering procedure that opposes the function of somatic learning by attempting to reduce the repertoire of voluntary consciousness. Conditioning neither requires focusing of awareness nor does it result in the learning of conscious somatic actions. Rather, their aim is to create an automatic response that is outside the range of volition and consciousness.

But we should be aware of the fact that this same form of conditioning can also take place in uncontrived ways by the fortunes of environmental forces that impinge upon our lives. Environmental situations that impose a constant stimulus on deep survival reflexes will, with sufficient repetitions, make them habitual—the reflex becomes learned and "potentiated."

Reflexes, like all other organic events, are both sensory and motor; and, thus, when they become habituated and involuntary, there is a dual loss of both conscious control of that area of motor action and conscious sensing of that motor action.

We should refer to this as a state of *sensory-motor amnesia.* It is a state that occurs universally in the human species as the predictably conditioned result of long-term stress conditions. Constant repetition of stressful stimuli will cause loss of conscious voluntary control of significant areas of the body's musculature, usually predominating at the center of gravity, i.e., the musculature at the juncture of pelvis and rib cage.

Once sensory-motor amnesia occurs, these areas of musculature can be neither voluntarily sensed nor controlled. The victim can attempt to relax his amnesic lumbar muscles voluntarily, for example, but he no longer has the ability of doing so; both the sensing and movement of these muscles are beyond the reach of his voluntary control. The muscles remain rigid and immobile, as if they belonged to someone else.

Because such reactions to constant stress can build up over sustained periods of time, the resultant chronic muscular contractions are associated with aging. But age is not a causative factor. Time, in itself, is neutral. It is what happens during our lifetime that causes muscular reflexes to habituate. Accumulated stress and trauma are the causes of sensory-motor amnesia, and what we mistakenly ascribe to the effects of "old age" are the direct effects of sensory-motor amnesia.

There is no bodily "cure" for sensory-motor amnesia. The chronic muscular rigidities habituated during aging are impervious to medical remedies. Third-person manipulations are of no avail.

There is, however, a way of releasing the involuntary restrictions of sensory-motor amnesia: it is somatic learning. If one focuses one's awareness on an unconscious, forgotten area of the soma, one can begin to perceive a minimal sensation that is just sufficient to direct a minimal movement, and this, in turn, gives new sensory feedback of that area which, again, gives a new clarity of movement, etc.

This sensory feedback associates with adjacent sensory neurons, further clarifying the synergy that is possible with the associated motor neurons. This makes the next motor effort inclusive of a wider range of associated voluntary neurons, thus broadening and enhancing the motor action and, thereby, further enhancing the sensory feedback. This back-and-forth motor procedure gradually "wedges" the amnesic area back into the range of volitional control: the unknown becomes known and the forgotten becomes relearned.

In another writing it was remarked that "... all forms of somatic education use this human ability to enlarge and improve the degree of our somatic awareness. Like two knitting needles, the sensory system and motor system are made to intertwine, creating a greater sensory awareness of our internal activities and a greater activity of our internal sensory awareness."[1]

Somatic learning is evoked by the teaching methods of Moshe Feldenkrais, but it is of central concern in the methods of Elsa Gindler, F. Mathias Alexander, Gerda Alexander and a host of contemporary practitioners. The techniques of somatic education taught by these teachers are applicable to any form of sensory-motor amnesia, including motor paralysis.

Somatic learning could be a response to amnesia, or it could just as well be an activity that is practiced all one's life, so as to avoid the habituating effects of stress. In whichever case, it is a learning that expands the human soma's range of action as well as perception. As a consequence, the more that is learned in this manner, the greater will be the range of voluntary consciousness for the constant task of adaptation with the environment.

A soma that is maximally free is a soma that has achieved a maximal degree of voluntary control and a minimal degree of involuntary conditioning. This state of autonomy is an optimal state of individuation, i.e., one having a highly differentiated repertoire of response possibilities to environmental stimuli.

The state of somatic freedom is, in many senses, the optimal human state. Looked at from a third-person, bodily viewpoint, somatic freedom is a state of maximal efficiency and minimal entropy. Looked at from a first-person somatic viewpoint, somatic freedom is what I would term a "fair" state—the ancient English word *fair,* meaning a temporal progress that is unblemished and without distortions or the befoulment of inhibition.

The Fair State of the human soma is a state of optimal synergy, wherein any intentional action evokes the spontaneous coordination of the entire somatic process, without any unconscious, involuntary inhibition. This can also be expressed from the third-person viewpoint which would view the Fair State of the soma as a condition of optimal mental and physical health.

In summary, somatics is study of the soma, which is not only first-person perception of the living body but is its first-person regulation.

The involuntary functions can be incorporated into the volitional system by the selective use of awareness to isolate the unlearned function and, by association, to *learn* it—that is, make it part of the conscious functioning of the sensory-motor system.

Notes

1. Hanna, Thomas. *The Body of Life*. New York: Alfred A. Knopf, 1979, p. 198.

Deane Juhan

*L*ike the late Thomas Hanna, Deane brings a considerable background *of intellectual work to bear on thinking through practical methods of embodiment. Originally a literary scholar, he became one of the leading teachers of the Trager Method, and presently conducts trainings throughout the world.* Job's Body *has become a fundamental text for body-workers.*

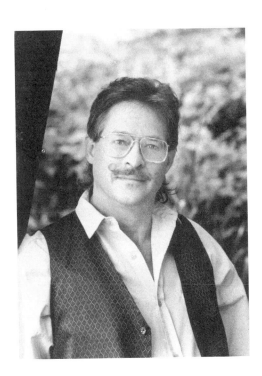

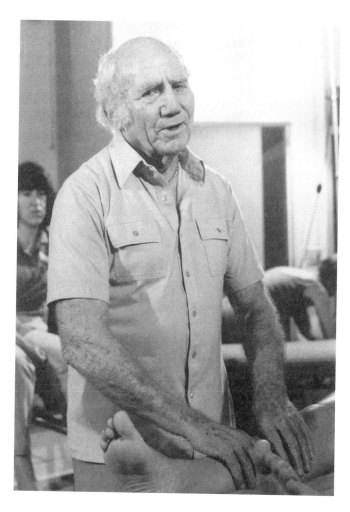

Milton Trager

Job's Body: A Handbook for Bodywork (Excerpts)

Deane Juhan

Introduction

"Having a body," commented Marcel Proust, "constitutes the principle danger that threatens the mind." My body is my means of having or doing anything whatever, necessary not only for all my activities but for life itself. And, paradoxically, its malfeasances can repeatedly thwart my aspirations, dash my hopes, and destroy my comfort.

Often these painful difficulties are unforeseen and apparently undeserved, very like the legendary torments of Job. Job was one of God's favorites, but this benevolent relationship did not prevent Him from accepting a diabolical wager from Lucifer, a ruthless testing of Job's loyalty with betrayal and grievous suffering. The very source of Job's happiness and strength becomes the goad of his pain. Faith, enthusiastic, meets Fate, implacable.

In fear and dismay he consults the "experts"—the legalists, physicians, and counselors of his day. Their answer has a familiar contemporary ring to it. They blame the victim: You have obviously sinned, or you would not be suffering. What Job is forced to discover is that in order to get more satisfactory insight, he must himself confront the powers that be, search out the forces that knit his body and his life together. "I desire to reason with God," he declares, and thereby begins an entirely new relationship with his physical and mental reality.

A good deal of the language of the *Book of Job* suggests provocative clues about where his search must lead him—towards "wisdom in the inward parts." I must, he realizes, "take my flesh in my own

Barrytown, NY: Station Hill Press, 1987.

teeth," and "take my life in my own hands." The resolution of his difficulties will not come from on high, but must be painstakingly unraveled from his own guts. And in the midst of his inquiry he finds a very different sort of sustaining power, not transcendent and capricious, but imminent and contingent, not all-knowing and arbitrary but growing, developing, and responsive. Not rooted in vision and myth, but like all vision and myth, rooted in biology. And when he can finally say, "I have heard of thee by the hearing of the ear. But now mine eye doth see thee," his revelation comes from casting his eye in a quite different direction than towards the blue heavens: "Deep in my skin it is marked, and in my very flesh do I see God."

~•~

Bodywork, somatic education, has long seemed to me to be one of the most potent tools for this sort of research. Sensory awareness is our primary source of defining information about objects and events within me as well as without, and there is simply no way of overstating the significance of heightening its acuity and attending to its constant fluctuations. A detailed, accurate, and continually updated body image is one of the indispensable elements of that most fundamental of dictums, "Know thyself." And, in turn, this knowing is the only reliable perspective from which to examine whatever else is knowable.

And even more compelling than that, without touch you die. Tactile input is of primary significance to the organization and successful function of a wide variety of physiological functions and psychological processes, and if it is stinted in our development, gross distortions of our genetic heritage are the inevitable result. *Job's Body* is an exploration of the clinical literature bearing on the subject of touch and its impact upon our physical and mental lives.

Of course, any selection like this one always leaves almost everything out. What I have tried to include are the principal themes that have sparked my curiosity and the theoretical conclusions which my experiences as a bodyworker and a student of biology have led me. In the body of the book itself, these themes are fleshed out and these conclusions are supported by much more detailed examinations and illustrations of the functional nature of our skin, connective tissue, muscle, bone, and nervous system. Naturally, it is my hope that this condensation will provoke the reader into a deeper exploration of the stories to be read in the flesh.

~ • ~

Because there is something in the touch of flesh with flesh which abrogates, cuts sharp and straight across the devious intricate channels of decorous ordering, which enemies as well as lovers know because it makes them both—touch and touch of that which is the citadel of the central I-am's private own: not spirit, soul; the liquorish and ungirdled mind is anyone's to take in any darkened hallway of this earthly tenement. But let flesh touch with flesh, and watch the fall of all the eggshell shibboleth of caste and color too.
—William Faulkner, *Absalom! Absalom!*

A Phenomenon Needing Explanation

The genesis of this book has been the attempt to explain to myself a phenomenon that I have observed again and again during the twelve years that I was a professional bodyworker at Esalen Institute in Big Sur, California. I had the opportunity to see many people arrive, suffering from various kinds of mental and physical distress, stay for a brief period, and then go back home relieved of significant amounts of pain and conflict. Both according to my own observations and by their own accounts, the bodywork they received during their stays was substantially—sometimes it seemed exclusively—responsible for these happy changes. And often these improvements have proven to be not just temporary ones; many individuals have come back for more, but they usually have not returned in their original conditions. It is clear that something set them off in new and more positive directions, and that they were interested in coming back to learn more about these changes, to be able to take them further, make them faster, more complete.

What these people have experienced is not a temporary analgesia or placebo effect, but rather a cumulative process of getting to know their own bodies and their own sensations from a fresh perspective, a process that continues to help them discover who and what they are and to learn to exercise some measure of self-control over many of the vagaries of their physical and emotional symptoms. I have seen stoops straighten, gnarled deformities become more comfortable and functional, injuries heal more quickly and more completely. I have seen dozens of imminent surgeries averted, medications reduced or eliminated, eyeglasses upgraded or even occasionally discarded, chronic pain diminish or disappear, various degenerative conditions slow to a halt and even reverse. And I have hard those that returned to Esalen talk enthusiastically about the positive changes they had experienced at home in their relationships with fellow workers, their employers, their friends, their lovers, spouses, children, parents. And with themselves.

Why should such a few sessions of bodywork, often accompanied by a minimum of verbal dialogue, affect so dramatically these people's symptoms, their relationships with themselves, and their relationships with others? Most of the bodywork techniques I have observed and practiced are neither rigidly systematic nor forceful. The usual impression is that the client is being gentled and pleasured, not being "fixed" or "cured." By what possible mechanisms, then, could something so simple as soothing touch alleviate painful and long-standing physical conditions, quell anxieties, foster more productive attitudes? And if simple touching indeed provided some sort of key, they why were some practitioners so much better at achieving these kinds of results than were others? These questions, and many more that come in their train, have led me to the explorations in this book.

Some of the practitioners who frequently achieve these sorts of results have had a great deal of formal training of various kinds to develop their skills. Some have had much less, and some little or none at all. Almost all of them, including those with the most formal training, insist that regardless of what specific technique they may be pursuing, the actual details of the placement and manipulation of their hands are largely guided by some intuitive process, and that very often they cannot pinpoint precisely which movements or pressures precipitated a dramatic change in the client. And yet the results are there for anyone to see.

If in fact a thing occurs repeatedly, then it must be in some way explainable. And if it is not explainable in currently acceptable terms, then whatever terms do explain it must be sought out, and the categories of what is currently acceptable will have to adjust themselves accordingly. It is the goal of this book to explore some of the verifiable relationships between the body and the mind in search of data that might contribute toward some concrete understanding of what is happening when skillful touching alters the structure, the chemistry, the feelings, and the behavior of a human being. I would like to find concrete reasons for the obvious successes of a largely intuitive process, a process which seems able to use very different specific techniques in order to arrive at the same results of relief from discomfort, dysfunction, and anxiety.

Looking about, I have discovered to my delight that there is indeed already a rich supply of hard experimental data which does support some concrete suggestions as to what is at the bottom of these phenomena. Some of the data, in fact, is so commonly available, so clear and unequivocal, that one can only wonder why medical science has not clamored more enthusiastically for the development and application of these kinds of skills. Therapeutic bodywork is presently relegated almost exclusively to the departments of physical therapy, and is often so hedged in there by procedural rules imposed by administrators and physicians—many of whom have no special training in bodywork—that the crucial intuitive element in their success is rendered very nearly inoperable. It is the investigation of available data from the perspective of the bodyworker who is having real success with the intuitive use of his or her hands that particularly interests me.

What Can Bodywork Do?

One of the debates that has accompanied bodywork throughout its history has been about what specific things various manipulations actually accomplish, and to what conditions it can therefore be applied with some expectation of success. Almost all of the physicians and practitioners just mentioned have agreed on one or two fundamental points. One is that most of the body's processes rely upon the appropriate movement of fluids through our systems, and that bodywork can be an effective means of promoting these circulations. Whether it is blood in the arteries, capillaries, and veins, the contents of the digestive tract, lymph in its vessels, secretions in their glands, or the fluids that fill all of the spaces in between our cells, manipulation can move them around much like I can push water back and forth in a rubber tube; and with a clear knowledge of these fluid pathways and some practice, I can become quite sophisticated in the ways in which I can stimulate their flows.

Now these flows, or the lack of them, can have far-reaching consequences upon many tissues and functions. Nutrients, oxygen, hormones, antibodies, and other immunizers, and of course water, must be delivered to every single cell continually if it is to survive and respond the way it should, and all kinds of toxic wastes must be borne away. There is no tissue in the body that cannot be weakened and ultimately destroyed by chronic interruptions of these various circulations.

Another argument frequently made for the efficacy of bodywork is that both our musculature and the connective tissues which hold us together often become stiffened or shortened or thickened, distorting our posture and limiting our movements. These tissues can be especially troubling after surgery or any other trauma, when the muscles are either tightening up in order to brace an injured area or are contracting in a general withdrawal reflex, and when the connective tissues are scarring over a wound.

These bracing and healing mechanisms often overdo their functions, and it is very common that individuals never recover their full range of motion or their normal levels of comfort after an operation or a serious injury. And these stiffenings, shortenings, and thickenings can also happen as a result of a wide array of overuse, disuse, spasm, injury, illness, fatigue, aging, poor habits, or the innumerable physical strains that various occupations demand of us. Bodywork has been used for thousands of years to relax muscles, eliminate spasm, diminish fatigue, soften connective tissue to make it more supple, and so free up the joints, restoring a fuller range of painless movement.

These kinds of effects upon our fluids and upon our solids have

been rightfully cited as benefits of any number of approaches to bodywork throughout its history. They would certainly be enough to establish its therapeutic value. But it is my feeling that they do not go half
far enough in describing the positive changes that can happen as a
result of skillful touching. Even though they are accurate identifications of benefits, they reflect almost exclusively the *mechanical* aspects
of bodywork and of our own system's responses—the laws govern-
ing hydraulics, the elasticity and tensile strength of tissues, and so on.

We are, of course, mechanical in many of our physical aspects, so
there is a great deal of justification for focusing upon these sorts of
effects and explanations, as far as they go. But we are much more than
mechanical. We are a confluence of physics, chemistry, and consciousness, streams and quanta of energies that interpenetrate one
another in enormously complex ways, that moment by moment create layers and layers of effects, and in which the subtle and the gross
are always inextricably intertwined.

In my experience, the plasticity of the body goes far beyond such
matters as the mechanics of the circulation of fluids, the local contractions of muscles, the stiffening of connective tissue here and there,
and so on. There is something in the actively organized relationships
between all of the body's various tissues which is more interesting—
and more relevant to our overall health—than are local tissue changes
in and of themselves. The skin, the connective tissues, and the muscles are vital organs, organs with multiple functions which profoundly
affect each other and all of the other parts of the body, and which are
affected by these other organs in turn. Every part of us is continually
undergoing dynamic changes from liquid sol states to solid gel states
and back again as we grow, move, learn, and age, and no single part
every changes its state without sending reverberations out to all the
other parts. Our organic life is an interconnectedness that goes far
beyond the mechanical relationships between fluids, tubes, levers,
cables, and springs. If we can genuinely affect one level of this interaction, then through it we can reach many levels, and the more sophisticated our sense of these interpenetrations are, then the more varied
and precise the manipulative facilitations used in bodywork can be.

And no matter how hydraulic, mechanical, or chemical we may

be in many respects, the physical laws which govern these kinds of relationships among our elements are only a part of the organization that forms and sustains human beings. Our other great principle of organization is neural, mental. And regardless of how hard purely mechanistic theorists try to explain the basic functions and the subtle nuances of our mental lives in terms of elementary physical laws, there is still a great deal about our states of mind and the consequent states of our tissues, about our experience and our consequent behavior, that so far at least has utterly resisted satisfactory explanation in those terms. The belief that such mechanistic explanations will one day prove to be adequate, once we have discovered and quantified all the details, is a philosophical stance, not a scientific one. Given the array of evidence before us at the present time, there is perhaps equal justification for maintaining that a great deal in our mental lives may *inherently* resist mechanical explanation. Indeed, the behavior of organic chemical compounds sometimes suggests that even they have some kinds of "feelings" for one another, rather than that they combine in some complex way to produce "feelings."

Neural activity is the most pervasive organizing principle in the body. There is no cell whose environment is not directly sustained or adjusted by the activities of the nervous system. It ultimately determines the plasticity of all other tissues and systems, and it is itself the most radically plastic of all the systems in the organism. There can be no movement, neither free nor limited, without muscular activity; there can be no muscular activity without neural stimulation; and the specific quality of every muscular action—its timing, duration, style, effectiveness—is a summation of all the activities of both the central and peripheral nervous systems at that moment. These muscular actions, in turn, are absolutely of the essence in our mental and physical development.

Organizing Mind

It is the mind that is the organizer of our health and our strength, of our associations and responses, of our thoughts, our feelings, and our tissues. The laws of physics and chemistry dictate the conditions which it has at its disposal, but so far no one has been even remotely successful in identifying any combination of these laws as the motivating factor behind the development of consciousness and behavior. How then might we successfully influence this organizer, without risking a major disturbance of the delicate chemical and physical balances upon which it unquestionably relies on for its continuing vitality? With what can we intervene that will not spoil the soup while we are adjusting the recipe?

Why not try the very thing that the nervous system uses to adjust its own organization, a thing which is neither chemical nor structural—tactile stimulation? It is the touching of the body's surfaces against external objects and the rubbing of its own parts together which produce the vast majority of sensory information used by the mind to assemble an accurate image of the body and to regulate its activities. "Only contact with the outside world," says Dr. Paul Schilder, "provides sufficient regulating sensations."[1]
We do not feel our body so much when it is at rest; but we get a clearer perception of it when it moves and when new sensations are obtained in contact with reality, that is to say, with objects.[2]

Not only is it true that the nervous system stimulates the body to move in specific ways as a result of specific sensations; it is also the case that all movements flood the nervous system with sensations regarding the structures and functions of the body. Movement is the unifying bond between the mind and the body, and sensations are the substance of that bond.

Friction on the skin, pressure on the deeper tissues, distortion of the tissues surrounding the joints—these are the media through which the organism perceives itself and through which it organizes its internal and external muscular responses. As we develop and mature, most of us build up and reinforce a reliably consistent sense of our selves by carefully selecting and maintaining a specific repertoire of movement habits—which generate a specific repertoire of sensations—and by surrounding ourselves with a stable environment with which to interact. This careful process of selection is largely unconscious, and so as long as we are comfortable we are rarely aware of any limitations or potential dangers our cultivated habits may entail. And even if a disturbing symptom appears, we generally do not suspect that our well-worn, tried-and-true behavior might be its cause. In fact, the very consistency of our normal patterns frequently prevents us from changing our ways long enough to obtain such an insight.

It is exactly this circular relationship between our habitual behaviors and the chronic conditions of our tissues that skillful touching can so usefully penetrate. New frictions, new pressures, and new movements of the limbs necessarily create new sensations, volumes of new data which the mind can scan in search of clues for new habits, new modifications, more constructive conditions. And here we are close to putting our finger on the possible reason why touch therapies can sometimes produce positive results so quickly, almost "miraculously." No matter how much I move myself around, my strongest tendency is to move in the same ways that I have always moved, guided by the same deeply seated postural habits, sensory cues, and mental images of my body; but if I can succeed in surrendering to the movements that another person imposes on my body, without my own system of cues and responses interfering, it is possible to treat my mind to a flood of sensations that may well be able to indicate what things I have been doing that have produced my aches and pains at the same time as they have reinforced my normal sense of self.

And even more important, this moment of surrender and new sensation can demonstrate to me that I am not permanently obliged to continue acting out a habitual compulsion. I can see that the habit is a habit, that I am something else, and that for the moment at any rate I can choose to repeat it or not. And if I can drop a compulsive behavior or attitude for a moment without causing a crisis, then perhaps I can dispense with it altogether. As every physician knows, this kind of insight can often be worth more than any number of drugs or procedures for the reversal of a chronic condition.

In other words, just as the mind organizes the rest of the body's tissues into a life process, sensations to a large degree organize the mind. They do not simply give the mind material to organize; they are themselves a major organizing principle. As we shall see, severe touch deprivation leads inevitably to psychological derangement and death—in a surprisingly short period of time. The sheer *quantity* of tactile stimulation that an organism receives, in addition to any considerations of the quality of that stimulation, bears a direct relation to that organism's success in sorting out both its relationship to the surrounding world and its own physiological processes. As it turns out, I learn about my body in exactly the same way that I learn about any other object, by feeling it. Without this active and continual tactile exploration, the organism literally loses its sense of where it is in all its pieces and parts, and rather quickly begins to fail to regulate appropriately its many complexly interwoven systems.

In bodywork, what is being felt is of major importance. This does not oppose it to science; rather, it puts bodywork in a position to add important dimensions of information to those of weight and measure. A painful spasm, or a chronic contraction which limits movement, or a destructive habit are not only specific neuromuscular events. They also include the feelings that preceded them, the feelings that accompany them, and the feelings that follow as consequences and condition future neuromuscular events. These feelings are not extraneous to physiology. On the contrary, in a large number of instances they can be demonstrated to be the precipitating factors of specific physiological conditions. Sensations and mental responses alter our chemistry and our structure just as frequently as it happens the other way around.

Furthermore, the dangers of fantasy and chicanery notwithstanding, it is not inherently impossible to be honest, accurate, and consistent in our assessment of these feelings and to use them systematically for therapeutic ends. What are the sensory and emotional conditions surrounding the generation of a muscular distortion? And what are the sensory and emotional conditions necessary for its lasting release? These are questions that can be of enormous significance to the individual suffering from such distortions, regardless of whether or not these sensory and emotional conditions can be weighed or chemically analyzed. These are questions that I would have the study and practice of bodywork address.

Sensorimotor Education and Self-Awareness

Bodywork, then, is a kind of sensorimotor education, rather than a treatment or a procedure in the sense common to modern medicine.

Nothing material is added or taken away, so there are no dosages to be strictly adhered to, no statistical rates of success for particular manipulations. If a student is having learning difficulties in school, I cannot effectively tutor him by simply pouring into his eyes and ears the information that will appear on the exam. The very nature of his problem is that he is not assimilating these things as he should. I must first find out something about what he does know, and then I must find what stops him from acquiring the things that he does not. I must enter into an active relationship with him, feel him out, discover what forms information must take before he can successfully absorb it, sort it out, and apply it appropriately. This process is not an exact one. It is partly objective and partly subjective, and the effective tutor is the one who knows how to find the balance between the two for each individual. This is the manner in which bodywork proceeds, first finding the reflex patterns of response that are presently active, and then searching for the quality of sensory input that will begin to alter those patterns for the better.

A point worth remembering here is that in this educational experience it is not the bodyworker who is "fixing" the client. The bodyworker is not attacking a localized problem with specialized tools, confident of achieving certain results. Instead, he or she is carefully generating a flow of sensory information to the mind of the client, information that is not being generated by the client's own limited repertoire of movements—new information that the mind can use to fill in the gaps and missing links in its appraisal of the body's tissues and physiological processes. It is then the mind of the client that does the "fixing"—the appropriate adjustment of postures, the more efficient and judicious distribution of fluids and gases, the fuller and more flexible relationship between neural and muscular responses.

The bodyworker is not an interventionist; he is a facilitator, a diplomatic intermediary between the physiological processes that have lost track of one another's proper functions and goals, between a mind that has forgotten what it needs to know in order to exert harmonious control and a body politic which increasingly utilizes disruptive demonstrations, terrorist tactics, and even the threat of all-out civil war to regain its governor's attention. Touching hands are not like pharmaceuticals or scalpels. They are like flashlights in a darkened room. The medicine they administer is self-awareness. And for many of our painful conditions, this is the aid that is most urgently needed.

There are hundreds and hundreds of conditions that do not threaten our lives, but only our comfort and our productiveness. There are conditions that lead up to crises, and conditions to deal with after the crises. There are functional disorders that are unquestionably created by habits and attitudes, not faulty parts or chemical deficiencies. There are conditions that do not reveal their causes to conventional diagnosis. There are scores of psychosomatic symptoms that refuse to be cleared up by conventional procedures. In short, our minds and our bodies face many bad situations between the womb and the grave which cannot be resolved by surgical or chemical intervention, but which just might be resolved—or even avoided altogether—by stimulating more self-awareness, restoring more of a sense of self-control, igniting a little bit of will power and aiming toward feelings that are more conducive, attitudes that are more positive, habits that are more productive. To develop these things we need sensory education, not physical intervention.

Self-awareness, self-control, and the active application of the will to the processes of growth and development are the major themes of this education. Bodywork can get us in touch with our present situation, give us a feel for possible alternatives, help us to grasp the forces that form us, put our fingers on the elements that have been missing in our ways of doing things, give us a renewed sense of our organic strength and intelligence. It can be a tremendous catalyst in the assertion of our self-responsibility for much of what we have become and much of what we can become. It can help us recall that we are living, growing systems, and not just genetic blueprints for engines doomed to begin wearing out the moment that they begin running, that we are an interweaving of processes and not just collections of parts, and that those processes are ultimately open-ended and creative, not mechanically deterministic. It can demonstrate to us that we neither have to collapse before the forces of gravity, disease, and decay, nor exhaust ourselves in a blind struggle against them, that it is possible to enter into active relationships with these forces, to match their insidiousness with our own cleverness, and to live a very satisfactory life in the midst of their threatening waves. It can give us clues about how to disentangle ourselves from widening vicious circles that threaten to engulf us because of our own unwitting compliance. It can be instrumental in putting a large measure of our lives back into our own hands.

These things can come about as a result of clarifications and improvements in our body image and through the discovery of the strengths and joys that coexist with our weaknesses and pains. Far from being mere hedonism, "the improvement of our sensual pleasure" is self-serving in the broadest, most enlightened and responsible sense of the word. It implies an intimate embrace of the good things that both the physical and mental sides of life have to offer, and a desire to enjoy those goodnesses with others.

Of course, for the purposes of evoking these improvements it is not touch *per se*, but the knowledgeable development of the quality of touch that is the important thing. A rigorous scientific education does not in any way insure this quality. And a merely intuitive grasp of it may be very limited in the uses to which it can be successfully applied. But neither of these objections should obscure for us the tremendous potential for relief that resides in effective touching.

Skin as Sense Organ

The Mother of the Senses

Touch is the chronological and psychological Mother of the Senses. In the evolution of sensation, it was undoubtedly the first to come into being. It is, for instance, rather well developed in the ancient single cell amoeba. All the other special senses are actually exquisite sensitizations of particular neural cells to particular kinds of touch: compressions of air upon the ear drum, chemicals on the nasal membrane and taste buds, photons on the retina. In the human embryo, the sense of touch develops in the sixth week, when we are less than an inch long. Light stroking of the upper lip at this time causes a strong withdrawal, a bending back of the entire neck and trunk.

Touch, more than any other mode of observation, defines for us our sense of reality. As Bertrand Russell observed, "Not only our geometry and our physics, but our whole conception of what exists outside us, is based upon the sense of touch."[3]

It is a remarkable testimony to this paramount place which it has in our sense of reality that touch is the longest single entry in the unabridged dictionaries of many languages, attesting to its wealth of associations in human thought and expression. In the Oxford English Dictionary, for instance, its ramifications continue for fourteen full columns, and if we include the immediately following entries of "touchable," "touching," and "touchy," the entry extends to twenty-one columns. Its metaphorical meanings run the gamut from "pure" to "tainted," from "sensitive" to "deranged," from "contact lightly" to "run through with a sword." Even painting, art for the eyes, and music, art for the ears, can "touch us deeply."

No other sense gives us so much of the world. Helen Keller and Laura Bridgeman, after all, spent their lives blind and deaf; their remarkable educations and achievements were accomplished through no other medium than that of touch. We can compensate for blindfolds, earplugs, or nose plugs with relative ease, but the blockage of all tactile sensations produces a profound and unresolvable disorientation, one that leads rapidly to psychosis.

Sensing Self

And information about object is not all that they give us. Every time that I touch something, I am as aware of the part of me that is touching as I am of the thing I touched. Tactile experience tells me as much about myself as it tells me about anything that I contact. I am constantly using the world to explore my reactions just as much as I am using my reactions to assess the world. My sense of my own surface is very vague until I touch; at the moment of contact, two simultaneous streams of information begin to flow: information about an object, announced by my senses, and information about my body announced by the interaction with the object. Thus I learn that I am more cohesive than water, softer than iron, harder than cotton balls, warmer than ice, smoother than tree bark, coarser than fine silk, more moist than flour, and so on.

We could even say that this role of the tactile senses in establishing a fuller and fuller sense of self is their primary function. An infant approaches objects not with an initial idea of research into and manipulation of externals, but with an idea of self-stimulation; and it discovers its own anatomical parts in exactly the same way (and at the same moments) that it discovers other objects. We can never touch just one thing; we always touch two at the same instant, an object and ourselves, and it is in the simultaneous interplay between these two contiguities that the internal sense of self—different from both the collection of body parts and the collections of external objects—is encountered.

Since [my ideas of] both the body and the world have to be built up, and since the body in this respect is not different from the world, there must be a central function of the personality which is neither world nor body. There must be a more central sphere of the personality. The body is in this respect periphery compared with the central functions of the personality.[4]

That is to say, my tactile surface is not only the interface between my body and the world, it is the interface between my thought processes and my physical existence as well. By rubbing up against the world, I define myself to myself.

This dialectic is life-long, and its formative power can hardly be overstated. It establishes preferences and aversions, habits and departures, becomes the very stuff in which attitudes are ingrained. The "feel" in my skin and the "feelings" in my mind, what I "feel" and how I "feel" about it, become so confounded and ambiguous that my internal "feelings" can alter what my skin "feels" just as powerfully as particular sensations can shift my internal states.

It is not too much to say that the sensory activity of the skin is a major element in the development of disposition and behavior, an element with enough sophistication and plasticity to account for wide divergences of experience and observation:

The skin itself does not think, but its sensitivity is so great, combined with its ability to pick up and transmit so extraordinarily wide a variety of signals, and make so wide a range of responses, exceeding that of all other sense organs, that for versatility it must be ranked second only to the brain itself.[5]

Skin as Surface of the Brain

The Ectoderm

This close association between the skin and the central nervous system could not have more concrete anatomical and physiological connections. All tissues and organs of the body develop from three primitive layers of cells that make up the early embryo: The endoderm produces the internal organs, the mesoderm produces the connective tissues, the bones, and the skeletal muscles, while the ectoderm produces both the skin and the nervous system.

Skin and brain develop from exactly the same primitive cells. Depending upon how you look at it, the skin is the outer surface of the brain, or the brain is the deepest layer of the skin. Surface and innermost core spring from the same mother tissue, and throughout the life of the organism they function as a single unit, divisible only by dissection or analytical abstraction. Every touch initiates a variety of mental responses, and nowhere along the line can I draw a sharp distinction between the periphery which purely responds as opposed to a central nervous system which purely thinks. My tactile experience is just as central to my thought processes as are language skills or categories of logic.

The "skin" portion of the ectoderm, then, does not really separate from the "neural tube" portion and migrate outward at all. The neural tube expands by means of trunks, axons, and endings, with the skin as its advancing boundary. And it is the chemical and sensory make-up of the skin which provides the "template" for the connections and reflex patterns within the brain, not the other way around.

The skin is no more separated from the brain than the surface of a lake is separate from its depths; the two are different locations in a continuous medium. "Peripheral" and "central" are merely spatial distinctions, distinctions which do more harm than good if they lure us into forgetting that the brain is a single functional unit, from cortex to fingertips to toes. To touch the surface is to stir the depths.

There is a great deal of stress and discomfort and discord in our world that clearly do not yield to traditional medical procedures, but which require rather a coaxing into existence of new habits, new attitudes, new ways of relating to self and to others.

Indeed, inside every failed individual there is a potentially warm, loving creature struggling to get out. The trick is so to interact with the individual who has been tactually failed as to release that potentiality for something resembling the kind of humanizing experiences he should have enjoyed in infancy and childhood.[6]

It is difficult to imagine a more direct way to rectify these failures than by supplying the touch that was missing in the first place.

It is the burden of the bodyworker to discover and to develop within himself or herself that quality of touch which will provide the emotional comforting, the tactile information, and the integrating experience so acutely needed by the distressed individual. This is not an easy task, but the developing therapist may take some comfort in the fact that the surface he most directly stimulates, the human skin, has a marvelous intelligence of its own, and possesses the means of carrying his efforts to the very core of the person being touched.

Movement and Learning

It is only the sensations associated with movement that allow me to explore random movements and to begin to select those that approximate the skill I am trying to learn, and it is by means of sensations that I continue to refine my selected movements until my efforts produce the precise effect I want. Thus it is that we call acquiring new skills, or modifying old habits to fit new situations "getting the feel" of the activity.

In addition to these physical sensations, there is a mental feeling of "rightness" that comes to be associated with the specific manner of movement which produces satisfactory results. This sense of "rightness" is a large part of the pleasure of learning a skill, and is also one of the main reasons why habits become so ingrained, why my behavior takes on such recognizable personal patterns. So much of my sense of psychological and physical continuity, my sense of unity and security, depends upon my ability to repeat appropriate and predictable actions, that this feeling of "rightness" can scarcely be overestimated in its importance as an element of my psychic integration as a whole. Each time I "get the feel" for a new response, I also get a new feel for myself and for my relation to the world of objects at large. The activities of my muscles play an enormous role in my relationship to internal and external reality.

The Sense of Normalcy

This system of sensorimotor integration is marvelously adaptive, and its simple elements can be manipulated to produce the entire range of complex human skills. Unfortunately, the sense of "rightness" which comes about through repetition may not necessarily correspond to movement and habits that are "optimal" in their efficiency. "Rightness" in this context only means "familiarity," grooves that are well-worn. It is often strongly associated with movements and habits that are merely "satisfactory" in some limited way, or "normal" in the sense of "like before."

We all stand and walk differently, but we all stand and walk with an identical internal sense of "normalcy" associated with our own way of doing it; and this sense of norm has for each of us an equal feeling of "rightness" to it. Yet, in spite of each individual's own sense of "rightness," some of us stand and walk with far more ease and efficiency than others, while some have accustomed themselves to doing it so poorly that their posture and manner of walking undermine the health of the whole system.

Astonishingly enough, once a sense of normalcy has been established in connection with a way of doing something, perceived inefficiency or even pain are usually not enough to alter our behavior. We will tend to continue to do a thing the way we learned it, the way in which we first established our "feel" for it, in spite of the fact that subsequent problems develop as a result.

The security offered by the "normal," the familiar, is so powerful that it typically prevents us from achieving improvements. Often the truth is that if we stopped standing the way we have learned to do so over the years, we would be able to stand much more easily. But the constant illusion is that if I stop standing the way I have learned to do, I will not be able to stand at all.

Bodywork and the Sensations of Movement

This conservative tendency inherent in the feeling of normalcy has a great force of inertia. By maintaining learned patterns, it contributes much to my sense of continuity, the stability of my body image, and the firmness of my sense of self. On the other hand, it can prevent constructive changes and refinements just as much as it preserves learned patterns.

The central role played by the tactile sensations in the development and maintenance of this familiarity, this normalcy, provides bodywork and movement therapy with an extremely useful means of confronting the limitations of this protective conservatism.

Just as the individual utilized muscular movements and the sensations they evoked to select and establish his present patterns of behavior, so can the therapist induce new movements and new sensations to begin the selection and establishment of new patterns. If the individual tries to move in new ways on his own, his overwhelming tendency is to favor patterns of movement that feel "normal" to him—movements that he has characteristically used before. But by remaining passive and allowing the therapist to create movements and sensations *for* him, the individual can begin to "get the feel" for patterns of movements that might take laborious weeks and months for him to master on his own, and can experience a new sensory norm that would have been impossible for him to establish as quickly by himself. Then once this *feeling for* a new, more graceful, more efficient gesture is a conscious reality for him, he can move quite rapidly towards establishing for himself the muscle contractions that will reproduce the corresponding sensations.

It is possible for bodywork to be effective, and often to be so rapidly effective, because in fact it utilizes the same principles that guide the learning of motor responses in the first place. It is the motions and pressures of the muscles which create sensations, and it is the selection and repetition of specific sensations which condition the learned patterns of motor activity. It is the task of the bodyworker to provide movement and sensations which more nearly approximate "optimal," so that the conservatism of what is merely "normal" may be transcended in the learning processes of the individual.

Relaxation does not merely allow the bodyworker to move the client's joints more freely for the moment; it considerably increases the suggestive potency of those freer movements; it creates a neutral ground where the information of new sensations can be introduced into a system normally locked into its old patterns; it produces a palpable hint of what it would be like to respond differently.

The Role of Bodywork

The physical sensations—particularly the large variety of tactile sensations—are the foundations of self-awareness. Whenever I contact an object, two streams of information are opened up: one that gives me impressions about the object, and another that gives me impressions about the body part that is doing the contacting and its relationship to the rest of me. Likewise, whenever I make a movement I also initiate a double stream of sensory impressions: one that register the shape of the movement as a whole, and another that registers the size, shape, and specific qualities of all the body parts that are rubbed and pressed and distorted against one another in the course of the movement. And unless I am either touching an external object or moving my internal parts against one another, I do not generate any concrete sensory impressions about myself for the mind to entertain.

Descartes' fundamental principle—"I think, therefore I am"—is in this regard a false beginning upon which to base our reflections. It begs innumerable questions because it fails to address the sources of consciousness that are in fact primary in the formation of my sense of existence and identity. Far more to the point in our actual modes of self-perception would be the assertion that "I *feel*, and therefore I am." *Thinking* about those primary sensory realities comes later, and always introduces a host of variables and complications.

And what is most significant about these physical sensations in the context of bodywork is that tactile stimulation does not only announce the presence of and delineate the condition of our various tissues; it also crucial to the successful *organization* of those tissues. Without an adequate amount of continual sensory impressions, the mind very quickly loses track of the body's myriad activities and so loses control over their regulation and coordination. This organizing role of sensory impressions is so central to the managing of our complex organisms that psychosis and death are the inevitable sequels to sustained sensory isolation. Sensation is information, information without which the mind simply cannot make accurate and timely judgments about the legions of factors that continually affect our well being. In situations where adequate physical contact and movement are impossible, or even problematical, the sensory input of skilled bodywork can be invaluable to the mind as a source of the necessary data.

The flow of sensory information useful to the mind is the operative principle in effective bodywork. Self-awareness is obviously dependent upon this flow; and the constructive exertion of our will power relies completely upon it as well. Until we have some concrete knowledge about how things are situated, and until we know in what ways and to what degrees they can change, we are generally not motivated to initiate those changes; nor do we know how to make meaningful, helpful changes even if we want to. We are literally feeling our way along the course of our lives, and until we have *felt* something more complete, more harmonious, we don't know how to be *be* more complete and harmonious.

This is not by any means to suggest that the quality of pleasurableness is the only quality significant to effective bodywork. Touch can be superficial or penetrating, general or quite precise; it can evoke particular feelings or be quite neutral; it can mimic to a high degree the sensations that would accompany unrestricted and pain-free movements, or it can be merely an incoherent jumble of pressures and stretches. It can provoke in us altogether new concepts about our bodies, or it can just riffle over familiar territory. After all, any number of people can stroke us pleasantly without prompting us to refer to their touching as "bodywork."

It is in these distinctions that the intent, the training, and the experience of the practitioner become crucial. How to reach the depths without causing discomfort, how to focus pressure to produce particular sensations in particular places, how to manipulate a limb in such a way as to convey a sense of optimal movement rather than random or restricted movement, how to bring into the sensory foreground areas long since forgotten, how to alleviate compensations without worsening the original injury—these, and not simple pleasure *per se,* are the specific qualities that can contribute to increased awareness, enhanced organization, improved health.

Practiced touch can not only deliver a collection of sensory impressions, but it can also impart those impressions in such a way as to convey a smoother style, a larger repertoire, a greater flexibility, and a finer appropriateness to our movements. It can help us to learn—in ways that our upbringing did not—a whole new manner of sensing and behaving. It can help us to learn to more accurately assess our condition, to identify and resolve stress, to reverse vicious circles, to move towards health rather than towards increasing involvement with our infirmities. It can help us to establish the new sensory engrams and master the new conditioned responses that are necessary for successfully breaking out of our ingrained patterns and our compulsions.

Let us not suppose that bodywork can ever be anything like a "cure-all." There are many physical and mental misfortunes that do in fact result from genetic anomalies, many kinds of severe accidental traumata, many external mechanisms of disease that invade us. For these we need to continually improve the devices and procedures of modern medicine.

But there is also a vast array of ills that cannot improve until our conscious relationship to our bodies improves, until we learn to sense more exactly what we are made of and how we undergo internal change. True, there are amputations we cannot replace, damages we cannot fix, diseases we cannot cure; but there are ways in which we might more successfully *manage* their results and make life more productive and more comfortable in spite of them. There are recoveries that can be more complete, degenerations that can be slowed down, pitfalls in the courses of chronic illnesses which can be avoided. And there are intractable sufferings that can be mitigated in important ways even when we cannot give the promise, or even the hope, of a final cure.

In short, we can expect bodywork to be helpful in any situation where heightened self-awareness and improved control over conditioned responses might be of constructive use. These kinds of situations include a variety of human ills that is wide indeed. Bodywork will not replace the resources of the modern physician, nor should it seek to do so. But there is certainly no reason for it not to be a part of these resources. It can offer the patient a kind of information about himself and a depth of insight into his personal involvement with his problem that no lecturing, no prescription, and no surgery could ever impart.

Awareness is the only medicine that accomplishes its healing without disrupting the natural functions of the organism. In the face of his adversities Job cried, "Is not my help within me?" The answer is yes. But it is up to each of us to seek this help out, recognize it, develop it, and learn to use it successfully. We inhabit—we are—the most complex and marvelous manifestation of nature that we know. The more we inform ourselves about those marvels and complexities, the more success we can expect in utilizing our inheritance. And the more we distance ourselves from the organic intimacies that comprise us, the more problems we can be sure of encountering.

"Before the bar of nature and fate, unconsciousness is never accepted as an excuse; on the contrary, there are severe penalties for it."[7] Bodywork is one of the readiest and most effective antidotes to this unconsciousness.

Notes

1. Schilder, P., *The Image and Appearance of the Human Body,* International Universities Press, Inc., New York, 1950. P. 70.

2. Ibid., p. 87.

3. Russell, B., *The ABC of Relativity,* Harper Brothers, New York, 1925. (Quoted in Montagu, A., *Touching: The Human Significance of the Skin,* p. 6)

4. Schilder, p., op. cit., p. 124.

5. Montagu, A., *Touching: The Human Significance of the Skin,* Harper and Row, New York, 1971, p. 230.

6. Ibid., p. 257.

7. Jung, C., *An Answer to Job*

5.
Resources

Bibliography

This bibliography is primarily of texts related to practices of embodiment. The second volume will include an extensive bibliography of how such practices have been used to revision psychotherapy. The third volume will include more theoretical literature related to the philosophical and social significance of these practices.

Alexander, F. M. *The Use of the Self: Its Conscious Direction in Relation to Diagnosis, Functioning and the Control of Reaction*. With an Introduction by John Dewey. New York: E. P. Dutton, 1932.

_____. Edward Maisel, ed. *The Resurrection of the Body* (Boston: Shambhala, 1986).

Alexander, Gerda. *Eutony*. Great Neck, NY: Felix Morrow, 1985.

Bartenieff, Irmgard, with Dorothy Lewis. *Body Movement: Coping with the Environment*. New York: Gordon and Breach, 1990.

Brady, Genevieve. *The Human Form Divine: Or the Highest Physical Expression by the Use of Spiritual and Mental Forces*. Boston: The Four Seas Company, 1920.

Brooks, Charles. *Sensory Awareness: Rediscovering of Experiencing Through the Workshops of Charlotte Selver*. Great Neck, N.Y.: Felix Morrow, 1986.

Chodorow, Joan. *Dance Therapy and Depth Psychology: The Moving Imagination*. NY: Routledge, 1991.

Cohen, Bonnie Bainbridge. *Sensing, Feeling, and Action: The Experiential Anatomy of Body-Mind Centering*. Northhampton, MA: Contact Editions, 1993.

Davis, Martha and Janet Skupien. *Body Movement and Nonverbal Communication: An Annotated Bibliography, 1971–1981*. Bloomington: Indiana Univ. Press, 1982.

Ehrenfried, L. *De L'Éducation du Corps A L'Équilibre de L'Esprit*. Paris: Aubier, 1956.

Feldenkrais, Moshe. *Awareness Through Movement: Health Exercises for Personal Growth*. New York: Harper and Row, 1972.

_____. *Body and Mature Behavior: A Study of Anxiety, Sex, Gravitation and Learning*. New York: International Universities Press, 1970.

_____. *The Case of Nora: Body Awareness as Healing Therapy* Berkeley: Frog Ltd., 1993.

_____. *The Elusive Obvious*. Capitola, CA: Meta Publications, 1981.

_____. *The Potent Self*. New York: Harper Collins, 1992.

Gindler, Elsa. "Gymnastik for Everyone." *Somatics*. Vol. VI, Autumn/ Winter, 1986–87, pp. 35–39.

Grossinger, Richard. *Planet Medicine*. Berkeley, California: North Atlantic Books, 1995.

_____. *Embryogenesis: From Cosmos to Creature: The Origins of Human Biology*. Berkeley: North Atlantic Books, 1986.

Hewes, Gordon. "The Anthropology of Posture." *Scientific American* 196. February 1957, pp. 123–132.

_____. "World Distribution of Certain Postural Habits." *American Anthropologist*. Vol 57, 1955, pp. 231–244.4

Hanna, Thomas. *Bodies in Revolt*. Novato: Freeperson Press, 1986.

_____. *The Body of Life*. New York: Knopf, 1979.

_____. *Somatics: Reawakening the Mind's Control of Movement, Flexibility, and Health*. New York: Addison-Wesley, 1988.

Johnsen, Lillemor. *Integrated Respiration Therapy: The Breathing Me*. Privately published in 1981, translated from the original Norwegian.

Johnson, Don Hanlon. *Body, Spirit and Democracy*. Berkeley, CA: North Atlantic Books, 1994.

_____. "Sensitive Inquiry." *Revision*. Winter 1994/95.

_____. "Towards a Multi-Directional Spirituality." *Contact Quarterly*. 19, no. 1, Winter/Spring 1993. 35–44.

_____. "Verticality and Enlightenment." *Somatics*. 9, no. 3. 4–9. 1993

_____. *Body: Recovering our Sensual Wisdom*. Boston: Beacon Press, 1983. 2nd edition: Berkeley, CA: North Atlantic Books, 1992.

_____. "Body-Work and Being." *New Realities*. Vol. VIII. September/October, 1987, pp. 20–23.

_____. "Ideal Bodies and Social Conformity." *Yoga Journal*. March/ April, 1985, pp. 16–20.

_____. "Principles versus Techniques: Towards the Unity of the Somatics Field." *Somatics*. Vol. VI, Autumn-Winter, 1986–87. 4–8.

_____. *The Protean Body*. New York: Harper and Row, 1977.

_____. "Somatic Platonism." *Somatics*, vol. 3, no.1 (Autumn, 1980), 4–7.

Johnson, Will. *Balance of Body, Balance of Mind: A Rolfer's View of Buddhist Practice in the West*. Atlanta, GA: Humanics, 1993.

Juhan, Deane. *Job's Body: A Handbook for Bodywork*. Barrytown, NY: Station Hill, 1987.

Keleman, Stanley. *Emotional Anatomy*. Berkeley: Center Press,1985.

Kofler, Leo. *The Art of Breathing As the Basis for Tone Production*. 7th Revised Edition. New York: Edgar S. Warner and Co., 1901. (Available in the Lincoln Center Libary.)

Ladd, Valerie, ed. *Rhythm for Dance and Art: The Exact Notes Taken of the Teaching in Action of Florence Fleming Noyes*. Portland, CT: Noyes School, 1982.

Lober, Irene. *Auf eigenen Füßen gehen: Somato-psychologische Erfahrungen einer ehemals Querschnittsgelähmten*. Lohrbach: Der Grüne Zweig 131, 1989.

Mauss, Marcel. "The Techniques of the Body." Trans. B. Brewer. *Economy and Society*. Vol. 2, 1973, pp. 70–88.

Mayland, Elaine L. *Rosen Method: An Approach to Wholeness and Well-Being Through the Body*. Printed privately. E. Mayland, 616 University Avenue, Palo Alto, CA 94301. 1991.

Middendorf, Ilse. *The Perceptible Breath*. Trans. Gudula Floeren and Dieter Eule. Paderborn, Germany: Junfermann Verlag, 1990.

Murphy, Michael. *The Future of the Body: Explorations into the Further Evolution of Human Nature*. Los Angeles: Jeremy Tarcher, 1992.

Olsen, Andrea, with Caryn McHose. *BodyStories: A Guide to Experiential Anatomy*. Barrytown, NY: Station Hill Press, 1991.

Rolf, Ida, *Rolfing: The Integration of Human Structures*. Santa Monica, CA: Dennis-Landman, 1977.

_____. *Ida Rolf Talks About Rolfing and Physical Reality*, ed. Rosemary Feitis, New York: Harper and Row, 1978.

Rubenfeld, Ilana. "An Interview with Charlotte Selver and Charles Brooks." *Somatics*. Vol. I, Spring 1977, pp. 14–20.

Seem, Mark. *Bodymind Energetics: Toward a Dynamic Model of Health.* Rochester, VT: Thorsons Publishers, 1987.

Somatics: Magazine-Journal of the Bodily Arts and Sciences (1516 Grant Avenue, #220, Novato, CA 94947

Speads, Carola. *Ways to Better Breathing.* Great Neck, NY: Morrow, 1986.

Steinman, Louise. *The Knowing Body: The Artist as Storyteller in Contemporary Performance.* Berkeley, CA: North Atlantic Books, 1995.

Still, A.T. *Philosophy of Osteopathy.* Indianapolis, IN.: American Academy of Osteopathy, 1899.

Stone, Randolph. *Polarity Therapy.* Sebastopol, CA: CRCS Publications, 1986.

Sutherland, W.G. *Teachings in the Science of Osteopathy.* A. Wales, ed. Cambridge, MA: The Rudra Press, 1990.

Sweigard, Lulu E. *Human Movement Potential: Its Ideokinetic Facilitation.* New York: Harper and Row, 1974.

Teeguarden, I.M. *The Joy of Feeling Body-Mind: Acupressure—Jin Shin Do.* Briarcliff Manor, NY: Japan Publications USA, 1987.

Todd, Mabel Elsworth. *The Thinking Body: A Study of the Balancing Forces of Dynamic Man.* New York: DanceHorizons, 1972.

Upledger, John, and Vredevoogd, Jon. *Craniosacral Therapy.* Seattle: Eastland Press, 1983.

Upledger, John. *Your Inner Physician and You: Craniosacral Therapy and SomatoEmotional Release.* Berkeley, CA: North Atlantic Books, 1991.

Empirical Studies

1. Austin JH, Pullin JS. Improved Respiratory Function after Lessons in the Alexander Technique. *Amer Rev of Respiratory Disease* 1984: 129(2):275.

2. Austin JH, Ausubel P. Enhanced Respiratory Muscular Function in Normal Adults after Lessons in Proprioceptive Musculoskeletal Education without Exercises. *Chest* 1992: 102(2).

3. Bach-y-Rita E. New Pathways in the Recovery from Brain Injury Part I. *Somatics* 1981: 3(2).

4. Bach-y-Rita E. New Pathways in the Recovery from Brain Injury Part II. *Somatics* 1981 3(4).

5. Barlow W. An Investigation Into Kinaesthesia. *Med Press and Circular* 1946: 215: 60.

6. Barlow W. Postural Homeostasis. *Annals of Phys Med* 1952: 1:77–89.

7. Barlow W. Psychosomatic Problems in Postural Re-education. *The Lancet* 1955: 9(2):659.

8. Beringer E. A Common Thread. *The Feldenkrais J* 1986: 2.

9. Brown E, Kegerris S. Electromyographic Activity of Trunk Musculature During a Feldenkrais Awareness through Movement Lesson. *Isokinetics and Exer Sci* 1991: 1(4):216–21.

10. Fisher K. Early Experiences of a Multidisciplinary Pain Management Programme. *Holistic Medicine* 1988: 3:47–56.

11. Garlick D. Comparison of Respiratory Movements and Frequencies in Normal and Trained Subjects. *Proceeding of Austrail Phys and Phar Society* 16(2):256.

12. Ginsburg C. On Plasticity and Paraplegia. *Somatics* 1980: 3(1).

13. Ginsburg C. A Foot is to Stand On: Some Reflextions from a Feldenkrais Perspective. Part I. *Reflextions: The J of the Reflex Res Proj* 1981: 2(3).

14. Ginsburg C. A Foot is to Stand On: Some Reflextions from a

Feldenkrais Perspective. Part II. *Reflextions: The J of the Reflex Res Proj* 1981: 2(4).

15. Gutman G. Herbert, Brown. Feldenkrais vs. Conventional Exercise for the Elderly. *J of Gerontology* 1977: 32(5).

16. Hunt V, Massey W. Electromyographic Evaluation of Structural Integration Techniques. *Psychoenergetic Sys* 1977: 2:199–210.

17. Jones FP. Method for Changing Stereotyped Response Patterns by the Inhibition of certain Postural Sets. *Psych Rev* 1965: 72:196–214.

18. Jones FP. The Influence of Postural Set on Pattern of Movement in Man. *International J of Neurology* 1963: 4(1):60–71.

19. Jones FP. Postural Set and Overt Movement: A Force-Platform Analysis. *Perceptual and Motor Skills* 1970: 30:699–702.

20. Jones FP. Voice Production as a Function of Head Balance in Singers. *Journal of Psych* 1972: 82:209–15.

21. Kaplan M. Eye Movements and Respiratory Function. *Visual Training Series* 1988: 60(9).

22. Lake B. Acute Back Pain: Treatment by the Application of Feldenkrais Principles. *Austrailian Fam Phys* 1985: 14(11).

23. Ruben P. A Case Study. *The Feldenkrais Journal* 1988: 4.

24. Silverman J, Rappaport M, Hopkins HK, Ellman G, Hubbard R, Belleza T, Baldwin T, Griffin R, Kling R. Stress Stimulus Intensity Control and the Structural Integration Technique. *Confinia Psychiatrica* 1973: 16:210–19.

25. Soames RW, Atha J. The Role of the Antigravity Musculature during Quiet Standing in Man. *Euro J of Applied Phys* 1981: 47:159–67.

26. Solit M. A Study in Structural Dynamics. *The J of the Amer Osteo Assoc* 1962: 62:30–40.

27. Stevens CH, Bojsen-Moller F, Soames RW. Influence of Initial Posture on the Sit-to-Stand Movement. *Euro J of Applied Phys* 1989: 58:687–92.

28. Weinberg R, Hunt V. Effects of Structural Integration on State-Trait Anxiety. *J of Clinical Psych* 1979: 35(2):319–22.

29. Wildman F. The Feldenkrais Method: Clinical Applications. *PhysTherapy Forum* 1986: 5(8).

30. Wildman F. Learning—The Missing Link in Physical Therapy. *Phys Therapy Forum* 1988: 7(6).

Resources

Alive and Well: Institute of
Conscious BodyWork
  100 Shaw Drive
  San Anselmo, CA 94960
  415-258-0402

American Center for the
Alexander Technique
  129 West 67th St
  New York, NY 10023
  212-799-0468

The School for Body-Mind
Centering
  189 Pondview Drive
  Amherst, MA 01002

Aston-Patterning
  P. O. Box 3568
  Incline Village, NV 89450
  702-831-8228

The Authentic Movement
Institute
  PO Box 11410
  Oakland, CA 94611
  510/237-7297

Gerda Alexander
  14 Frederiksgade, DK 1265
  Copenhagen, Denmark

California Institute of Integral
Studies
  Somatics Program
  765 Ashbury
  San Francisco, CA 94117
  415-753-6100, ext. 219

Center for BodyMind
Integration
  450 Hillside
  Mill Valley, CA 94941
  415-383-4017

Center for Energetic Studies
  2045 Francisco
  Berkeley, CA 94709

Contact Quarterly: A Vehicle for
Moving Ideas
  P.O. Box 603
  Northhampton, MA 01061
  413-586-1181

Continuum
  P. O. Box 6574
  Woodland Hills, CA 91365

Core Energetics
  Siegmar Gerken
  P. O. Box 806
  Mendocino, CA 95460
  707-937-1825

Esalen Institute
  Big Sur, CA 93920
  408-667-3000

Feldenkrais Resources
  830 Bancroft Way
  Berkeley, CA 94710
  510-540-7600

Hakomi Institute
  Richard Heckler
  2059 15th Ave
  San Francisco, CA 94953
  415-753-2266

Hellerwork
  406 Berry St
  Mt Shasta, CA 96967
  916-926-2500

Lomi Somatic Education
  4101 Middle Two Rock Rd
  Petaluma, CA ZIPCODE?
  707-778-9422

The Middendorf Breath Institute
  435 Vermont Street
  San Francisco, CA 94107
  415-255-2174

Moving on Center: School for
Participatory Arts and Research
  1609 Virginia St
  Berkeley, CA 94703

Naropa Institute
  Somatics Program
  2130 Arapahoe Ave
  Boulder, CO 80302

Ohio State University
  Somatics Studies
  Prof. Seymour Kleinman
  317 Pomerene Hall
  1760 Neil Ave
  Columbus, OH 43210
  614-292-4311

Study Project in
Phenomenology of the Body
  Elizabeth Behnke
  P. O. Box O-2
  Felton, CA 95018.

The Rolf Institute
  P. O. Box 1868
  Boulder, CO, 80306
  800-530-8875

Rubenfeld Synergy Training
  115 Waverly Place
  New York, NY 10011
  212-254-5100

The Guild for Structural
Integration
  P. O. Box 1559
  Boulder, CO 80306
  800-447-0150

The Rosen Institute
  825 Bancroft Way
  Berkeley, CA 94710
  510-845-6606

The Sensory Awareness
Foundation
  1314 Star Rte
  Muir Beach, CA 94965

The Somatics Society and
Journal
    1515 Grant Avenue, #220
    Novato, CA 94945
    415-892-0617

Tamalpa Institute
    Box 794
    Kentfield, CA 94914
    415-461-9479

The Trager Institute
    33 Millwood
    Mill Valley, CA 94941
    415-388-2688